Society and Health

Society and Health

Benjamin C. Amick III, Ph.D.
Sol Levine, Ph.D.
Alvin R. Tarlov, M.D.
Diana Chapman Walsh, Ph.D.

New York   *Oxford*   OXFORD UNIVERSITY PRESS   1995

Oxford University Press

Oxford   New York
Athens   Auckland   Bangkok   Bombay
Calcutta   Cape Town   Dar es Salaam   Delhi
Florence   Hong Kong   Istanbul   Karachi
Kuala Lumpur   Madras   Madrid   Melbourne
Mexico City   Nairobi   Paris   Singapore
Taipei   Tokyo   Toronto

and associated companies in
Berlin   Ibadan

Library of Congress Cataloging-in-Publication Data
Society and health / Benjamin C. Amick III ... [et al.].
p. cm.   Includes bibliographical references and index.
ISBN 0-19-508506-X
1. Social medicine—United States.   2. Medical policy—United
States.   I. Amick, Benjamin C.
RA418.3.U6S64   1995
306.4'61—dc20   95-30314

5 7 9 8 6 4
Printed in the United States of America
on acid-free paper

PREFACE

Although the recent growth of interest in the relationship between society and health has been concentrated in the academic sphere, the concept has also captured the attention of an increasing number of journalists and popular writers. The increased focus on the social determinants of health resulted from the confluence of: (1) developments in social epidemiology, (2) the globalization of health and social data, and (3) national introspection and self-assessment.

Developments in social epidemiology. Worldwide, many individual scientists and groups have made important research and training contributions to the study of the social determinants of health. In the post World War II era, one major figure whose influence still persists is John Cassel who, with his colleague Herman Tyroler at The University of North Carolina School of Public Health, inspired and directed the attention of medical and epidemiological colleagues to the importance of societal factors in the etiology of health. Cassel emphasized the importance of social science concepts and methods in the study of health and illness, and directed attention to how social variables may affect psychophysiological pathways in resisting illness.

Subsequently, interest in quantitative methods in sociology, social epidemiology, and health promotion/disease prevention converged in the research of Leonard Syme, at the University of California, Berkeley, and Lester Breslow, then State Director of Public Health. The Alameda County Study, launched in the mid 1960s, was a longitudinal study of health, health behaviors, and social circumstances in 10,000 residents of Oakland and environs. This study and research on similar themes continues to this day and has been contributed to by students of Syme and Breslow, including Lisa Berkman, Michael Marmot, George Kaplan, Mary Haan, Nancy Krieger and dozens of others working in universities around the world. Their research on populations showed that health status, including life expectancy and prevalence of chronic disease and disability, is related to one's marital status, social supports, and social class as well as to simple health habits such as hours of sleep, eating breakfast, and physical activity.

Michael Marmot, Geoffrey Rose, and colleagues at University College London, demonstrated in the longitudinal Whitehall Study that health status was directly and linearly related to position in the occupational hierarchy (a co-variate of education and income level), and that position in the social structure imposed an independent effect on health that was separate from the effects of adverse health habits.

Sociologists, anthropologists, and psychologists at other academic centers have deepened our knowledge of the influences and interactions of such variables as social class, race, age, and stress in different social and cultural contexts. They have provided a body of rich empirical data and have posited different conceptual schemes and hypotheses to explain some of the epidemiological findings on social factors and health. Particularly noteworthy have been the contributions of the behavioral science departments and divisions at the Johns Hopkins School of Hygiene and Public Health, the Columbia School of Public Health, and the University of Michigan's Institute of Social Research.

Globalization of health and social data. Advances in electronic communication, transportation, and international trade, governance, and regulation in the past half century have led to improvements in health and social data collection for purposes of monitoring health, providing essential health services, preventing world-wide epidemics, and decision making relative to international aid and capital investments. The United Nations, The World Health Organization, and the World Bank provide acceptable quality information on every nation of the world, information which is becoming increasingly standardized. The Organization for Economic Cooperation and Development (OECD), a Paris-based research organization supported by twenty-four wealthy industrialized nations, collects and provides standardized health, social, and economic data on each of the member countries.

The net result is wide accessibility at relatively low cost of large and continuously updated data sets on health, economics, and social indicators for most of the nations of the world. This allows for analyses of the relationship between health, economic, and social factors not only within a nation but also comparisons among nations. For example, Richard Wilkinson of the University of Sussex and the International Centre for Health and Society at University College London has reported that relative health status among OECD nations is related to neither total national income nor income per capita. Wilkinson has discovered that among industrialized nations the relative steepness of the income distribution is highly correlated with the relative ranking of health among those nations. He has also discovered, however, that within a nation the degree of unevenness of income across social layers is strongly correlated with the health of the population. Relative, rather than absolute, wealth within a population is decisive.

National Introspection. The collapse of socialism in the communist nations and the ending of the cold war five years ago has permitted more openness in assessing the interaction of governmental policies, economic factors, and the well-being of the population. There is international awareness that under communism's authoritarian government and controlled economies, health has deteriorated at least as measured by life expectancy from birth. The widened disparity of life expectancy between East and

West Germany is startling, as are the relatively stagnant figures over forty years for Hungary, Rumania, and the other nations.

On the other hand, unregulated market economies in the Western nations are being openly criticized for their lack of compassion and for their concentration of wealth among the rich with the progressive shrinking of real income for both the middle and lower economic classes (*The Economist*, November 5, 1994). There are reasons to expect that wider public attention to the details of social organization as a health determinant will grow in the years ahead. There are at least three formally established research units that are attempting to build knowledge and to raise social factors and social processes into sharper scientific, as well as public, focus as determinants of disease.

The Canadian Institute for Advanced Research in Toronto was founded in 1982 by Fraser Mustard and continues under his leadership. " Population Health,'' one of the Institute's programs, is directed by Robert Evans, Professor of Economics at the University of British Columbia, Vancouver. In 1994, the Population Health group published *Why Are Some People Healthy and Others Not? The Determinants of Health of Populations*.

The International Centre for Health and Society was established four years ago at University College London and is directed by Michael Marmot. This group is largely responsible for developing the certain relationship between two gradients: social strata as defined by job, education, or income, and health as defined by life expectancy or morbidity and mortality rates from almost any chronic disease. Richard Wilkinson of the International Centre has developed the concept of within-nation patterns of income distribution as correlates of health.

In 1991, the Henry J. Kaiser Family Foundation's Functional Outcomes Program established through a grant the Society and Health Program in Boston, which is a joint undertaking of the Harvard School of Public Health and the Tufts-New England Medical Center. Diana Chapman Walsh and Sol Levine were cofounders and codirectors of the Program until 1993 when Walsh became president of Wellesley College. To formally launch the program a conference was held in Boston on October 15–17, 1992. Approximately forty scientists from several nations were invited to submit manuscripts or to participate as discussants. The conference was officially opened by Harvey Fineberg, Dean, Harvard School of Public Health, and Jerome Grossman, Chairman of the Board and Chief Executive Officer, Tufts-New England Medical Center. This book contains most of the papers presented at the conference, subsequently revised and edited.

Our goal in this volume is to raise social factors and social processes into sharper focus as determinants of health. We have asked the authors to highlight what they believe to be the most compelling questions they confront in analyzing their topic. Individual chapters range from the effects on health of such proximal factors as the family, the work situation, and the community environment, to the more pervasive and distal influences of social stratification (based on gender, racism, and social class), political economy, and culture. The book concludes with some policy considerations.

One perennial question in the health literature is, Why are there such dramatic gender differences in health? Walsh, Sorensen, and Leonard offer an intriguing model of how the social structure expresses itself in daily life and differentially impinges on the health of men and women. To illustrate this connection, the authors describe how the structure of power, the division of labor, and definitions of masculinity and femininity are manifest in the everyday life of women. In applying their perspectives to gender and smoking, they observe that part of the health advantage enjoyed by women can be attributed, paradoxically, to early patriarchal structures that prevented women from imitating men in their smoking habits. The authors challenge us to consider how we conceptualize and measure power arrangements and incorporate them into our research and intervention strategies.

Historically, many lay people and scholars treated race as a measure of innate biological endowment to explain a large proportion of the health differences between blacks and whites. King and Williams offer a different formulation to explain the marked racial disparities in health. The authors argue that to understand the health of African-Americans demands an appreciation of their marked heterogeneity in the United States. They examine the concept of race in the light of American history and view race as a socially constructed category which has served to maintain the inferior social status of blacks. The authors challenge us in our studies of race and health to encompass the broader social fabric or African-American life including the pervasive presence of racism.

A selective review of the literature on family and children's health is provided by Schor and Meneghan who highlight the significance of parental support in children's development. With changing economic conditions over the last 20 years, women have had to enter the labor force resulting in less time spent with their children. The authors show that improving children's health requires that schools and other social institutions change in concert with dramatic developments in the family. Providing women with appropriate work environments and child care are two policies worthy of consideration.

Patrick and Wickeizer, in their chapter on the community, reveal that social factors not only influence a population's health status, but also constitute the contexts within which organized efforts can be made to promote health. Thus, for example, the social organization of the community can limit or facilitate strategies to improve the health of the community. The authors synthesize a diverse literature and provide us with a framework to understand the changing community and its relationship to health. Today, as community residents struggle with the location of hazardous waste dumps, the closing of factories, and the growth of violence, Patrick and Wickeizer offer useful suggestions for ways of building better communities.

What is distinctive about Johnson and Hall's chapter on work is their conceptualization of how class structure forges the division of labor and the environments within which workers function. They show that work may affect the health of working class and middle class people through different causal mechanisms. For lower class workers the physical and toxic hazards of work may interact with control on the job to create health problems. For upper class workers the psychosocial demands of the job may interact with the hard driving personalities of some to produce health problems for them. In making this important differentiation, Johnson and Hall are encouraging a new direction in research on social class, work, and health.

Marmot, Boback, and Smith focus directly on the relationship between social class and health. Reviewing extensive data from the United Kingdom, the European continent, and Japan, the authors provide an ambitious agenda for research on social class and health. In attempting to explain health differentials across the life course, the authors draw attention to differences across social strata in material conditions, early life experiences, behaviors, and various psychosocial factors.

Ellen Corin demonstrates that we cannot assume that the concepts and variables we develop and the classifications we employ are true reflections of reality, especially when we are studying health and illness in social and cultural settings very different from our own. The variables used in research investigations are constructed by people whose fundamental assumptions are shaped by the social and cultural context in which they live. Even seemingly robust, well established variables such as stress and social support, whose impact on health are well established, may manifest their influence in diverse ways depending on the settings and contexts in which they occur. Thus, we may have to reformulate our thinking about the variables and the indicators we employ as we move our studies from one social and cultural setting to another. Corin, arguing for more meaning-centered research, challenges us to scrutinize the constructs used in social epidemiology.

Harvey Brenner focuses on factors of economic growth and stability and their effects on such variables as family income, unemployment rates, and sources of industrial toxicity. Using historical data, he assesses the effects of the larger political economy on socioeconomic status, which he treats as a dynamic concept intervening between the larger society and the health of the population. Building on prior research and presenting new analyses, Brenner demonstrates the beneficial health consequences of stable and equitably-distributed economic growth. His new theoretical propositions provide rich materials for research on how economic and social arrangements affect the socioeconomic circumstances within which health is produced.

One of medical care's distinctive functions, and one that has not been emphasized sufficiently, is its potential to enhance the patient's quality of life. Bunker, Frazier, and Mosteller offer an initial effort to quantify the effects of medical care on the overall health of the population. They find that no more than one-sixth of the extension of longevity in the United States in this century can be attributed to medical care. However, the authors extend this line of inquiry established by McKeown to consider health-related quality of life as an important criterion in assessing the contribution of health care. Their analysis provides valuable data and raises important questions about the tradeoffs between quality and length of life.

S. M. Miller contends that to promote health it is vital to advance educational, industrial, and economic policies that would redress three main inequalities—resource inequality (one's material means), relational inequality (one's connection with others), and relative inequality (the power or status we have). Miller's framework for examining policy provides health professionals with new insights into how important it has become to reintegrate social and health policy. Providing a new perspective on the health care debate, Miller argues that the nation should pay greater attention to promoting employment and changing employment policies to produce equity in wages, benefits, and assets to improve health.

The chapters of this volume are filled with policy and political implications. As editors who emphasize the need to delineate the causal linkages between society and health and to uncover strategic points for intervention, we recognize that some important areas have not been covered. Other topics deserving attention include the role of the school and other educational organizations in the production of health, the relationship of the health sector to other sectors, the role of religion and the church, and the societal determinants of health in the developing world.

We hope that this book stimulates further research and inspires other scientists to study social determinants. The field needs a coherent conceptual framework, more creative integration of existing knowledge, and more reliable evidence of how social factors impinge on human organisms and are translated into the biology that is antecedent to disease. Progress in these areas will permit us to develop a quantitatively supportable explanation of the relative influences on health of social and environmental characteristics, genetic factors, nutrition, and medical care.

ACKNOWLEDGMENTS

In developing this volume we were informed and stimulated by the members of the Joint Program on Society and Health—the New England Medical Center and the Harvard School of Public Health. This book and the broader efforts of the Joint Program on Society and Health have been supported by a grant from the Henry J. Kaiser Family Foundation. Dr. Jerome H. Grossman, Chairman and CEO of the New England Medical Center, and Dr. Harvey V. Fineberg, Dean of Harvard's School of Public Health, have supported our efforts to understand how society influences health, to learn how risks to health are generated and experienced, and to ascertain what steps can be taken to protect and foster the health of populations.

Three members of the program have been especially helpful. Debra Lerner, Ichiro Kawachi, and Rima Rudd have made valuable suggestions at different stages in the preparation of the volume and have provided extensive critical reviews of several chapters. Four Society and Health Post-Doctoral Fellows—Chloe Bird, Steve Ren, Eunice Rodriguez, and Jenny Ruducha—also reviewed multiple drafts of individual chapters.

Drafts of each chapter were presented by the authors for formal review and comment at a two-day conference in Boston during October 1992. The chapters were critically reviewed by experts in the field. Paul Cleary, Richard Cooper, Julio Frenk, Alan Harwood, James House, Robert Kuttner, Fraser Mustard, Alonzo Plough, Michael Reich, Töres Theorell, and Lois Verbrugge engaged the authors in challenging and incisive discussions and supplied the authors with detailed comments about their work. Edward Schiller, who was unable to attend the conference, contributed valuable comments on Harvey Brenner's chapter.

We are also fortunate to have been able to enlist strong support from members of a "Society and Health Working Group'' in Boston. While several members of this group participate as authors, others provided valuable input at different points in the extensive editing of each chapter. We would also like to thank Hortensia Amaro, Susan Bell, Phil Brown, Graham Colditz, Peter Conrad, Elizabeth Goodman, Susan Gore, Steve

Gortmaker, Jonathan Howland, Kathryn Lasch, Jean Baker Miller, Pat Rieker, and Rosemary Taylor for their valuable comments and suggestions.

We are grateful for the help and stimulation provided by our colleagues in Canada at The Population and Health Program of the Canadian Institute for Advanced Research (CIAR), and those in the United Kingdom at The International Centre for Health and Society based at University College London Medical School. Ellen Corin's chapter on culture is based on work she had done at the CIAR, and Michael Marmot's chapter is based on his work at University College London Medical School.

The production of this book was itself a cooperative effort of members of the Division of Health Improvement of the Health Institute at The New England Medical Center. Susan Haff nurtured the book from its inception to fruition. She has been the hub of all activity around the book and with her intelligence and diligence managed to make this volume a reality. Constance Kelley, Sheila Scott, and Carole Walsh have spent many hours typing and retyping drafts of chapters, responding in good nature to continual time pressures from us to get the book completed. They deserve special thanks for their understanding and tireless support of the authors. Teresa Celada's research and editorial skills contributed to many of the chapters in the book. Susan Malspeis helped navigate several stormy statistical issues. Jesse Saletan worked with Susan Haff in organizing the 1992 conference and provided every author with edited transcripts of all discussions of their chapter. Jamie Kudera at the Harvard School of Public Health worked closely with Susan Haff in the coordination of the conference.

We would like to thank Stewart Wolf, Judith Lasker, and Brenda Egolf for their informative comments on the history of research in Roseto, Pennsylvania. Barbara Rosencrantz offered a historian of medicine's perspective on the section on the history of public health in the Introduction. We are deeply grateful for her helpful and discerning counsel.

We were fortunate to have a talented and patient editor of the book. Ann Goodsell edited each chapter, some twice, providing the authors with suggestions for improvements. Her gentle hand is evident throughout the book. Finally, we would like to express our gratitude to Jeffrey House at Oxford University Press for the valuable suggestions he provided and for his wisdom, patience, and support.

CONTENTS

Contents

CONTRIBUTORS

Benjamin C. Amick, III, Ph.D.
Research Scientist
The Health Institute
New England Medical Center
    Lecturer
Department of Health and Social
    Behavior
Harvard School of Public Health

Martin Bobak, M.D.
Joint Wellcome Trust Fellow
London School of Hygiene and
    Tropical Medicine

M. Harvey Brenner, Ph.D.
Professor of Health Policy and
    Management
The Johns Hopkins University

John P. Bunker, M.D.
CRC Clinical Trials Centre
King's College School of Medicine
    and Dentistry
Rayne Institute

Ellen Corin, Ph.D.
Director
Psychosocial Research Unit
Douglas Hospital

George Davey Smith, M.D.
Senior Lecturer
Epidemiology and Public Health
University of Glasgow

Howard S. Frazier, M.D.
Professor of Health Policy and
    Management
Harvard School of Public Health

Ellen Hall, Ph.D.
School of Hygiene and Public Health
The Johns Hopkins University

Jeffrey V. Johnson, Ph.D.
School of Hygiene and Public Health
The Johns Hopkins University

Gary King, Ph.D.
Associate Professor
Department of Community Medicine
    and Health Care
The School of Medicine
University of Connecticut Health
    Center

Lori Leonard, M.S., Sc.D. Cand.
Department of Health and Social
    Behavior
Harvard School of Public Health

Sol Levine, Ph.D.
Senior Scientist
Director
Joint Program in Society and Health
The Health Institute
New England Medical Center
Professor
Department of Health and Social
  Behavior
Harvard School of Public Health

Michael G. Marmot, M.D.
Professor and Head
Department of Community Medicine
University College and Middlesex
  School of Medicine
University College London

Elizabeth G. Menaghan, Ph.D.
Professor
Department of Sociology
Ohio State University

S. M. Miller, Ph.D.
Senior Fellow
Commonwealth Institute

Frederick Mosteller, Ph.D.
Professor Emeritus
Department of Health Policy and
  Management
Harvard School of Public Health

Donald Patrick, Ph.D., M.S.P.H.
Professor and Director
Social and Behavioral Science Program
Department of Health Services
University of Washington

Edward L. Schor, M.D.
Director
Functional Outcomes Program
The Health Institute
New England Medical Center

Glorian Sorensen, Ph.D.
Director
Community Based Programs
Division of Cancer, Epidemiology, and
  Control
Dana Farber Cancer Institute

Alvin R. Tarlov, M.D.
Senior Scientist
Director
Division of Health Improvement
The Health Institute
New England Medical Center
Professor of Health Promotion
Department of Health Policy and
Management
Harvard School of Public Health

Diana Chapman Walsh, Ph.D.
President
Wellesley College

Thomas M. Wickizer, Ph.D.
Associate Professor
Department of Health Services
University of Washington

David R. Williams, Ph.D.
Associate Professor
Associate Research Scientist
Institute for Social Research
Survey Research Center
The University of Michigan

Society and Health

1

Introduction

BENJAMIN C. AMICK III, SOL LEVINE, ALVIN R. TARLOV, and DIANA CHAPMAN WALSH

Although many people throughout history have believed that social conditions affect health, it was not until the twentieth century that researchers established a body of knowledge concerning the social determinants of health and their pathways. In the United States, especially after World War II, the federal government and private foundations launched major training programs and research projects in the health and social sciences (Freeman and Levine, 1989a). Medical sociology, health psychology, and health economics achieved specialties within their larger respective disciplines. And within epidemiology and other public health disciplines investigators incorporated social variables in designing their studies. Generations of research have now documented the impact on health of social factors like class, race, education, sex, marital status, employment, and the quality of jobs (cf Ostfeld and Eaker, 1985; Susser et al., 1985; Freeman and Levine, 1989b).

Before examining some of the intellectual currents in the study of social determinants of health, we will consider briefly the rise of social medicine and the development of public health in the nineteenth century. For it was during this period that the pervasive influence of social factors on health began to be widely appreciated.

The Emergence of Public Health and Social Medicine

Noxious health conditions accompanied the massive growth of urban industrial society in Europe and the United States. The state had to confront the dramatically high rates of disease among the poor as well as the squalor in which they lived. In Germany the government asked the physician Rudolph Virchow (1849) to study the typhus epi-

3

demic in Upper Silesia and to make recommendations to control the spread of the disease. Before the epidemic the population had increased substantially without a concomitant increase in housing. From 1834 to 1847 only 852 new domiciles had been built while the population increased by 17,017. This increase resulted in an average of almost ten persons living in each household. It was crowded conditions and nutritional deprivation, according to Virchow, that made the working classes more susceptible to typhus. Wealthier Germans, by contrast, had larger houses with fewer inhabitants and more money to purchase food.

Virchow assigned some importance to the role of the weather in the epidemic: rain destroyed crops and this led to malnutrition or starvation and to the presence of decaying organic matter which gave rise to the disease. But Virchow took pains to emphasize the central role of social conditions:

> Do we not always find the diseases of the populace traceable to defects in society? No matter whether meteorological conditions, general cosmic changes and such are inculpated, never do these in themselves make epidemics, they only induce them whenever, through poor social conditions, the people have lived under abnormal conditions for a long time. (Virchow, 1849, p. 117)

He went on to argue that the focus of medicine should shift from changing the individual to the society:

> Let it be well understood, it is no longer a question of treating one typhus patient or another by drugs or by the regulation of food, housing and clothing. Our task now consists in the culture of 1 1/2 millions of our fellow citizens who are at the lowest level of moral and physical degradation. (Virchow, 1848, p. 311)

In France, the physician Louis Villerme examined differences in mortality between the poor and the affluent (Villerme, 1828, 1830). In analyses of the 12 geographic districts of Paris, he found that the 12th district, with an average per capita income of 36 francs, had a 37 percent greater risk of mortality than the first district, which had an average per capita income of 120 francs. The risk varied with age but was consistently higher for those living in the poorer 12th district. The affluent, Villerme observed, enjoyed better health because of good housing, food, and sanitation, and freedom from excessively arduous work. He recommended improved schooling and working conditions as social interventions that would reduce class differences in mortality.

Across the English Channel, Edwin Chadwick, a civil servant was promoting sanitation measures to improve the health of the working poor in his report, *An inquiry Into The Sanitary Condition of the Labouring Population of Great Britain* (Chadwick, 1842). This report led to the passage of the Public Health Act of 1848 that ushered in the sanitation movement (Flinn, 1965). The cornerstones of the sanitation movement fostered by Chadwick and his followers were improvement in the quality of drinking water, inspection of food, reduction in pollution, better management and treatment of sewage, and improvement in housing. These measures, later listed in *The Royal Sanitary Commission Report of 1871* (Royal Sanitary Commission, 1871), indicate that the public health awakening in Great Britain was concerned mainly with environmental sanitation in order to improve the social conditions of the poor (Winslow, 1923). The control of disease among the impoverished was defined as a problem of the physical environment rather than, as portrayed by Louis Villerme and Rudolph Virchow, a sociocultural problem.

In the United States, Lemuel Shattuck, a civil servant and statistician like Chadwick, laid the foundation for public health in his *Report of the Massachusetts Sanitary Commission* (1850). The report discussed sweeping sanitary measures and eventually led to the creation of the State Board of Health in Massachusetts. In order to assure that the public health would be protected, Shattuck stressed the need to improve the health of all state residents including the poor and immigrant populations.

In Great Britain, Germany, and France, as well as in the United States, there was a growing belief among governmental leaders that society bore some responsibility for the health problems of its people. This served as an impetus to the creation of the State Boards of Public Health (Rosen, 1992). By the end of the nineteenth century, doctors assumed greater responsibility in working with the state to investigate the social causes of diseases and to prescribe ameliorative social and medical measures. These collaborations fostered the development in Europe of the fields of social medicine (Guerin, 1848a, b, c) and social hygiene (Grotjahn, 1915). While social medicine, with its emphasis on social class differences, did not obtain a foothold in the United States until much later (Hanlon, 1974; Rosen, 1948; Wolff, 1952), various physicians and other private citizens with social concerns joined with governmental leaders to confront fundamental social problems associated with excess mortality among the poor (Schmeckebier, 1923). It was becoming more apparent that the overall improvement in life expectancy and success against infectious diseases, like tuberculosis, had masked the more intractable nature of illness and disease amongst the poor (Bates, 1992; DuBos and DuBos, 1987).

The foundations for public health were established by Lemuel Shattuck and such successors as Alice Hamilton (1943), C.-E. A. Winslow (1923), and Edgar Sydenstricker (1926). A critical step was the recognition that medical and sanitary engineering training were not adequate to address the multifactorial social and health problems and that new programs had to be established. By 1920 public health study programs had been started at the University of Michigan, the University of Pennsylvania, MIT, Harvard University, the University of Chicago, and Johns Hopkins University (Hanlon, 1974; Rosen, 1992). The founders of these programs such as William Sedgwick and Milton Rosenau at Harvard, William Welch at Johns Hopkins, and Alexander Abbott at Pennsylvania established new schools of public health during this period, beginning with the School of Hygiene and Public Health at Johns Hopkins (Fee, 1987, 1991; Porter, 1994).

Public health, with a firm foundation in environmental sanitation and infectious disease control, began to incorporate the methods of the social sciences. The early employment of these methods was evident in governmental efforts to uncover the social factors related to disease. At the US Census Bureau, Sydenstricker and colleagues (1926) employed the methods of social demography and social surveys to describe the health of community residents in Hagerstown, Maryland, and, with Goldberger (1920) and colleagues in the US Public Health Service, to describe the economic conditions that fostered the development of pellagra.

Research on social factors in health in the twentieth century is much too extensive to be summarized here. What may be useful, however, is to present some of the dominant frameworks that have guided research in this field.

Exploring Social Pathways to Health

Social Integration

A useful perspective in the study of society and health was provided by one of the fathers of modern sociology, Emile Durkheim (1897), who advanced our understanding of the social determinants of health by directing our attention beyond individual economic circumstances to the measurement and description of the social system or collectivity. For example, in his study of suicide, Durkheim argued that rates of suicide varied with the degree of social integration or solidarity of different social groups, viewing rising suicide rates as an indicator of the decline in social cohesion.

Durkheim's representation of society received one of its clearest expressions in the studies by Leighton and his colleagues of mental health in Stirling County, Nova Scotia (Leighton et al., 1959; Hughes et al., 1960; Leighton et al., 1963), as well as in other communities (Leighton, 1969). For Leighton, too, the social system was the main causal variable in health. The Stirling County studies sought to compare rates of mental illness between communities and to identify the pathways by which sociocultural conditions influence mental health. Leighton conceptualized the community as an organism regulated by a web of reciprocal relationships that integrate individuals within the community. Shared attitudes and sentiments provide an important source of integration and social cohesion. "The systems of sentiment formulate for each person what he ought to be doing, what he wants to be doing, and what he can be doing; and how to perceive, interpret and react to events and to the behavior of others" (Leighton, 1959, p. 210). When the community could no longer perform its integrative functions, mental health problems increased among its members. Residents in communities with increased "cultural confusion," "occupational disadvantage," and "secularization" were reported to exhibit much worse psychiatric symptoms than those seen in integrated communities (Leighton et al., 1963).

The same attention to the importance of social integration is evident in the work of Bruhn and Wolf (1979), who studied Roseto, Pennsylvania, an ethnically cohesive and egalitarian Italian-American community. Despite a significant level of high-risk lifestyle behavior in this community, its population had relatively low rates of heart disease compared with residents of two nearby communities, one primarily of English descent and the other German. The authors concluded that the strong traditional value structure and social equality within the community of Roseto protected individual members from some of the risks of modern life:

> From the beginning the sense of common purpose and the camaraderie among the Italians precluded ostentation or embarrassment to the less affluent, and the concern for neighbors ensured that no one was ever abandoned. This pattern of remarkable social cohesion, in which the family, as the hub and bulwark of life, provided a kind of security and insurance against any catastrophe, was associated with the striking absence of myocardial infarction and sudden death among those in the first five decades of life. (Bruhn and Wolf, 1979, p. 136)

Over time, with greater educational, work, and financial opportunities, the community experienced increased social differentiation and individual expression of wealth, as well as a concomitant weakening of social ties (Wolf and Bruhn, 1993). While there were methodological criticisms (Keys, 1966a, b) of the earliest reports of the Roseto research (Bruhn, 1965; Stout et al. 1964), more recent longitudinal investigations have indicated that as the sociocultural buffers dissipated (Lasker et al., 1994), the risk of myocardial infarction and total mortality increased in the next generation of Roseto residents (Egolf et al., 1992).

The Roseto research embodies a familiar trajectory in the social epidemiology of heart disease: the change to a more "modern" culture in which material achievement defines a person's status with the attendant dissolution of protective social ties. Other studies of the health effects of social change emphasize such factors as the role of increased life stress (e.g., moving from rural to urban areas), the weakening of social supports (e.g., the loss of friends and relatives), and the adoption of new lifestyles (e.g., a "more Western" diet) as explanations for the higher risk of developing hypertension, heart disease and other disorders (cf., Scotch et al., 1960; Syme et al., 1964, 1966; Tyroler and Cassel, 1964; Henry and Cassel, 1969; Marmot and Syme, 1976).

Social Structure

Another major approach studying the social determinants of health is to focus on the ways people's specific positions and roles in the social structure determine their behavior and experience. In the research of Srole et al. (1961), Langer and Michael (1963), Hollingshead and Redlich (1958), and Dohrenwend and Dohrenwend (1969), it is not the community or social system *per se* that is the object of study but the socioeconomic status or position that people occupy within the same community or even across communities. In this research tradition, one's social class position is viewed as determining one's prospects in life; one's access to social, educational, and economic resources; and one's exposure to life stresses. In the Midtown Manhattan study, Srole et al (1961) found that socioeconomic status (SES) accounted for differences in mental illness. To explain these differences, they reasoned ". . . that stress factors were more abundant in the lives of adults of low socioeconomic status, and of children born into families of low socioeconomic status" (Langer and Michael, 1963, p. 15). Similarly, Dohrenwend and Dohrenwend (1969) postulated a greater number of "undesirable" life events among people in the lower social classes as the reason for their higher rates of mental illness.

Investigators have also tried to explain differences in the health status of people who occupy the same socioeconomic status but who vary with regard to their role require- ments as parents, spouses, workers, and friends. Some work or family roles, for exam- ple, may cause stress-related health problems because they are defined ambiguously; the person may be unclear as to what is expected, may be overloaded and unable to manage everything, may be experiencing role conflict and feel that significant others have different expectations as to how one should perform, or may have little discretion or latitude on the job (Kahn et al., 1964; Croog, 1970; Caplan et al., 1975; Karasek and Theorell, 1990).

On the other hand, when people are able to perform roles that are valued, they are likely to achieve a greater sense of well-being and even experience better physical health. An increasing number of studies have shown that women who are able to do in- teresting work outside the home have a greater sense of control and report better health (Verbrugge, 1989). Investigators have found the study of multiple roles and their inter- action a fertile area for deepening their understanding of social influences on health (Pearlin, 1983). There is evidence that women who work in jobs with little substantive complexity, such as data entry clerks, may tend to interact less with their children (Menaghen and Parcel, 1991) and that tensions at work can contribute to arguments at home with one's spouse (Bolger et al., 1989).

Methodological Improvements

One salutary development in the study of society and health has been the marked im- provement in our methods for gathering, storing, and analyzing large amounts of social and health data. More sophisticated survey methods, advances in the statistical sci- ences, and greater computing capacities have provided powerful new techniques to ex- amine the multicausal origins of chronic disease (Afifi and Breslow, 1994; Lilienfeld and Stolley, 1994). Multivariate statistical techniques have allowed simultaneous com- parison of a range of independent factors, including measures of SES, social ties, so- cial support, stress, lifestyles, and biological factors. Prospective epidemiological stud- ies in Framingham Massachusetts (Haynes and Feinleib, 1980; Haynes et al., 1980), in Alameda County, California (Berkman and Breslow, 1983; Kaplan and Haan, 1986), Tecumseh, Michigan (House et al., 1982), and London, England (Marmot et al., 1978; 1991), to name but a few, have demonstrated the influence of particular social conditions on health after partialling out the influence on the health outcome of lifestyle factors, psychological factors, traditional biomedical risk factors, and biological factors. While some of the assumptions underlying multivariate approaches have been questioned, and the limitations of multiple regression techniques in particular have been pointed out (Dutton and Levine, 1989), there is little question that we have strengthened our capacity to analyze large data sets efficiently. In addition, laboratory techniques permit easier measurement of neurohormones associated with psychological arousal, while physiological monitoring instruments permit more precise measurement of the biological sequelae of high-risk lifestyles (Weiner, 1992). These various methodological developments have given researchers many opportunities to extend their empirical inquiries, but we need further conceptual clarification of social variables and the pathways by which they influence health.

Current Perspectives and Emerging Concerns

Distinguishing Proximal from Distal Social Factors

In thinking about the social determinants of health, analysts find it useful to distinguish between proximal and distal social factors (House and Mortimer, 1990). Proximal social factors include the readily identified settings and institutions in which we live and participate on a day-to-day basis such as the family, work organization, school, neighborhood, and community. Distal social factors include the more pervasive forces in society—such as the political economy, culture, social stratification, and systems of gender, race and ethnic relations—which change slowly over time.

The distinction focuses attention on the different levels of influence of various factors and the links by which broader social forces affect people's daily lives and well-being. For example, fluctuations in the larger economy may shape relations in the family, workplace, and community, and these, in turn, may affect people's health. What usually is treated as an independent variable, i.e., the work setting, family, or community, thus can be fruitfully analyzed as a dependent variable. Similarly, it is useful to reexamine and treat such standard independent variables as sex, class, and race as dependent variables since they are deeply embedded in larger systems of social relations.

In studying the relations between gender and health, analysts try not only to uncover mechanisms by which gender correlates with health but also to explore the broader social forces that shape gender relations within a given society. Researchers try to learn how the division of labor and systems of power relations in a society affect the everyday roles and experiences of men and women, the ways in which they are socialized, and the kinds of jobs into which they are recruited. For example, women who work outside the home are still expected to do most of the housework (Shelton, 1992). But since the jobs most women hold give them little latitude or control in when and how they work, they experience difficulties in reconciling the competing demands of home and work (Hall, 1989).

Researchers have considered the links between distal and proximal factors in trying to explain the persistent social class gradient in health. A number of studies have documented improved levels of health at each successively higher social class level (for reviews see Haan et al., 1989; Adler et al., 1994). Investigators know that poverty is related to health but they find it more difficult to explain the social class gradient in health status and how it operates. Differences in working conditions have been proposed as one plausible pathway by which the larger system of social stratification influences health (Marmot and Theorell, 1988). Lower-class workers tend to occupy jobs where they confront more physically hazardous working conditions, and more boredom and overall stress; they also have less leeway in managing demands or hazards on the job.

Even more difficult to explain than the existence of this social class gradient are findings from Britain, the United States, India, and elsewhere that the the degree of inequality in a society—the distance in income and wealth between those at the top of the social hierarchy and those at the bottom—is itself related to the health status of the people in that society (Kawachi et al., 1994; Marmot and Davey Smith, 1989; Sen, 1993; Wilkinson, 1992). It is first necessary to ascertain whether this relationship will hold up in future studies. If so, it will be necessary to address not only the population's general standard of living but also the gap between the top and the bottom of the social hierarchy.

Investigators interested in understanding the strong and almost ubiquitous relationship between race and health are critically examining the ways in which race has been defined and measured. Researchers have characteristically compared the health differences between blacks and whites without paying attention to the social basis of racial differences (Cooper, 1991; Jones et al., 1991). More recently, various researchers have summoned a range of historical, epidemiological and public health data to demonstrate the ambiguity and inconsistency in the use of race as a variable in research on health. Racial designations have been shown to reflect differences in socioeconomic, political, and cultural as well as biological factors (King and Williams, 1992; Laviest, 1994). Researchers are now examining the contribution of these factors to racial disparities in health.

Concern About Culture and Meaning

Although social and behavioral scientists have long stressed the importance of cultural factors in people's health behavior—in perceiving symptoms, seeking health care, adhering to medical regimens, and responding to health promotion programs—they are now directing attention to the role of cultural factors in determining health status (Mishler et al., 1981). The increasing racial and ethnic minority population in the United States and in several other developed countries has enhanced professional interest in the relation between cultural factors and health. One emerging concern, among those who conduct cross-cultural studies of health, is how to interpret the statements of people from different cultural backgrounds. What do they really mean when they provide answers to questions posed by interviewers (Good et al., 1992)? We cannot assume that measures used in epidemiological research are equivalent across cultures. Even seemingly robust, well-established variables such as stressful events and social support, whose impact on health is well documented, may have variable meanings and may manifest their influence in diverse ways depending on the context. For example, social support is imbedded in a broader social context with attendant social norms and expectations. The acceptance of help may be interpreted in some cultural settings as incurring a heavy obligation that can constitute a source of stress rather then serve as a buffer against it. New approaches and more intensive qualitative methods are being designed to address these concerns (Charmez, 1991).

Definitions of Health

What constitutes health and how to measure it are old questions that have not yet been resolved. In health services research, health-related quality of life, sometimes designated as functional performance and well-being, is emerging as a major criterion to assess the impact of health care (Levine, 1987). Investigators are going beyond the traditional paradigm that views health only in terms of adherence to or deviation from physical or biochemical markers. Instead, they are including in their assessment of health people's own reports of their sense of well-being and their ability to perform valued social roles (Levine, 1987; Ware, 1993).

Although the World Health Organization (1948) and various scholars (DuBos, 1959) have long urged a broadening of the concept of health to include how well people are able to perform their daily tasks, only recently has daily functioning begun to be included routinely in the assessment of people's health status. A number of recent developments, including the dramatic rise of chronic disease, the burgeoning of new technologies to prolong life, and the emergence of cost as a critical concern, have served to foster the inclusion of functional performance as a criterion in assessing health status (Croog and Levine, 1989).

Will those who study the health effects of social factors be as hospitable to the social definition of health as their colleagues in the health services field? Will they include health-related quality of life along with morbidity and mortality in assessing the influence of social factors? A qualified positive response can be given to these questions. There is already evidence that some major investigations, such as the landmark *Whitehall II Study of Civil Servants* (Marmot et al., 1991) in the United Kingdom and the *Nurse's Health Study* (Colditz, 1990) in the United States, are making use of functional outcome and well-being as well as standard morbidity and mortality measures in their longitudinal research on population health.

Specific or General Influences

To discern the effects of social factors on health is it more fruitful to study people's vulnerability to a specific disease or to consider their general susceptibility to any one of a number of health outcomes (Najman, 1980)? Epidemiologists have generally maintained that a demonstrable relationship between a specific social factor and a specific disease outcome is a necessary condition for establishing causality (see Berkman and Breslow, 1983, Chapter 1, for a discussion of causality in epidemiology); however, restricting our focus to the relationship between a specific social factor and a specific outcome may not adequately capture the more pervasive influence of that factor on health.

Consider, for example, the frequently employed social variable, work stress. It may be related to a wide range of such conditions as hypertension (Schnall et al., 1990), myocardial infarction (Theorell et al., 1991), upper extremity musculoskeletal injuries (Bongers et al., 1993), drinking (Amick, 1993), and mental illness (Sauter et al., 1990). If investigators focus only on the relation of work stress to the etiology of heart disease, and not to general health, the relationship may be found to be significant statistically, but small in magnitude.

Those who emphasize the notion of general susceptibility do not necessarily deny the need to document specific etiologic pathways linking social, psychological, and biological mechanisms that produce specific pathologies. Rather, they emphasize the need to consider a range of different pathways. Syme and Berkman (1976) and Cassel (1976) have argued that social factors have nonspecific influences on the natural history of a range of diseases. Cassel (1970), Dohrenwend and Dohrenwend (1970), and others suggest that stress may weaken individuals and make them more susceptible to the onset of health conditions to which they are naturally prone.

Conclusion

The scientific community has become more accepting of the importance of social factors and of the need to learn the mechanisms by which they affect health. The chapters in this book testify to the range of different disciplines that are contributing to our growing body of knowledge on the relationship between society and health. Research on health is moving away from narrow parochialism and becoming more interdisciplinary. Our task is to integrate the relevant concepts, methods, and findings from various disciplines to enhance and deepen our understanding of the cause of health and illness.

References

Adler, N., T. Boyce, M. Chesney, S. Cohen, S. Folkman, R. Kahn, and S. Syme. 1994. Socioeconomic status and health: The challenge of the gradient. *Am. Psychol.* 49:15–24.
Afifi, A., and L. Breslow. 1994. The maturing paradigm of public health. *Annu. Rev. Public Health* 15:223–235
Amick, B. 1993. *Work Organization and Drinking: A Review and Synthesis.* Paper Presented at the Social Determinants of Drinking Conference, Nov. 23–25, Kiawah Island, SC.
Bates, B. 1992. *Bargaining for Life: A Social History of Tuberculosis 1876–1938.* Philadelphia: University of Pennsylvania Press.
Berkman, L., and L. Breslow. 1983. *Health and Ways of Living: The Alameda County Study.* New York: Oxford University Press.

Bolger, N., A. DeLongis, R. Kessler, and E. Wethington. 1989. The contagion of stress across multiple roles. *J. Marriage Fam.* 51:175–183.

Bongers, P., C. deWinter, M. Kompier, and V. Hildebrandt. 1993. Psychosocial factors at work and musculoskeletal disease. *Scand. J. Work Environ. Health* 19:297–312.

Bruhn, J. 1965. An epidemiological study of myocardial infarctions in an Italian-American community: A preliminary study. *J. Chron. Dis.* 18:353–357.

Bruhn, J., and S. Wolf. 1979. *The Roseto Story.* Norman, OK: University of Oklahoma Press.

Caplan, R., S. Cobb, J. French, R. Harrison, and S. Pinneau. 1975. *Job Demands and Worker Health.* DHEW Pub. No. (NIOSH) 75-160. Washington, DC: U.S. Government Printing Office.

Cassel, J. 1970. Physical illness in response to stress. In S. Levine and N. Scotch (eds.), *Social Stress*, pp. 189–209. New York: Aldine Publishing.

Cassel, J. 1976. The contribution of the social environment to host resistance. *Am. J. Epidemiol.* 104:107–123.

Chadwick, E. 1842. *Report to Her Majesties principal Secretary of State for the Home Department, from the Poor Law Commissioners, on an inquiry into the Sanitary Conditions of the Labouring Classes of Great Britain.* London: W Clowse & Son.

Charmaz, C. 1991. *Good Days, Bad Days: The Self, Chronic Illness and Time.* New Brunswick, NJ: Rutgers University Press.

Colditz, G. A. 1990. The Nurses' Health Study: Findings during 10 years of follow-up of a cohort of U.S. women. *Curr. Probl. Obstet. Gynecol. Fertil.* 13:129–174.

Cooper, R. 1991. Celebrate diversity—or should we? *Ethnicity and Disease* 1:3–7.

Croog, S. 1970. The family as a source of stress. In S. Levine and N. Scotch (eds.), *Social Stress*, pp. 19–53. New York: Aldine Publishing.

Croog, S., and S. Levine. 1989. Quality of life and health care interventions. In H. Freeman and S. Levine (eds.) *Handbook of Medical Sociology*, pp. 508–528. Prentice Hall: New York.

Dohrenwend, B., and B. Dohrenwend. 1969. *Social Status and Psychological Disorder.* New York: Wiley.

Dohrenwend, B., and B. Dohrenwend. 1970. Class and race as status related sources of stress. In S. Levine and N. Scotch (eds.), *Social Stress*, pp. 111–140. New York: Aldine Publishing.

DuBos, R. 1959. *Man Adapting.* New Haven: Yale University Press.

Dubos, R., and J. Dubos. 1987. *The White Plague: Tuberculosis, Man, and Society.* New Brunswick: Rutgers University Press.

Dutton, D., and S. Levine. 1989. Overview, methodological critique, and reformulation. In J. Bunker, D. Gomby and B. Kehrer (eds.), *Pathways to Health: The Role of Social Factors*, pp. 29–69. Menlo Park, CA: The Henry J. Kaiser Family Foundation.

Durkheim, E. 1897. *Suicide: A Study in Sociology.* (Translated by J. Spaulding and G. Simpson from *Le Suicide* and reprinted in 1951). New York: Free Press.

Egolf, B., J. Lasker, S. Wolf, and L. Potvin. 1992. The Roseto effect: A 50-year comparison of mortality rates. *Am. J. Public Health* 82:1089–1092.

Fee, E. 1987. *Disease and Discovery: A History of the Johns Hopkins School of Hygiene and Public Health*, 1916–1939. Baltimore: Johns Hopkins University Press.

Fee, E. 1991. Designing schools of public health for the United States. In E. Fee and R. Acheson. (eds.), *A History of Education in Public Health*, pp. 155–194. New York: Oxford University Press.

Flinn, M. 1965. *Report on the Sanitary Condition of the Labouring Population of Great Britain by Edwin Chadwick 1842.* Edinburgh: University Press.

Freeman, H., and S. Levine. 1989a. The present status of medical sociology. In H. Freeman and S. Levine (eds.), *Handbook of Medical Sociology*, pp. 1–13. New York: Prentice Hall.

Freeman, H., and S. Levine. 1989b. *Handbook of Medical Sociology*. New York: Prentice Hall.

Goldberger, J., G. Wheeler, and E. Sydenstricker. 1920. A study of the relation of family income and other economic factors to pellagra incidence in seven cotton-mill villages of South Carolina in 1916. *Public Health Rep.* 35:2673–2714.

Good, M., P. Brodwin, B. Good, and A. Kleinman. 1992. *Pain as Human Experience: An Anthropological Perspective*. Berkeley: University of California Press.

Grotjahn, A. 1915. *Soziale Pathologie*. Berlin: August Hirschwald Verlag.

Guerin, J. 1848a. Medecine sociale: Au corps medicale de France. *Gazette Medicale de Paris* (March 11):203.

Guerin, J. 1848b. Medicine sociale: La medicine sociale et la medecine socialiste. *Gazette Medicale de Paris* (March 18):203.

Guerin, J. 1848c. Medecine Sociale: De l'association medicale au point de vue de la situation actuelle. *Gazette Medicale de Paris* (March 18):211.

Haan, M., G. Kaplan, and S. Syme. 1989. Old observations and new thoughts. In J. Bunker, D. Gomby, and B. Kehrer (eds.), *Pathways to Health: The Role of Social Factors*, pp. 76–117. Menlo Park, CA: The Henry J. Kaiser Family Foundation.

Hall, E. 1989. Gender, work control, and stress: A theoretical discussion and empirical test. *Int. J. Health Serv.* 19:725–745.

Hamilton, A. 1943. *Exploring the Dangerous Trades: The Autobiography of Alice Hamilton, MD*. Boston: Little, Brown.

Hanlon, J. 1974. *Public Health Administration and Practice*. St. Louis, MO: C.V. Mosby.

Haynes, S., and M. Feinleib. 1980. Women, work and coronary heart disease: Prospective findings from the Framingham Heart Study. *Am. J. Public Health* 70:1331–1341.

Haynes, S., M. Feinleib, and W. Kannel. 1980. The relationship of psychosocial factors to coronary heart disease in the Framingham Study, III. Eight year incidence of coronary heart disease. *Am. J. Epidemiol.* 111:37–58.

Henry, J., and J. Cassel. 1969. Psychosocial factors in essential hypertension. *Am. J. Epidemiol.* 90:171–200.

Hollingshead, A., and F. Redlich. 1958. *Social Class and Mental Illness*. New York: Wiley.

Holmes, T., and R. Rahe. 1967. The social readjustment rating scale. *J. Psychosom. Res.* 11:213–225.

House, J., C. Robbins, and H. Metzner. 1982. The association of social relationships and activities with mortality: Prospective evidence from the Tecumseh Community Health Study. *Am. J. Epidemiol.* 116:123–140.

House, J. S., and J. Mortimer. 1990. Social structure and the individual: Emerging themes and new directions. *Soc. Psychol. Q.* 53:71–80.

Hughes, C., M.-A. Tremblay, R. Rapoport, and A. Leighton. 1960. *People of Cove and Woodlot: Communities from the Viewpoint of Social Psychiatry*. New York: Basic Books.

Jones, C., T. LaViest, and M. Lillie-Blanton. 1991. "Race" in the epidemiologic literature: An examination of the American Journal of Epidemiology 1921–1990. *Am. J. Epidemiol.* 134:1079–1084.

Kahn, R., D. Wolfe, R. Quinn, and J. Snoek. 1964. *Organizational Stress*. New York: Wiley.

Kaplan, G., and M. Haan. 1986. *Socioeconomic Position and Health: Prospective Evidence from the Alameda County Study*. Presented at the 114th Annual Meeting of the American Public Health Association, Las Vegas, NV.

Karasek, R., and T. Theorell. 1990. *Healthy Work: Stress, Productivity, and the Reconstruction of Working Life*. New York: Basic Books.

Kawachi, I., S. Levine, S. M. Miller, K. Lasch, and B. Amick. 1994. *Income Inequality and Life Expectancy—Theory, Research and Policy*. Society and Health Working Paper Series No. 94-2. Boston: Harvard School of Public Health.

Keys, A. 1966a. Arteriosclerotic heart disease in Roseto, Pennsylvania. *JAMA* 195:137–139.

Keys, A. 1966b. Arteriosclerotic heart disease in a favored community. *J. Chron. Dis.* 19:245–254.

King, G., and D. Williams. 1992. *Race and Health: A Multidimensional Approach to African-American Health.* Paper presented at the Society and Health Conference, Oct. 12–15, Boston, MA.

Langer, T., and S. Michael. 1963. *The Midtown Manhattan Study: Life Stress and Mental Health,* Vol. II. London: Free Press.

Lasker, J., B. P. Egolf, and S. Wolf. 1994. Community social change and mortality. *Soc. Sci. Med.* 39:53–62.

LaViest, T. 1994. Beyond dummy variables and sample selection: What health services researchers ought to know about race as a variable. *Health Serv. Res.* 29:1–16.

Leighton, A. 1959. *My Name is Legion: Foundations for a Theory of Man in Relation to Culture.* New York: Basic Books.

Leighton, A. 1969. A comparative study of psychiatric disorder in Nigeria and rural North America. In S. Plog and R. Edgerton (eds.) *Changing Perspectives in Mental Illness,* pp. 179–199. New York: Holt, Reinhart & Winston.

Leighton, D., J. Harding, D. Macklin, A. Macmillan, and A. Leighton. 1963. *The Character of Danger: Psychiatric Symptoms in Selected Communities.* New York: Basic Books.

Levine, S. 1987. The changing terrains in medical sociology: Emergent concern with quality of life. *J. Health Soc. Behav.* 28:1–6.

Lilienfeld, D., and P. Stolley. 1994. *Foundations of Epidemiology,* 3rd edn. New York: Oxford University Press.

Marmot, M., G. Rose, M. Shipley, and P. Hamilton. 1978. Employment grade and coronary heart disease in British civil servants. *J. Epidemiol. Community Health* 32:244–249.

Marmot, M., G. Davey-Smith, S. Stansfeld, C. Patel, F. North, I. White, E. Brunner, and A. Feeney. 1991. Health inequalities among British civil servants: The Whitehall II Study. *Lancet* 337:1387–1393.

Marmot, M., and L. Syme. 1976. Acculturation and coronary heart disease in Japanese-Americans. *Am. J. Epidemiol.* 104:225–247.

Marmot, M., and T. Theorell. 1988. Social class and cardiovascular disease: The contribution of work. *Int. J. Health Serv.* 18:659–674.

Marmot, M., and G. Davey-Smith. 1989. Why are the Japanese living longer? *Br. Med. J.* 299:1547–1551.

Menaghan, E., and T. Parcel. 1991. Determining children's home environments: The impact of maternal characteristics and current occupational and family experience. *J. Marriage Fam.* 53:417–431.

Mishler, E., L. Amarasingham, S. Osherson, S. Hauser, N. Waxler, and R. Liem. 1981. *Social Contexts of Health, Illness, and Patient Care.* New York: Cambridge University Press.

Najman, J. 1980. Theories of disease causation and the concept of general susceptibility: A review. *Soc. Sci. Med.* 14:231–237.

Ostfeld, A., and E. Eaker (eds.). 1985. *Measuring Psychosocial Variables in Epidemiologic Studies of Cardiovascular Disease.* USDHHS PHS NIH Pub. No. 85-2270. Washington DC: US Government Printing Office.

Pearlin, L. 1983. Role strains and personal stress. In H. Kaplan (ed.), *Psychosocial Stress: Trends in Theory and Research,* pp. 3–32. New York: Academic Press.

Porter, D. (ed.). 1994. *The History of Public Health and the Modern State.* Atlanta: Rodopi Press.

Rosen, G. 1948. Approaches to a concept of social medicine: A historical survey. *Milbank Q.* 26:7–21.

Rosen, G. 1992. *A History of Public Health*, 3rd edn. Baltimore: Johns Hopkins Press.

Royal Sanitary Commission. 1871. *Second report of the Royal Sanitary Commission of Great Britain*. London: Eyre & Spottiswoode.

Sauter, S., L. Murphy, and J. Hurrell. 1990. Prevention of work-related psychological disorders. *Am. Psychol.* 45:1146–1158.

Schmeckebier, L. 1923. *The Public Health Service: Its History, Activities and Organization*. Baltimore: Johns Hopkins Press.

Schnall, P., C. Pieper, J. Schwartz, R. Karasek, Y. Schlussel, and T. Pickering. 1990. The relationship between "job strain,": workplace diastolic blood pressure and left ventricular mass: Results of a case-control study. *JAMA* 263:1929–1935.

Scotch, N. 1960. A preliminary report on the relation of socio-cultural factors to hypertension among the Zulu. *Ann. NY Acad. Sci.* 86:1000.

Sen, A. 1993. The economics of life and death. *Sci. Am.* (May):40–47.

Shattuck, L. 1850. *Report of the Sanitary Commission of Massachusetts 1850*. Dutton & Wentworth: State Printers. Reissued by Harvard University Press: Cambridge, MA, 1948.

Shelton, B. A. 1992. *Women, Men and Time: Gender Differences in Paid Work, Housework and Leisure*. New York: Greenwood Press.

Srole, L., T. Langer, S. Michael, M. Opler, and T. Rennie. 1961. *Mental Health in the Metropolis*, Vol. 1. New York: McGraw-Hill.

Stout, C., J. Morrow, E. Brandt, and S. Wolf. 1964. Study of an Italian community in Pennsylvania. Unusually low incidence of death from myocardial infarction. *JAMA* 188:845–849.

Susser, M., W. Watson, and K. Hopper. 1985. *Sociology in Medicine*, 3rd edn. New York: Oxford University Press.

Sydenstricker, E. 1926. A study of illness in a general population group Hagerstown Morbidity Studies No. 1: The method of study and general results. *Public Health Rep.* 41:2069–2078.

Syme, S., M. Hyman, and P. Enterline. 1964. Some social and cultural factors associated with the occurrence of coronary heart disease. *J. Chron. Dis.* 17:277–289.

Syme, S., N. Bohrani, and R. Buechley. 1966. Cultural mobility and coronary heart disease. *Am. J. Epidemiol.* 82:334–346.

Syme, L., and L. Berkman. 1976. Social class, susceptibility and sickness. *Am. J. Epidemiol.* 104:1–8.

Theorell, T., A. Perski, K. Orth-Gomer, A. Hamsten, and U. deFaire. 1991. The effect of returning to job strain on cardiac death risk after a first myocardial infarction before age 45. *Int. J. Cardiol.* 30:61–67.

Tyroler, H., and J. Cassel. 1964. Health consequences of culture change II. The effect of urbanization on coronary heart disease in rural residents. *J. Chron. Dis.* 17:167–177.

Verbrugge, L. 1989. The twain meet: Empirical explanations of sex differences in health and mortality. *J. Health Soc. Behav.* 30:282–304.

Villerme, L. 1828. Memoires sur la mortalite en France, dans la classe aisee et dans la classe indigente. *Annales d'Hygiene Publique* 1:51–98.

Villerme, L. 1830. De la mortalite dans le divers quartiers de la ville de Paris, et des causes qui la rendent tres differente dans plusieurs d'entre eux, ainsi que dans les divers quartiers de beaucoup de grande villes. *Annales d'Hygiene Publique* 3:294–341.

Virchow, R. 1848. Report on the typhus epidemic in Upper Silesia. *Archiv. f. pathol. Anatomie. u. Physiologie u.f. klin. Medicin* Vol II, No. 1 & 2:143–317. Reprinted in Gesammelete Abhandlungen aus dem Gebiete der offentlichen Medicin und der Seuchenlehre, 1879, Berlin: August Hirschwald Verlag. Translated and Reissued as *Rudolf Virchow: Col-*

lected Essays on Public Health and Epidemiology, Vol. 1. L. J. Rather (ed.). Canton, Mass: Science History Publications, 1985.

Virchow, R. 1849. The epidemics of 1848. *Archiv. f. pathol. Anatomie. u. Physiologie u.f. klin. Medicin* Vol III, No. 1:3–10. Reprinted in Gesammelete Abhandlungen aus dem Gebiete der offentlichen Medicin und der Seuchenlehre, 1879, Berlin: August Hirschwald Verlag. Translated and Reissued as *Rudolf Virchow: Collected Essays on Public Health and Epidemiology*, Vol. 1. L. J. Rather, (ed.). Canton, Mass: Science History Publications, 1985.

Ware, J. 1993. *SF-36 Health Survey Manual and Interpretation Guide*. Boston: Nimrod Press.

Weiner, H. 1992. *Perturbing the Organism: The Biology of Stressful Experience*. Chicago: The University of Chicago Press.

Wilkinson, R. 1992. Income distribution and life expectancy. *Br. Med. J.* 304:165–168.

Winslow, C.-E.A. 1923. *The Evolution and Significance of the Modern Public Health Campaign*. New Haven: Yale University Press.

Wolf, S., and J. Bruhn, with the collaboration of B. Egolf, J. Lasker, and B. Philips. 1993. *The Power of the Clan: The Influence of Human Relationships on Heart Disease*. New Brunswick: Transaction Publishers.

Wolff, G. 1952. Social pathology as medical science. *Am. J. Public Health* 42:1576–1582.

World Health Organization. 1948. The Constitution of the World Health Organization, April 7, Geneva, Switzerland: World Health Organization.

2

Family Pathways to Child Health

EDWARD L. SCHOR
and ELIZABETH G. MENAGHAN

Children's physical and emotional health and their cognitive and social functioning are strongly influenced by how well their families function. A family's functioning reflects its composition and the characteristics of its members—their talents and dispositions, their daily activities, their beliefs and values, and their experiences together and apart. Families are also shaped by the world in which they live and their positions and roles within it. As intermediaries between society and their children, parents may be buffeted or supported by external forces. This chapter will explore how changes in the composition and activities of families in the United States are affecting their abilities to safeguard and promote their children's health. We will give particular attention to how family composition and parents' economic roles affect children, and how family patterns of action and interaction shape the health of children, their youngest and most vulnerable members. In tracing the roots of family characteristics and behavior that alter children's life chances and health status, we will consider the extent to which social factors—particularly parents' education, employment and income—explain variations in what families do. We will assess the extent to which such variations in behavior directly affect children's health even when social influences are statistically controlled. We will also explore the interaction between societal and family influences.

Children's health outcomes include early mortality and morbidity, functional status and emotional well-being, and the formation of lifestyles and attitudes with implications for later health; the conclusions one reaches about the quality of children's health depend in part on one's choice of outcomes to assess and on comparison groups. Viewed historically, the health of children in the United States is better than it has ever been (Zill et al., 1983). Neonatal, postneonatal, and childhood mortality rates, for instance, have all declined progressively over the past three decades (Golden, 1985).

Compared to other developed nations, however, children's health in the United States ranks at or near the bottom, despite the nation's standing as world leader in per capita health expenditure (Grant, 1992). There are also large and sometimes increasing disparities in mortality and morbidity among American children according to race, ethnicity, and income (Golden, 1985; Rosenbaum et al., 1991). And while some health problems have been virtually eliminated through immunization programs and public provision of safe water and waste disposal, other problems—termed "the new morbidity" by Haggerty (1975) and "social morbidity" by others—are increasing. Such problems include parental aggression, physical and sexual abuse, and neglect; developmental and learning disabilities, emotional distress, and behavioral and psychosomatic disorders; and high-risk behaviors such as experimentation with alcohol and other substances, acts of delinquency, and impulsive or unprotected sex that leaves children vulnerable to disease, unplanned pregnancies, and premature parenthood.

Parents are often blamed for such problems. It is evident, however, that much of children's compromised potential has its origins outside the family. This failure has its roots in social, economic, and environmental circumstances that affect children's health and well-being directly, and in circumstances that affect children indirectly by undermining the salutary influence of their families. Families function in an environment not entirely of their own making, and they must try to assure their children's well-being in an often hostile milieu of economic pressures and changing social values. Parents are expected to protect their children's physical health and safety, to foster their emotional well-being, and to provide socialization and education that imparts the life skills necessary for success. Parents are also expected to teach skills and inculcate beliefs and attitudes that will shape children's subsequent health behavior. In carrying out these functions, parents are influenced by external forces acting on the family, by their own individual resources, and by the structural, demographic, and developmental characteristics of the family itself. Thus, as we will emphasize, family interactions need to be interpreted not only as manifestations of the family system but also as responses and adaptations to social forces (Fig. 2–1). To improve the health and well-being of children in the United States today, we need a more thorough understanding of how families influence their children's health, and how various social factors operate on and through families to alter children's health. Such a grasp of specific processes is essential if our family policies are to have the intended effects.

It is increasingly clear that access to medical treatment and utilization of health-care services, while important, are not the primary contributing factors to reducing the new morbidity among children and adolescents. In fact, several reviews of factors in adult health argue that health care contributes less to health outcomes at all ages than has been assumed. Williams (1990) asserts that equality of access to medical care is unlikely to eliminate inequality in health status. Socioeconomic inequality, he argues, operating in part via SES-linked differences in living conditions and lifestyle characteristics, would produce significant inequality in health outcomes even if access to medical care were equalized. Socioeconomic status in childhood also has lifelong effects; even

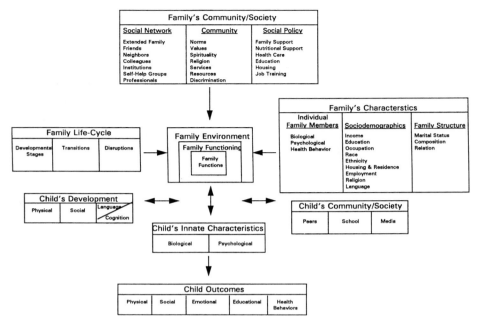

Figure 2-1 Social context of child health.

if children improve their situation later in life, negative health effects persist. Williams cites Forsdahl's 1977 study of Norwegian mortality data, which found that despite the subsequent disappearance of county-level differences in standard of living, very strong correlations persisted between infant mortality rates in the county of birth and mortality from all causes at ages 40 to 69.

Nor is access to traditional health care particularly pertinent to the epidemiology of the "new" and social morbidity, in which social forces are dominant influences on child and adolescent health. Children's own resilience and vulnerability, and the support provided by their families, are important mediators of social forces' influence on children's emotional and social well-being. For adults as well as children, it is as important to understand how social circumstances shape emotional well-being and risk behaviors as it is to study patterns of health-care utilization.

Social Factors and Children's Health

In most studies of child and adult health in the United States, social factors—among which socioeconomic status (SES) is the most prominent—account for the majority of variation. Thus it is important to understand how changes in the family over the last few decades have altered the economic and interpersonal resources available to children.

Trends in Employment and Earnings: Men, Women, and Families

Large and growing numbers of American children live in families whose incomes are below the official poverty level; after dropping in the 1960s and 1970s, the proportion of children who are poor reverted in the 1980s to the high levels of the 1940s and 1950s. But because trends in family income and changes in family composition are interrelated, we need to look separately at trends in employment status and earnings and in family formation and dissolution during the same time period.

For the past two decades, young men have experienced a decline in earning power when employed and an increase in vulnerability to layoff and job loss. Both diminished wages and declining participation in the workforce have hit black men particularly hard (Wilson and Neckerman, 1987). As Coontz (1992) has noted, the decline in American men's earnings over the last two decades has little to do with changing preferences or commitments to work; instead it reflects nationwide changes in the structure of employment opportunities. Hamburg (1992) has described a scientific, technologic, and economic transformation of the world that in its wake has caused social dislocations, many of which are inimical to family functioning. As agricultural jobs have been mechanized, manufacturing jobs have moved abroad, and lower-wage service jobs have burgeoned, the distribution of opportunities for men has shifted. Young men with limited educations are particularly hard-hit, when jobs that require physical strength and hard work become scarce and jobs that require technical skills and advanced training become more numerous.

Meanwhile, young women have experienced some improvement in their earning power. Their attachment to the labor force has grown, and they return to the labor force fairly rapidly after childbirth. Three decades ago, about one quarter of mothers of children worked; today about half of children under age one (Zigler and Black, 1989) and preschool-age children, and over 70 percent of school-age children, have mothers who work outside the home (U.S. Department of Labor, 1988). It is estimated that by 1995 the mothers of 80 percent of all school-age children will be employed. Two-parent families have thus avoided some of the economic consequences of men's declining earning power by means of maternal employment, but at a cost in maternal time spent with children (Hochschild, 1989). Single mothers' earnings are even more critical to their children's economic well-being, but more severely constrain direct maternal care, and increase time pressure. Furthermore, the gender gap in earnings means that even when single mothers are employed full-time year-round, their families have far fewer economic resources than do dual-earner or male-earner married couples or single-father families.

For all U.S. families except non-Hispanic whites, median family income in constant dollars declined in the 1980s. Furthermore, in 1993, the disparity between the top and bottom quintiles was greater than ever before; the top quintile received 48.2 percent of the total income and the bottom quintile less than 4 percent (DeParle, 1994). Children are now more likely than any other age group to be living in poverty: more than one in five children is poor. The poverty rate is especially high in female-headed households, hovering around 51–56 percent since 1970; but poverty rates have climbed among married-couple families as well (Coontz, 1992).

Trends in Family Composition

Meanwhile pervasive changes have been occurring in family structure and composition. The proportion of family households with children that are headed by married couples has been decreasing, and mother-stepfather and father-stepmother families make up a growing share of the family households that include two parents.[1] The proportion of children living with never-married and formerly married parents, particularly mothers, has been increasing over the same time period.

Typical age at marriage, very low in the 1950s, has been increasing steadily in the ensuing decades. One explanatory factor is the declining proportion of premarital pregnancies that are resolved by early marriage. Instead, increasing numbers of women choose abortion, and a large majority of those giving birth now raise their babies as unmarried mothers (Cooksey, 1990). Births to unmarried women increased from 5 percent to 22 percent between 1960 and 1985, and the proportion of mothers who were unmarried quadrupled from 5 percent to 23 percent (Moore et al., 1987). As Furstenberg has pointed out, pregnant teenagers who elect to carry their babies to term are, on average, a particularly disadvantaged group: they tend to be from poorer families of origin, to be members of ethnic minorities, to be low in educational attainment, and to have poor occupational prospects. Unsurprisingly, these never-married mothers are particularly likely to be poor, and analyses of their earnings prospects—given their educational and cognitive skills, prevailing wage rates in jobs accessible to poorly educated women, and the costs of quality child care—suggest that few could support their families adequately even if they worked full-time year-round.

Meanwhile the marriages that did occur between the mid-1960s and the early 1980s became increasingly unstable. Between 1960 and 1985 the divorce rate more than doubled, from 9.2 to 21.7 per thousand. (The annual divorce rate seemed to level off in the early 1980s, and the 1987 rate of 18 divorces per 1000 married women represented a slight decline from previous highs.) Since over half of divorces involve families with children (54 percent in 1984), it is estimated that approximately 25 percent of children growing up in this decade will have experienced a divorce (Furstenberg and Cherlin, 1991). Fewer children were living with two parents in 1989 (75 percent) than in 1971 (83 percent), and many more were living with a divorced parent (10 percent vs. 4 per-

1. The U.S. Census defines family households as those containing two or more members linked by blood/kinship, marriage or adoption, while households of individual adults living alone, as well as those containing members not linked by blood, marriage, or adoption, are considered non-family households. Our focus here is on family households with at least one child under 18; these may be headed by married couples, unmarried mothers, unmarried fathers, and other adults such as grandparents, aunts or siblings of the children.

cent) (U.S. Bureau of the Census, 1971, No. 225; 1990, No. 445). In 1988, 61 percent of children lived in a household with both biological parents, 19 percent with the mother only, 9 percent with mother and stepfather, and 11 percent in some other family arrangement (Mincy, 1992; National Center for Health Statistics, 1988, No. 178). The rate of increase in the proportion of single-parent families has slowed since the early 1970s (U.S. Bureau of the Census, 1990, No. 447), but the proportion of female-headed families with children has still increased.

Not all single-mother families are single-adult households. Overall, only 6 percent of U.S. children live with one or more of their grandparents (Moore et al., 1987), but children living with a single parent are more than four times as likely to have a grandparent present as are those in two-parent families (14 percent vs. 3 percent). Still, these numbers are low in an absolute sense, and most single parents cannot count on the assistance of another adult in the household.

The typical composition of white and black families differs strikingly. A much higher proportion of black households is maintained by a single parent, usually a woman (34 percent of black households vs. 12 percent of white households in 1988), and the trend is for that difference to widen. Between 1970 and 1988 the number of black single-parent households in the United States increased by 127 percent; while in the same period, white single-parent households increased by 83 percent. The prime factor contributing to this disparity was the higher rate of childbearing out of wedlock by black women. In a 1981 survey, white parents were more likely than blacks to be married or permanently cohabiting (83 percent vs. 51 percent), while black children were more likely to be living in a household where the adults had never been legally married and in which the mother was present but the father absent (15 percent vs. 0.8 percent) (Collins, 1984). In 1988, 51 percent of black children and 16 percent of white children lived with their mother only (Eggebeen and Lichter, 1991).

Depending on their age, 40–46 percent of black children had experienced a disruption (divorce or remarriage), a rate much higher than that experienced by white children (Collins, 1984). White children, however, are more likely to face adjustment to a remarriage. At the rates of a decade ago, 4 in 7 white children will have joined stepfamilies within 5 years of parental divorce, compared to 1 in 8 black children (Furstenberg et al., 1983). But remarriage does not necessarily mean stability; 37 percent of remarriages end in divorce (Furstenberg et al., 1983). And mother-stepfather families resemble single-parent families more than they do biological two-parent families in both interaction patterns and child outcomes (Astone and McLanahan, 1991; Thomson et al., 1992).

Alongside these massive changes in marital formation and dissolution, the timing and magnitude of childbearing has also changed. Maternal age at childbearing reached a historic low in the 1950s: women's median age at the birth of their first child was under 20. In subsequent decades, median age has increased sharply for whites and less dramatically for nonwhites. The rate of first births to women aged 15–19 and 20–24 has been decreasing since 1970, while the rate of first births to women aged 25–29 and

30–34 has been increasing (National Center for Health Statistics, June 1989). Socio-economic and ethnic differences in the timing of childbearing have persisted: low-SES women and minority women begin childbearing earlier. Family size has been declining, however, among all groups (Eggebeen and Lichter, 1991). The percentage of married couples with four or more children decreased from 11 percent in 1966, to 3 percent in 1975 (U.S. Bureau of the Census 1967, No. 164; 1976, No. 291). Racial and ethnic differences in family size, while evident, have decreased over time.

There are clear links between economic changes and these changes in family formation and stability. As men's ability to support children has declined, their commitment to marriage has waned. Marriages stressed by economic uncertainties have been more likely to disrupt. As South and Lloyd (1992) have documented, using data from the 1990 U.S. Census, high rates of male unemployment depress marriage rates and increase the rate of births to unmarried women among both blacks and whites. South and Spitze (1986) have shown that, among married couples, a husband's nonemployment increases the likelihood of marital disruption; other studies suggest this occurs because men react to employment loss and the associated economic hardship it entails with anger, irritability, and withdrawal from interaction (Conger et al., 1990). Thus, declining economic conditions make marital formation less likely and marital disruption more common.

Meanwhile, wives' employment and earning power have tended to call into question their undiluted responsibility for housework and child care, creating new sources of conflict in their marriages. Given marital dissatisfaction, their own employment makes women more likely to end their marriages. And never-married and divorced American fathers have proven relatively unlikely to share either income or time with their children. As a result, an unprecedented number of American children have employed mothers and experienced a variety of supplementary child-care arrangements; if their fathers are absent from the household, they also contend with limited economic resources and tenuous or nonexistent ties with their fathers.

Effects on Children of Employment, Occupation, and Income Patterns

Poverty is the best predictor of poor health outcomes for children, including mortality (McCormick, 1983; Wise et al., 1985), activity limitations (National Center for Health Statistics, 1986, No. 154; 1986, No. 156; 1986, No. 160) and utilization of health care (National Center for Health Statistics, 1986, No. 160). These clear-cut links call for more searching exploration of the mechanisms through which low income produces poor outcomes.

Effects of Parents' Educational Level

One such mechanism appears to be minimal education. Parents' educational level is significantly correlated with measures of child health and well-being (Zill et al., 1983), and education tends to vary with income. Maternal education level in particular is associated with higher rates of use of health services. In addition to better employment and higher incomes, educated parents bring more knowledge and, perhaps greater skills, to their role as parents, and thus have more options at hand as they interact with their children. Educational level is reflected in attitudes and assumptions: Mechanic (1964) found that mothers with less education tended to be more fatalistic about illness and less concerned about detecting it in their children, and took fewer precautions to protect their children's health. Parents' educational status also plays a role in their children's appropriate behavior (Lei et al., 1972) and educational achievement (Haveman et al., 1991).

Effects of Fathers' Unemployment and Mothers' Employment

Appraisal of the effects of parents' employment status have tended to focus on the potential negative effects of fathers' unemployment and of mothers' employment. A long line of studies suggests that a father's loss of employment or chronic unemployment erodes family functioning (see Moen et al., 1983). The effects on the family of a mother's employment are far less clear, and seem contingent on multiple factors, including the mother's marital status, and access to assistance with child care and housework and the parents' gender-role traditionalism. According to developmental theory, young children's physical, social, and psychological development is especially sensitive to their environment and to the quality of their relationships; partly for this reason, the dramatic increase in the proportion of mothers of young children who work outside of the home, and their presumed diminished presence in the lives of their children, has become an issue of social concern. Little of this research, however, has focused directly on the quality of mother-child interaction (Belsky, 1988; Goldston, 1988; Scarr et al., 1988; Zigler and Hall, 1988).

The relationship between maternal employment and patterns of health-care use is complex. During their study, Alexander and Markowitz (1986) found that children of working mothers were both less likely to be reported as ill (40 percent vs. 48 percent) and less likely to have visited a health-care facility (58 percent vs. 67 percent). Having a child in poor health was the strongest predictor of use of children's health-care services by working mothers. Cafferata and Kasper (1985) found that working mothers were less likely to seek medical care when their children had mild illnesses or needed well-child care, but equally likely to seek care in case of more serious illness. Mothers' employment influences health-care utilization; decreasing utilization by enhancing social support, but increasing it by adding to daily stress (Alexander and Markowitz, 1986). Others have noted a direct relationship between use of health-care services and the degree of stress mothers reported experiencing (Mechanic, 1964).

In any case, it is difficult to disentangle the effects of mothers' employment from other factors. Employment per se may not be decisive (Bronfenbrenner and Crouter, 1982) but only one among many variables that can influence developmental and behavioral outcomes for children of employed mothers. Other possible variables include the presence and employment status of another adult in the household, family income, the mother's working hours, the marital relationship (including role conflicts and agreement about the desirability of maternal employment), and the availability and quality of nonparental supervision of the children (Croog, 1970). Along with income and education, these employment-related aspects of family life are powerful influences on parents' abilities to carry out their functions on behalf of their children, as well as indicators of other circumstances that can undermine family functioning. Further complicating such investigations is the difficulty of finding "pure" groups of working and nonworking mothers. In the past decade the overwhelming majority of mothers have worked during their children's first few years, though very few have sustained continuous full-time full-year employment (Greenstein, 1990). As maternal employment has become more pervasive, researchers' attention has turned to assessing the consequences of variations in the nature and extent of that employment.

Effects of Workplace Conditions

Parents' employment can influence their childbearing in several ways. First, workplace conditions and job latitude—that is, one's degree of control over one's actions on the job—have predictable emotional effects, which color working parents' interactions with their spouses and children, and thus influence children's health and well-being. Unhappiness and stress at work can undermine the self-esteem and emotional well-being of parents, who then act out their dissatisfaction at home. They may become abusive, coercive, unresponsive, insensitive, withdrawn, or otherwise dysfunctional. Conversely, parents who are gratified by their work and find life satisfying are more likely to interact in positive ways at home. This favorable outcome may be contingent on the domestic division of labor: if the bulk of household and child-care responsibilities still falls to the working mother, the amount of unstructured "quality time" she has available for the family will be limited. When the division of labor in the household is equitably shared, however, Ross and Mirowsky find that employed mothers have greater satisfaction and emotional satisfaction than homemaking mothers. Finally, the absence of adequate child care can also color a mother's life satisfaction and emotional health.

Employment can also alter parenting behavior through the transfer to the home of modes of supervision and interaction that one learns, or learns to value, at work. People's styles of relating to others tend to reflect the degree of latitude and independence they exercise over work-related decisions. Thus parents who work in autocratic or coercive environments are unlikely to adopt a democratic or participatory form of parenting. Drawing on the work of Kohn (1977), Parcel and Menaghan (1990) found that parents, whose work involves self-regulation and initiative and who typically work with symbols and people more than with materials, are more likely to foster self-direction and independence in their children. These results hold even when researchers introduce statistical controls for the effects of education, which influences both the ability to obtain a white-collar position and styles of parenting. The corollary is that parents whose work typically involves relating to things rather than symbols or people, allows the worker little control, and requires conformity to externally-imposed standards and subordination to rules if not people will be more concerned with children's obedience than their inner motivation. Rogers et al. (1991) report more behavior problems among children whose mothers hold such jobs. This finding suggests that a narrow focus on obtaining children's behavioral compliance and conformity is not an optimal parental strategy; behavior problems are lower when parents promote self-regulation and internalization of norms and standards. The work parents perform also affects the nature of their interactions with their children. Mothers who do relatively complex work offer more cognitive stimulation and emotional support to their children, who in turn develop better verbal skills than the children of mothers employed at routine work (Parcel and Menaghan, 1990).

Effects of Family Composition

How have changes in the composition of children's families affected their well-being? The meaning of these changes for children's development and well-being is uncertain, in part because they are so intertwined with the effects of socioeconomic factors; some observers question whether there are any demonstrable differences in the health status of children in single-parent and two-parent families when related socioeconomic factors are taken into account (Jennings and Sheldon, 1985). Differences in family structure do have clear implications for the financial and personal resources available to children, though large racial differences in rates of poverty persist within each type of family structure (Eggebeen and Lichter, 1991). Two-parent black families, for instance, earned only 80 percent of the income of white two-parent families in 1984. Within racial groups, one-parent families have lower incomes. The mean income for female-headed white families, for example, was only about 40 percent of that of two-parent white families (Mincy, 1992). Sixty-six percent of children living with never-married mothers alone were poor, versus 11 percent of children living with both parents (Dawson, 1991). Children in female-headed families are three to four times more likely to live in relative poverty than children in married-couple families.

Family structure, then, is related to poverty: increases in single-mother families have contributed to increases in the poverty rate and vice versa. This relationship is especially pronounced among families headed by never-married mothers (Besharov, 1989). Eggebeen and Lichter (1991) estimate that changing family structure accounted for roughly 65 percent of the increase in official poverty among black children in the 1980s and for 37 percent of the growth in official and relative poverty between 1980 and 1988. The key question is how family composition, and changes in family composition, affect family functioning and health outcomes independent of economic deprivation.

Much recent research has focused on children whose parents divorce. Divorce is postulated to have adverse emotional effects on children for several reasons. First, the break-up of the family may convey to children that their world is unstable and undependable. Second, children may interpret the departure of the noncustodial parent as a personal rejection, a failure, and a loss. Third, continuing spousal conflict can force the child to take sides against one parent, or at best to live in a continually stressful environment. Fourth, divorce usually results in disruption of daily family routines, and the diminished economic situation of the mother—usually the custodial parent—shrinks the resources available to help cope with the changing family circumstances. The social and emotional resources of the custodial parent may also be diminished by divorce, rendering that parent less able to meet the child's needs. Finally, remarriage on the part of either or both parents changes family relationships further in ways over which the child has little or no control.

Recent studies have not found family intactness to be associated with utilization of pediatric services (Wingert et al., 1968) or with the personal health practices of children or adults, although health practices were more variable within single-parent families (Loveland-Cherry, 1986). Adverse effects on "new-morbidity" outcomes, including behavior problems, may be more common (Cherlin et al., 1991). The proportion of American adolescents aged 12 to 16 who had received professional psychological help within the previous 12 months nearly doubled between the late 1960s and 1981, from 2 percent to 4 percent, an increase essentially accounted for by adolescents in single-parent families and step-families (Zill, 1985). Psychological counseling or therapy for children is least common in intact families with both biological parents (4 percent), most common when the child lives with neither biological parent (16 percent), and substantial for other family forms: father and stepmother (11 percent), mother and stepfather (12 percent), and mother alone (11 percent) (Zill, 1985).

The effects of family disruption seem to depend somewhat on the child's age. The period before age 6 or 7 appears to be a developmentally sensitive period in which to experience a divorce: young children are at substantially greater risk of developing emotional, behavioral, and learning problems than older children who experience marital disruption (Zill, 1985). The most overt consequences occur within the first year or two following a divorce (Hetherington et al., 1978; Cherlin et al., 1991). On the other hand, McLanahan and Bumpass (1988) argue that children of all ages experience emotional turmoil when their parents separate, and that the consequences of a temporary period of acting-out, withdrawal, and depression may be more profound during adolescence than earlier.

Disruptions in roles, routines, and family functioning are most marked during the first year after separation. Family members are more likely to eat at irregular times and less likely to eat dinner together, though children's nutrition does not seem to suffer (Johnson et al., 1992). Bedtimes are more erratic and children are more likely to arrive at school late (Hetherington et al., 1978). Divorced parents make fewer maturity demands, communicate less well with their children, tend to be less affectionate, and are far less consistent in discipline and control of their children than married parents (Hetherington et al., 1978). By contrast, single mothers prematurely demand independence and self-reliance from their preschool children (Kriesberg, 1970). Divorced mothers of boys are likely to feel less competent and more anxious, angry, and externally controlled than married or divorced mothers of girls (Hetherington et al., 1978).

Children in disrupted (divorced and/or remarried) families in general, and in single-parent families in particular, seem to experience more stress (Sandler, 1980) and to function less well. These children are more likely to live in poverty, to perform poorly in school, and to exhibit emotional or behavioral problems (Moore et al., 1987; Dawson, 1991). However, few studies control for the adversity faced by such families, whether it be decreased income, lack of social support, or ongoing spousal conflict. Nor do many control for family functioning and children's emotional status prior to divorce. As research in the field has become more sophisticated, the previously identified powerful relationship between marital disruption and children's problem behavior is being called into question. High-conflict marriages produce the same negative effects on children as does marital disruption (Emery, 1988; Cherlin et al., 1991). Much of the emotional distress thought to be associated with divorce is accounted for when emotional status before divorce is taken into account.

The work of Roghmann and colleagues (1973) underlines the difficulty of separating family structure from function. They found that compared to well-functioning two-parent families, single-parent families and two-parent families that were functioning badly were similar in their self-reports of health and in their higher rates of chronic health problems. However, the number of parents in a family did not influence medical care-seeking and/or utilization or apparent ability to cope with illness. Roghmann and colleagues concluded that family structure is important in determining families' functioning only insofar as it hinders coping with the pressures of life. Chen and Cobb (1960) noted an increased rate of psychosomatic disorders in children deprived of adequate parenting. When families become less a place of protection and security, children become more vulnerable to problem behavior (Furstenberg and Condran, 1988). It is how well parents provide such support, rather than the particular family structure, that is critical. It seems likely, however, that single parents rearing children with little support from others will, on average, be handicapped in their parenting ability, even when economic disadvantages have been taken into account.

Other recent changes in family structure have less ambiguous implications. The decline in family size is expected to have positive effects on children's health. Family size has been found to be inversely related to rates of utilization of health-care services for illness (Tessler, 1980), although the pattern is less consistent when controlling for the age and sex of family members (Schor et al., 1987). Preventive health services are used more heavily by smaller families, but the effect of family size loses its power if the parents perceive the child's health as poor or worry a great deal about the child's health (Andersen and Kasper, 1973). Medical care for treatment of injuries is a unique circumstance, in that the number of medical visits for such problems increases with number of children in the family (Schor, 1987).

The growing tendency to delay childbearing beyond the teenage years also appears to be having a positive effect on children's health. Children of teenage mothers are more vulnerable to a variety of health and developmental risks (Hofferth and Hayes, 1987; Zigler and Black, 1989), although it is difficult to isolate maternal age from related educational and economic differences (Spivak and Weitzman, 1987). Maternal age does not have an independent effect on children's behavioral problems (Baldwin and Cain, 1980), and probably not on their physical or social health either. Most of the adverse outcomes for children associated with teenage motherhood, including intellectual deficits, can be attributed to the mothers' truncated education, poor employment, and lack of social support (Baldwin and Cain, 1980). Learning the needs of infants and meeting them is a complex task that may conflict with other tasks of adolescence. Good age-peer role models may be lacking, and teenage mothers' own parents, with whom most adolescent mothers live, may have poor parenting skills themselves. The effects of early childbearing also vary depending on how much support young mothers enjoy: Within single-parent homes, Kellum and colleagues (1977) found greater psychological well-being and better social adaptational outcomes among children of teenage mothers when a grandmother was present. Presumably the grandparent supplemented the single mother's ability to provide instrumental, cognitive, and affective support to the child.

Links Between Economic Activity, Family Composition, and Children's Health

Family composition and parents' employment and income affect the child-focused resources available in the household and consequently a child's health. These resources encompass more than sheer money; they include parental time, energy, and attention as well. Parents' efforts to offset shortages of money by increasing their participation in the labor force may shortchange childrearing in ways that harm family relationships and children's outcomes. Time, energy, and money shape the emotional climate within families, including harmony and conflict among the adults, as well as relations between parents and children—notably strategies of child socialization, support and control, and the consistency of parent-child interaction. Before looking at how shortages of economic resources can constrain both the social support available to parents and the support and control they can offer their children, let us characterize optimal functioning of families.

Ideally, parents provide their children a sense of being supported, and socialize and educate them to function in the family and in society. In doing so, they explicitly select, modify, and structure their children's physical and social environments and the time spent in them. They arrange social and learning opportunities, and monitor and supervise their children's interactions with their peers. Apart from transmitting heritable predispositions and qualities, parents influence children's health and well-being by providing instrumental and cognitive-affective support. Instrumental support includes food, clothing, and shelter, as well as supervision, safety, hygiene, and health care; cognitive and affective support encompass social support, including love, esteem and communication, socialization, and the inculcation of coping skills. The distinction between these two categories of support is somewhat artificial: the way in which parents carry out their instrumental tasks serves as a model of attitudes and behaviors toward family members, and thus becomes part of the process of socializing children.

American society considers children entitled to food, clothing, shelter, public education and, recently, health care. When parents fail to provide these entitlements, governments are likely to intervene. They may go so far as to take custody of the child, even when it is evident that social forces beyond the family's control have substantially contributed to its failure. Many parents fail to provide adequate material resources and supervision to their children. The Food Research and Action Center reported in 1991 that about 5.5 million American children had experienced hunger in the previous month (Community Childhood Hunger Identification Project, 1991). From 68,000 to 100,000 children are estimated to be homeless on any given night (Children's Defense Fund, 1991). Many homes are not safe for children: over 2.6 million children under 5 years old suffered injuries in their own homes in 1990, (National Center for Health Statistics, 1990, No. 181); residential fires are among the leading causes of death due to injury among children aged 1 to 5 in the United States (Baker et al., 1992). Nor are children necessarily safer elsewhere: large numbers of preschool children, especially poor children, spend their days in unsafe or developmentally inappropriate child-care arrangements (Children's Defense Fund, 1991, p. 38). About 2.4 million children are reported to be abused or neglected annually (Children's Defense Fund, 1991, p. 122), despite documented underreporting. Nor are parents uniformly able to provide needed health care: in 1988, 12 percent of children had no regular source of health care, and 36 percent had not received any routine health care during the previous year (National Center for Health Statistics, 1990, No. 181).

Parental inability to provide material and instrumental support due to limited resources is a major explanatory factor for poor health in children. Instrumental support has important secondary consequences for children's well-being. For example, a home in an unsafe neighborhood has obvious direct consequences for the child's physical health and safety. Secondarily, an unsafe neighborhood limits the child's autonomy in play and potential learning experiences, and restricts access to play areas, friends, and other sources of social support. By contrast, a safe neighborhood allows for easier access to friends, which in turn leads to greater social competence and greater acceptance of individual differences.

Family income also affects children's dependence on mass media as a source of entertainment. Children and adolescents vary greatly in the amount of television they watch, but average weekly viewing (21–28 hours) accounts for more time than any other activity except sleeping, including time spent in the classroom (Comstock et al., 1979). When the immediate neighborhood is dangerous, reliance on television tends to grow. In some households the TV becomes a substitute for friends and playmates, and occasionally for parental supervision. Extensive reliance on television as recreation has generally adverse effects. While some children's television shows enhance children's

abilities to do simple arithmetic and promote some prosocial attitudes such as appreciation of ethnic diversity, watching as little as 1–2 hours per day of television can lower
academic performance, especially in reading (Pearl, 1982). Television-viewing is also
associated with physical inactivity and obesity; the prevalence of obesity increases by
2 percent for every hour above the norm (Dietz and Gortmaker, 1985). There is also
evidence that heavy exposure to violence on television and in movies increases children's propensity for aggressive and antisocial behavior (Comstock and Strasburger,
1990).

As children grow older, the quality and safety of their neighborhoods, schools, and
recreation programs become increasingly important. Schools are powerful social institutions with the potential to influence children's physical and emotional health, and social competence, as well as their educational abilities and achievement. The climates
and experiences they provide differ; Rutter and colleagues (1979) demonstrated the
importance of those differences when they found that adolescents' behavior and attitudes—as exemplified by behavior in school, academic performance, dropout rates and
delinquency—were clearly tied to the schools they attended. In general, especially
when property taxes are the primary support for public education, more affluent families have access to better schools; at every income level, however, nonwhite families
face greater obstacles to access to safe communities than do whites (Massey et al.,
1987).

Many parents also fail to provide optimal cognitive and affective support, both essential to children's well-being. Children who feel loved and valued, and who have a
sense of belonging, are more likely to have positive self-concepts and to be able to
form meaningful relationships with others. Parents' abilities to transmit such messages
to their children are, as we shall see, heavily dependent on their own feelings of being
part of a system of social support.

Difficulties can occur at all income levels, but the overwhelming majority of families that are failing to carry out their essential functions are poor. How does poverty
undermine a family's ability to create a supportive environment for its children
(McAdoo, 1978)? Low-income families have to contend with more chronic stress and
with various forms of social discrimination that generate emotional distress and undermine self-esteem and self-confidence (Conger et al., 1984; Sandler, 1980). Heads of
families with low incomes are also disproportionately young, unmarried, and poorly
educated. Thus, in addition to minimal access to material and social resources related
to income, employment, and community residence, poor parents' lack of maturity and
experience, combined with meager support systems, weak self-esteem, and shaky emotional status, create a constellation of factors that are likely to compromise their competence at childrearing.

Low income and poor economic prospects also adversely affect children's health by
corroding the optimism and sense of control of the adults in the family (Elder, 1974).
Parents transmit their beliefs and values to their children, including beliefs about
health and illness. Gochman's review (1985) of families' contribution to children's

concepts of health and illness suggests that children adopt from their parents beliefs about how much control they have over their own health, reactions to illness, assessments of their own health, and values attached to health. Failure to act to promote one's health appears to be related to perceived susceptibility to illness and to a sense of lack of control over one's own health (Rundall and Wheeler, 1979; Tinsley and Holtgrave, 1989). In general, lower-SES individuals perceive themselves and their children to be in poorer general health but less susceptible to episodes of illness than individuals in higher-SES groups (Bush and Iannotti, 1990; Marshall et al., 1970). Lower-SES adults and children also perceive themselves as having less control over their health (Cockerham et al., 1986). This belief becomes self-fulfilling in that parents who consider themselves unable to influence whether their children will be injured are less likely to take preventive steps such as seat-belt use (Bowman et al., 1987). Shared health beliefs within families are demonstrable at an early age, and those beliefs have become relatively stable by grade 3 or 4 (Dielman et al., 1980).

Parents also model healthy and unhealthy behavior directly. Wittingly or unwittingly, parents educate their children about how to cope with stress, frustration, and adversity, and how to make their way through life and eventually provide for their own needs. Adults with lower education and income are most likely to engage in practices such as smoking and heavy drinking that jeopardize their health; they are also least likely to use preventive health services for themselves or their children (Rundall and Wheeler, 1979; Pill and Stott, 1985; Maiman et al., 1986; Tinsley and Holtgrave, 1989; Waller et al., 1990). Unhealthy behavior can be ascribed to a variety of social factors, including the relative expense of a healthy diet; access to stress-reducing drugs including alcohol, tobacco, and illegal substances; and limited access to recreational facilities. Neglect of disease-preventing activities such as self-exam for cancer and pursuit of preventive medical and dental care may be a matter of education or of access to care.

According to the theory of behavioral intentions, the likelihood that children will smoke can be predicted by their attitudes toward smoking, which seem to be established prior to adolescence (Fishbein and Ajzen, 1975). Parental influence on children's smoking has been well-documented: children whose parents smoke are more likely to smoke themselves, and smoking by the parent of the same sex is the more powerful predictor of the child's smoking (Graham, 1987; Murray et al., 1985). Parents' attitudes toward their child smoking are also very powerful. If neither parent opposes the child smoking, the child is approximately five times more likely to smoke than if both parents voice disapproval (Nolte et al., 1983).

While health-risk behavior seems to cluster in families—and specifically within generations—the evidence for familial patterns in health promotion and disease prevention is mixed (Baranowski and Nader, 1985; Perusse et al., 1988). Some researchers have found familial patterns in health-promoting behaviors such as regular physical activity, balanced diet, use of seatbelts and the like, and such patterns have been demonstrated in the use of preventive medical care (Baranowski and Nader,

1985; Schor et al., 1987; Grytten et al., 1989; Nutbeam et al., 1989). Tyroler and col-leagues (1965) found clustering of preventive behaviors among mother-child and wife-husband pairs. A Canadian fitness survey found that family members resembled one another in terms of physical fitness, and explored but did not report on family similari-ties in leisure and exercise (Perusse et al., 1987, 1988). It must be noted, however, that despite such patterns there is not much evidence for a general preventive orientation (Baranowski and Nader, 1985; Pill and Stott, 1985; Lau et al., 1990). Performance of a particular preventive activity cannot be expected to accurately predict the adoption of preventive behaviors (Pill and Stott, 1985).

Poverty can alter parents' affective behavior as well. In a review of the literature, Maccoby (1984) found that parents of different income levels did not differ very much in their acceptance of their children, but that middle-class parents interacted with their children more than working- or lower-class parents in ways known to improve chil-dren's cognitive and social development, self-esteem, and emotional well-being. Mid-dle-class parents were also more engaged in their children's day-to-day lives, more re-spectful of their children, and more likely to act to promote their children's maturity and independence. Maccoby argues that such parent-child interactions are the func-tional mediator between social status and various aspects of children's health and be-havior.

Relationships within families—between spouses and siblings, and between parents and children—serve as models or templates for future relationships (Cauce et al., 1990; Dubow et al., 1991). Parents' relationships with one another provide powerful models for children's interpersonal behavior, and can shape children's later choices of partners and ways of relating to them. Children whose families characterized by caring, sup-portive interactions will have a sense of belonging to and being happy in their families (Roghmann et al., 1973). Conversely, family discord and conflict erode children's sense of security and connection. When social and economic pressures increase marital conflict and erode marital commitment, children absorb negative lessons about the pos-sibilities of mutually satisfying adult relationships.

The quality and extent of social support available to parents also affect children's health. Parents' social relationships are reciprocal, reflecting both the nature of avail-able social resources and the parents' ability to engage them. The most crucial sources of support are personal relationships; there is evidence that impersonal substitutes such as public programs whose support is largely instrumental cannot compensate for defi-ciencies in personal relationships (Coyne et al., 1990). Parents, especially mothers, who have supportive friends and relatives feel more competent and act more compe-tently with regard to their children (Seybold, Fritz, and MacPhee, 1991). Support net-works provide alternative role models for parenting (Cochran and Brassard, 1979), en-abling mothers to adapt better to the problems of caring for children and promoting better interactions with their children (Crnic et al., 1983; Seybold et al., 1991). Moth-ers' social support can thus have important effects on children's development (Cochran and Brassard, 1979; Shonkoff, 1984). Conversely, mothers with the least support from their families and weakest ties to other sources have the highest levels of distress. Distressed mothers are in turn less emotionally available to their children; maternal depression in particular is associated with children's poor health outcomes (Billings and Moos, 1983). In addition to its adverse effects on parenting, social isolation is associated with poor preventive health behavior on the part of parents (Suchman, 1965; Moody and Gray, 1972) and consequently with less apt models for children.

Parents who themselves are socially isolated are more likely to have values and beliefs discordant with their community; they will feel alienated and will be less likely to adopt conventional child-rearing practices and health habits. Consistent with this, Coontz (1992) suggests that social isolation increases the likelihood of child abuse and incest, behaviors that are at variance with the values of the society at large.

Finally, the social support available to parents clearly affects the support parents provide their children (for reviews, see Cochran and Brassard, 1979; Belle, 1989; Sarason et al., 1990; Boyer, 1991). Parents' own experience with social networks, their social connections and skills are models and resources for their children. Mothers' social networks are a likely source of friends for their young children, and their kinship networks serve as models for their children's relationships with relatives (Parke and Bhavnagri, 1989).

Social support benefits children by providing them regular positive experiences and a set of stable, socially rewarded roles (Cohen and Wills, 1985); they are also likely to derive a clear and positive sense of personal identity and self-efficacy (Thoits, 1985). Mothers' ability to express affect and their overall supervisory competence are positively related to children's overall social competence and social behavior (Parke and Bhavnagri, 1989). Family support and affirming interactions with other adults can also have a continuing influence on children's ability to cope with stress (Werner and Smith, 1982). Adolescents whose families rated high on measures of affective-cognitive support exhibited fewer behavior problems and less delinquency, depression, and drug use (Zill and Rhoads, 1991). Conversely, adolescents who received little family support were more depressed (Barrera and Garrison-Jones, 1992). Parental warmth and acceptance also contributes to academic achievement and teacher-rated competencies (Dubow et al., 1991). Active parental involvement in their children's schools and education has been associated with both academic achievement and social maturity (Comer, 1991).

Support includes exercising control and supervision. Preschool-age children demonstrate more social competence when they are being supervised (Parke and Bhavnagri, 1989). Older children and adolescents whose parents monitor and supervise them actively (knowing their whereabouts, friends and activities) have lower rates of delinquent behavior (Parke and Bhavnagri, 1989). Clearly, social circumstances may limit the supervision parents can provide. In one study of 8th graders, those lacking after-school supervision for whatever reason were twice as likely to smoke and use alcohol and marijuana as those with adult supervision (Pinch et al., 1986).

To be effective in the long term, parental control and supervision must be age-ap-propriate and aimed at developing self-regulation in the child. Children whose families support their autonomy are likely to feel that their health-promoting behavior is being facilitated and affirmed (Gochman, 1985; Kaplan and Toshima, 1990); such children are more likely to adhere to health behaviors recommended by their family or physi-cian (Hanson et al., 1987). Conversely, when social support is excessive so that chil-dren feel emotionally enchained, when autonomy is excessive and inappropriate for the age of the child, or when support is contingent upon some behavior and used puni-tively, it can prolong a sick role by bestowing on it positive gain, can promote poor health habits, or can promote adolescent rebellion (Kaplan and Toshima, 1990; Love-land-Cherry, 1986).

Over time, children develop increasingly well-differentiated senses of social sup-port: they have an awareness of their own needs for support and are aware that people vary in their ability to meet those needs (Reid et al., 1989). Children whose parents are depressed or dissatisfied with their lives or marriages, have trouble with alcohol or other drugs, or are embroiled in conflict with the child, give lower ratings to the social support their families provide (Reid et al., 1989). Adverse effects on health of low so-cial support is evident in the increased rates of accidents, injuries, and poisoning among young children whose parents have divorced (Dawson, 1991). Adolescents with weak attachments to their families are more likely to smoke (Foshee and Bauman, 1992). Children are also acutely sensitive to differential treatment by their parents: dif-ferences in treatment are related to differences in children's self-esteem, well-being, and rates of delinquency (Dunn and Plomin, 1991).

When families fail to provide the necessary support, children seek alternative sources of cognitive and social stimulation, models of behavior, and even instrumental support. In some cases support surpasses what the family might have been able to pro-vide; the enduring interest of adults other than their parents can be the critical factor that allows children to succeed in life (Garbarino et al., 1978). But only for low-SES children have "institutional representatives" (teachers and recreation workers) been found to be influential figures. Ironically, children in this group reported fewer people outside the family who took an interest in them than did children in the highest-SES group; thus this "safety net" is not readily available (Garbarino et al., 1978). When nei-ther the family nor other adults provide the support they need, children often adopt the social norms of subgroups such as cliques, gangs, or cults whose beliefs and behaviors can jeopardize the child's health and well-being.

Conclusion

The causal pathways that link social factors like poverty, education, and employment to children's health are neither linear nor unidirectional. Individual families can be se-verely constrained by the broad societal forces impinging on them: for most outcomes pertinent to children, the parents' position in the larger social system is the key predictor. Parents' functioning and "choices" about childrearing are unavoidably shaped by the educational and economic resources they can bring to bear. Thus families' ability to provide adequately—not to mention optimally—for their children is dependent on their own social circumstances and on the larger social context in which they operate. An extreme response to these observations maintains that interventions aimed at altering individual families' patterns of interaction are misplaced: since the strongest determinants of patterns of interaction are extrafamilial, the best way to change families is to change the economic and social forces impinging on them (Wacquant and Wilson, 1989).

Without denying the powerful social forces affecting families, other theorists argue that there is wide variation among families, and in individual outcomes, within socioeconomic strata and within family types (Bradley, 1985). Families themselves constitute their members' main social context, and are unmatched in their domination of the time, attention, and emotions of their youngest members. Nor are parental actions and attitudes completely determined by economic factors. Parents' armamentaria of interactive and problem-solving techniques are learned, and reflect ethnocultural influences and experiences in their own families of origin. And if parental characteristics and choices impede or enhance children's development, interventions aimed at altering parental actions and attitudes are reasonable.

It seems unlikely, however, that interventions aimed at altering individual behavior will be sufficient. The main causes of children's morbidity and mortality are no longer those for which it is appropriate or efficacious to turn to the medical-care system for prevention. Today, the problems that most commonly endanger children and limit their accomplishments and potential have social origins and require social solutions. Their prominence reflects in part the success of medicine and public health in reducing the incidence and consequences of traditional health problems, but it is also a manifestation of the changing world in which children live: changing economic structures, changes in family composition, and greater poverty among families with children. Parents have less time for their children, fewer social supports for themselves, and more social and family disruptions with which to cope.

Children's well-being is also threatened by patterns that have failed to change: patterns of race-, class-, and gender-based inequality that leave many parents unable to provide for their children and unable to gain access to quality neighborhoods and school systems. Nonwhite and female-headed families continue to be disproportionately poor, and poor families continue to be consigned to less safe neighborhoods and poorer school systems. This pattern is unlikely to change without a national commitment to reducing such inequalities and altering the way in which school systems are funded.

Furthermore, social policy still provides little assistance to working parents with young children. While affluent parents have a range of options for supplemental child care, working parents with low earnings typically rely on informal arrangements with neighbors and friends that provide little continuity. Reductions in the extent of income inequality and increases in family support services and programs are needed to reduce related inequalities in children's health and well-being.

Helping families carry out their functions is not merely a matter of resource allocation or even redistribution. To meet the needs of children adequately, the staggering changes in the family that have characterized the latter half of the twentieth century would have to be matched by equivalent changes in the social institutions that play a central role in the lives of families. For example, schools could expand their role to provide a safe and nurturing environment before and after their hours of formal operation. They would have to modify their organizational structure and operations to facilitate the involvement of parents at times when they are available. Ideally, schools could serve as the locus for an array of integrated educational, social, health, and community services. Such an expanded definition of the role of the school represents a new paradigm for public education.

Similarly, employers would have to create gender-neutral pay structures and opportunities for advancement, and work schedules and benefits that allow workers to meet their parental and familial obligations without penalty. Businesses could also participate directly in activities for the social good of children and families, such as providing child care and supporting local schools.

To support today's families, communities may need to find new ways to provide socializing and social-support. Social isolation increases as families become smaller and more mobile, and as parents increasingly work away from the home. Parents still need networks of social support—formerly provided by friends and neighbors—and communities ought to facilitate the development of such linkages. Children's health and safety, social relationships, competence, and emotional well-being all benefit when their attainment is deemed a social responsibility and not merely the responsibility of their families.

Political leaders should begin to apply a family-impact assessment to legislation and regulation so that families are not inadvertently compromised by public policy in their ability to meet their responsibilities.

All these changes would require a change in public priorities, and an alteration in the way we as a society view our collective responsibilities to one another and especially to our children. We need to reconceptualize the roles and organization of major social institutions, such as schools, industry, and government, to help families cope with the social pressures on them and on their children, and to think afresh about what it is that families are supposed to accomplish and how they are to do so. New thought needs to be given to the values, beliefs, and expectations that both guide and limit families and other social institutions. A sense of community, an acknowledgement of our shared responsibility for the welfare of all children is essential to effect change. Given the strong link between adults' well-being and their ability to support the emotional and physical health of their children, one of the best ways to safeguard the health of America's children is to enhance the economic security and social support available to their parents.

References

Alexander, C. S., and R. Markowitz. 1986. Maternal employment and use of pediatric clinic services. *Med. Care* 24:134–147.

Andersen, R., and J. D. Kasper. 1973. The structural influence of family size on children's use of physician services. *J. Comp. Fam. Stud.* 4:116–130.

Astone, N., and S. McLanahan. 1991. Family structure, parental practices, and high school completion. *Am. Soc. Rev.* 56:309–320.

Baker, S. P., B. O'Neill, M. J. Ginsburg, G. Li. 1992. *The Injury Fact Book*, 2nd ed. New York: Oxford University Press.

Baldwin, W., and V. S. Cain. 1980. The children of teenage parents. *Fam. Plann. Perspect.* 21:34–43.

Baranowski, T., and P. R. Nader. 1985. Family health behavior. In D. C. Turk and R. D. Kerns (eds.), *Health, Illness, and Families: A Life-Span Perspective*, pp. 52–80. New York: John Wiley & Sons.

Barrera, M., Jr., and C. Garrison-Jones. 1992. Family and peer social support as specific correlates of adolescent depressive symptoms. *J. Abnorm. Child. Psychol.* 20:1–16.

Belle, D. 1989. Studying children's social networks and social supports. In D. Belle (ed.), *Children's Social Networks and Social Support*, pp. 1–12. New York: Wiley-Interscience.

Belsky, J. 1988. Infant day care and socioemotional development: The United States. *J. Child. Psychol. Psychiatry* 29:397–406.

Besharov, D. J. 1989. Targeting long-term welfare recipients. In P. H. Cottingham and D. T. Ellwood (eds.), *Welfare Policy for the 1990s*, pp. 146–164. Cambridge, MA: Harvard University Press.

Billings, A. G., and R. H. Moos. 1983. Comparisons of children of depressed and nondepressed parents: A social environmental perspective. *J. Abnorm. Child. Psychol.* 11:463–486.

Bowman, J. A., R. W. Sanson-Fisher, and G. R. Webb. 1987. Interventions in preschools to increase the use of safety restraints by preschool children. *Pediatrics* 79:103–109.

Boyer, E. L. 1991. *Ready to Learn: A Mandate for the Nation.* Princeton, NJ: The Carnegie Foundation for the Advancement of Teaching.

Bradley, R. H. 1985. The home inventory: Rationale and research. In J. Lachenmeyer and M. Gibbs (eds.), *Recent Research in Developmental Psychopathology, Book Supplement to the Journal of Child Psychology and Psychiatry*, pp. 191–201. New York: Gardner.

Bronfenbrenner, U., and A. C. Crouter. 1982. Work and family through time and space. In S. B. Kamerman and C. D. Hayes (eds.), *Families That Work: Children in a Changing World*, pp. 39–83. Washington, DC: National Academy Press.

Bush, P. J., and R. J. Iannotti. 1990. A children's health belief model. *Med. Care* 28:69–83.

Cafferata, G. L., and J. D. Kasper. 1985. Family structure and children's use of ambulatory physician services. *Med. Care* 23:350–360.

Cauce, A. M., M. Landesman, S. Reid, and N. Gonzales. 1990. Social support in young children: Measurement, structure, and behavioral impact. In B. R. Sarason, I. G. Sarason, and G. R. Pierce (eds.), *Social Support: An International View*, pp. 64–94. New York: Wiley-Interscience.

Chen E., and S. Cobb. 1960. Family structure in relation to health and disease: A review of the literature. *J. Chron. Dis.* 12:544–567.

Cherlin, A. J., F. F. Furstenberg, Jr., P. L. Chase-Lansdale, K. E. Kiernan, P. K. Robins, D. Morrison, and J. O. Teitler. 1991. Longitudinal studies of effects of divorce on children in Great Britain and the United States. *Science* 252:1386–1389.

Children's Defense Fund. 1991. *The State of America's Children 1991*, pp. 38, 109, 122. Washington, DC: Children's Defense Fund.

Cochran, M., and J. A. Brassard. 1979. Child development and personal social networks. *Child Dev.* 50:601–616.

Cockerham, W. C., G. Kunz, G. Leuschen, and J. L. Spaeth. 1986. Symptoms, social stratification and self-responsibility for health in the United States and West Germany. *Soc. Sci. Med.* 22:1263–1271.

Cohen, S., and T. A. Wills. 1985. Stress, social support, and the buffering hypothesis. *Psychol. Bull.* 98:310–357.

Collins, W. A. 1984. *Development During Middle Childhood: The Years from Six to Twelve*, pp. 1–23. Washington, DC: National Academy Press.

Comer, J. P. 1991. Parent involvement in schools: An ecological approach. *Elementary Sch. J.* 91:271–278.

Community Childhood Hunger Identification Project: A Survey of Hunger in the U.S. 1991. Washington, DC: Food Research and Action Center.

Comstock, G., S. Chaffee, N. Katzman, M. McCombs, and D. Roberts. 1979. *Television and Human Behavior*. New York: Columbia University Press.

Comstock, G. C., and V. C. Strasburger. 1990. Deceptive appearances: Television violence and aggressive behavior. *J. Adolesc. Health* 11:31–44.

Conger, R. D., J. A. McCarty, R. K. Yang, B. B. Lahey, and J. P. Kropp. 1984. Perception of child, child-rearing values, and emotional distress as mediating links between environmental stressors and observed maternal behavior. *Child Dev.* 55:2234–2247.

Conger, R. D., G. H. Elder, Jr., F. O. Lorenz, K. J. Conger, R. L. Simons, L. B. Whitbeck, S. Huck, and J. N. Melby. 1990. Linking economic hardship to marital quality and instability. *J. Marriage Fam.* 52:643–656.

Cooksey, E. C. 1990. Factors in the resolution of adolescent premarital pregnancies. *Demography* 27:207–218.

Coontz, S. 1992. *The Way We Never Were: American Families and the Nostalgia Trap*. New York: Basic Books.

Coyne, J. C., J. H. Ellard, and D.A.F. Smith. 1990. Social support, interdependence, and the dilemmas of helping. In B. R. Sarason, I. G. Sarason, and G. R. Pierce (eds.), *Social Support: An Interactional View*, pp. 129–149. New York: Wiley-Interscience.

Crnic, K. A., M. T. Greenberg, A. S. Ragozin, N. M. Robinson, and R. B. Basham. 1983. Effects of stress and social support on mothers and premature and full-term infants. *Child Dev.* 54:209–217.

Croog, S. H. 1970. The family as a source of stress. In S. Levine and N. A. Scotch (eds.), *Social Stress*, pp. 19–53. Chicago, IL: Aldine Publishing.

Dawson, D. A. 1991. Family structure and children's health and well-being: Data from the 1988 National Health Interview Survey on Child Health. *J. Marriage Fam.* 53:573–584.

DeParle, J. 1994. Census sees falling income and more poor. *NY Times*, Oct 6.

Dielman, T. E., S. L. Leech, M. H. Becker, I. M. Rosentstock, W. J. Horvath, and S. M. Radious. 1980. Dimensions of children's health beliefs. *Health Educ. Q.* 7:219–238.

Dietz, W. H., Jr., and S. L. Gortmaker. 1985. Do we fatten our children at the television set? Obesity and television viewing in children and adolescents. *Pediatrics* 75:807–812.

Dubow, E. F., J. Tisak, D. Causey, A. Hryshko, and G. Reid. 1991. A two-year longitudinal study of stressful life events, social support, and social problem-solving skills: Contributions to children's behavioral and academic adjustment. *Child Dev.* 62:583–599.

Dunn, J., and R. Plomin. 1991. Why are siblings so different? The significance of differences in sibling experiences within the family. *Fam. Process* 30:271–283.

Eggebeen, D. J., and D. T. Lichter. 1991. Race, family structure, and changing poverty among American children. *Am. Soc. Rev.* 56:801–817.

Elder, G. H., Jr., 1974. *Children of the Great Depression*. Chicago, IL: University of Chicago Press.

Emery, R. E. 1988. *Marriage, Divorce, and Children's Adjustment*. Beverly Hills, CA: Sage Publications.

Fishbein, M., and I. Ajzen. 1975. *Belief, Attitude, Intention, and Behavior: An Introduction to Theory and Research*, pp. 381–382. Reading, MA: Addison-Wesley.

Forsdahl, A. 1977. Are poor living conditions in childhood and adolescence an important risk factor for arteriosclerotic heart disease? *Br. J. Prev. Soc. Med.* 31:91–95.

Foshee, V., and K. E. Bauman. 1992. Parental and peer characteristics as modifiers of the bond-behavior relationship: An elaboration of control theory. *J. Health Soc. Behav.* 33:66–76.

Furstenberg, F. F., Jr., and A. J. Cherlin. 1991. *Divided Families: What Happens to Children When Parents Part*. Cambridge, MA: Harvard University Press.

Furstenberg, F. F., Jr., and G. A. Condran. 1988. Family change and adolescent well-being: A reexamination of U.S. trends. In A.J. Cherlin (ed.), *The Changing American Family and Public Policy*, pp. 117–137. Washington, DC: Urban Institute Press.

Furstenberg, F. F., Jr., C. W. Nord, J. L. Peterson, and N. Zill. 1983. The life course of children of divorce: Marital disruption and parental contact. *Am. Soc. Rev.* 48:656–668.

Garbarino, J., N. Burston, S. Raber, R. Russell, and A. Crouter. 1978. The social maps of children approaching adolescence: Studying the ecology of youth development. *J. Youth Adolesc.* 7:417–428.

Gochman, D. S. 1985. Family determinants of children's concepts of health and illness. In D. C. Turk and R. D. Kerns (eds.), *Health, Illness, and Families: A Life-Span Perspective*, pp. 23–50. New York: John Wiley & Sons.

Golden, P. M. 1985. *Charting the Nation's Health: Trends Since 1960*. Washington, DC: U.S. Public Health Service.

Goldston, S. E. 1988. Promoting mental health in early child care settings. In *Proceedings of the Second Annual UCLA National Conference in Preventive Psychiatry*. Neuropsychiatric Institute, November 13–14, pp. 85–115, Los Angeles, CA: University of California.

Graham, H. 1987. Women's smoking and family health. *Soc. Sci. Med.* 25:47–56.

Grant, J. P. 1992. *The State of the World's Children 1992*. New York: Oxford University Press (published for UNICEF).

Greenstein, T. N. 1990. Marital disruption and the employment of married women. *J. Marriage Fam.* 52:657–676.

Grytten, J., I. Rossow, and L. Steele. 1989. Aspects of the formation of dental health behaviours in early childhood. *Dent. Health* 28:6–10.

Haggerty, R. J., K. H. Roghmann, and I. B. Pless. 1975. *Child Health and the Community*, pp. 94–95. New York: John Wiley & Sons.

Hanson, C. L., S. W. Henggeler, and G. A. Burghen. 1987. Social competence and parental support as mediators of the link between stress and metabolic control in adolescents with insulin-dependent diabetes mellitus. *J. Consult. Clin. Psychol.* 55:529–533.

Hamburg, D. A. 1992. *Today's Children: Creating a Future for a Generation in Crisis*. New York: Random House.

Haveman, R., B. L. Wolfe, and J. Spaulding. 1991. Childhood events and circumstances influencing high school completion. *Demography* 28:133–157.

Hetherington, E. M., M. Cox, and R. Cox. 1978. The aftermath of divorce. In J. H. Stevens, Jr. and M. Mathews (eds.), *Mother/Child Father/Child Relationships*, pp. 149–175. Washington, DC: The National Association for the Education of Young Children.

Hochschild, A. R. 1989. *The Second Shift: Working Parents and the Revolution at Home*. New York: Viking Press.

Hofferth, S. L., and C. D. Hayes. 1987. *Risking the Future*, Vol. 2. Washington, DC: National Academy Press.

Jennings, A. J., and M. G. Sheldon. 1985. Review of the health of children in one-parent families. *J. R. Coll. Gen. Pract.* 35 [*Occas. Pap.*]:478–483.
Johnson, R. K., H. Smiciklas-Wright, A. C. Crouter, and F. K. Willits. 1992. Maternal employment and the quality of young children's diets: Empirical evidence based on the
   1987–1988 Nationwide Food Consumption Survey. *Pediatrics* 90:245–249.
Kaplan, R. M., and M. T. Toshima. 1990. The functional effects of social relationships on
   chronic illnesses and disability. In B. R. Sarason, I. G. Sarason, and G. R. Pierce (eds.),
   Social Support: An Interactional View, pp. 427–453. New York: John Wiley & Sons.
Kellum, S. G., M. E. Ensminger, and J. Turner. 1977. Family structure and the mental health of
   children: Concurrent and longitudinal community-wide studies. *Arch. Gen. Psychiatry*
   34:1012–1022.
Kohn, M. L. 1977. *Class and Conformity: A Study in Values With a Reassessment.* Chicago, IL:
   University of Chicago Press.
Kriesberg, L. 1970. *Mothers in Poverty: A Study of Fatherless Families.* Chicago, IL: Aldine
   Publishing.
Lau, R. R., M. J. Quadrel, and K. A. Hartman. 1990. Development and change of young adults'
   preventive health beliefs and behavior: Influence from parents and peers. *J. Health Soc.
   Behav.* 31:240–259.
Lei, T.-J., E. W. Butler, and G. Sabbogh. 1972. Family sociocultural background and the behav-
   ioral retardation of children. *J. Health Soc. Behav.* 13:318–326.
Loveland-Cherry, C. J. 1986. Personal health practices in single parent and two parent families.
   Fam. Relat. 35:133–139.
Maccoby, E. E. 1984. Middle childhood in the context of the family. In W. A. Collins (eds.), *De-
   velopment During Middle Childhood: The Years from Six to Twelve*, pp. 184–239. Wash-
   ington, DC: National Academy Press.
Maiman, L. A., M. H. Becker, and A. W. Katlic. 1986. Correlates of mothers' use of medica-
   tions for their children. *Soc. Sci. Med.* 22:41–51.
Marshall, C. L., K. M. Hassanein, R. S. Hassanein, and C .L. Paul. 1970. Attitudes toward health
   among children of different races and socioeconomic status. *Pediatrics* 46:422–426.
Massey, D. S., G. A. Condran, and N. A. Denton. 1987. The effect of residential segregation on
   black social and economic well-being. *Soc. Forces* 66:29–56.
McAdoo, H. P. 1978. Minority families. In J. H. Stevens, Jr. and M. Mathews (eds.),
   Mother/Child Father/Child Relationships, pp. 177–195. Washington, DC: The National
   Association for the Education of Young Children.
McCormick, M. 1983. The contribution of low birthweight infant mortality and childhood mor-
   bidity. *N. Engl. J. Med.* 312:82–90.
McLanahan, S., and L. Bumpass. 1988. Intergenerational consequences of family disruptions.
   Am. J. Soc. 94:130–152.
Mechanic, D. 1964. The influence of mothers on their children's health attitudes and behavior.
   Pediatrics 33:444–453.
Mincy, R. B. 1992. The effect of labor market trends on parenting and children. Presented at
   *Wingspread Conference on Successful American Families: Challenges and Opportuni-
   ties*, July 26–28. Racine, WI: The Urban Institute.
Moen, P., E. L. Kain, and G. H. Elder, Jr. 1983. Economic conditions and family life: Contem-
   porary and historical perspectives. In R. R. Nelson and F. Skidmore (eds.), *American
   Families and the Economy: The High Costs of Living*, pp. 213–259. Washington, DC:
   National Academy Press.
Moody, P. M., and R. M. Gray. 1972. Social class, social integration, and the use of preventive
   health services. In E.G. Jaco (ed.), *Patients, Physicians and Illness*, pp. 250–261. New
   York: Free Press.

Moore, K. A., J. L. Peterson, and N. Zill. 1987. *America's Children: What Are Their Families Like?* Washington, DC: Child Trends.

Murray, M., S. Kiryluk, and A. V. Swan. 1985. Relation between parents' and children's smoking behaviour and attitudes. *J. Epidemiol. Community Health* 39:169–174.

National Center for Health Statistics: Current Estimates from the National Health Interview Survey, U.S., 1983. Vital Health Statistics. June 1986. Series 10, No. 154. Washington, DC: U.S. Public Health Service.

National Center for Health Statistics: Current Estimates from the National Health Interview Survey, U.S., 1984. July 1986. Series 10, No. 156. Washington, DC: U.S. Public Health Service.

National Center for Health Statistics: Current Estimates from the National Health Interview Survey, U.S., 1985. Vital Health Statistics. September 1986. Series 10, No. 160. Hyatsville, MD: U.S. Department of Health and Human Services.

National Center for Health Statistics. Family Structure and Children's Health: United States 1988. D. A. Dawson. Vital and Health Statistics. 1988. Series 10, No. 178. Hyattsville, MD: U.S. Department of Health and Human Services.

National Center for Health Statistics: Current Estimates from the National Health Interview Survey. Vital and Health Statistics. June 1989. Trends and Variations in First Births to Older Women, 1970–86. Series 21, No. 47. Hyattsville, MD: U.S. Department of Health and Human Services.

National Center for Health Statistics: Current Estimates from the National Health Interview Survey, U.S., 1990, P.I. Adams and V. Benson, Vital and Health Statistics. 1991. Series 10, No. 181. Hyattsville, MD: U.S. Department of Health and Human Services.

Nolte, A. E., B. J. Smith, and T. O'Rourke. 1983. The relative importance of parental attitudes and behavior upon youth smoking behavior. *J. Sch. Health* 53:264–271.

Nutbeam, D., L. Aar, and J. Catford. 1989. Understanding childrens' health behaviour: The implications for health promotion for young people. *Soc. Sci. Med.* 29:317–325.

Parcel, T. L., and E. G. Menaghan. 1990. Maternal working conditions and children's verbal facility: Studying the intergenerational transmission of inequality from mothers to young children. *Soc. Psychol. Q.* 53:132–147.

Parke, R. D., and N. P. Bhavnagri. 1989. Parents as managers of children's peer relationships. In D. Belle (ed.), *Children's Social Networks and Social Supports,* pp. 241–259. New York: Wiley-Interscience.

Pearl, D. 1982. *Television and Behavior: Ten Years of Scientific Progress and Implications for the Eighties,* Vol. 1, No. ADH82-1195. Washington, DC: U.S. Department of Health and Human Services.

Perusse, L., C. LeBlanc, A. Tremblay, C. Allard, G. Theriault, F. Landing, J. Talbot, and C. Bouchard. 1987. Familial aggregation in physical fitness, coronary heart disease risk factors, and pulmonary function measurements. *Prev. Med.* 16:607–615.

Perusse, L., C. LeBlanc, and C. Bouchard. 1988. Familial resemblance in lifestyle components: Results from the Canada Fitness Survey. *Can. J. Public Health* 79:201–205.

Pill, R., and N.C.H. Stott. 1985. Preventive procedures and practices among working class women: New data and fresh insights. *Soc. Sci. Med.* 21:975–983.

Pinch, W. J., M. Heck, and D. Vinal. 1986. Health needs and concerns of male adolescents. *Adolescence* 21:961–969.

Reid, M., S. Landesman, R. Treder, and J. Jaccard. 1989. My family and friends: Six- to twelve-year-old children's perceptions of social support. *Child Dev.* 60:986–910.

Rogers, S. J., T. L. Parcel, and E. G. Menaghan. 1991. The effects of maternal working conditions and mastery on child behavior problems: Studying the intergenerational transmission of social control. *J. Health Soc. Behav.* 32:145–164.

Roghmann, K. J., P. K. Hecht, and R. J. Haggerty. 1973. Family coping with everyday illness: Self reports from a household survey. *J. Comp. Fam. Stud.* 4:49–62.

Rosenbaum, S., C. Layton, and J. Liu. 1991. *The Health of America's Children.* Washington, DC: Children's Defense Fund.

Rundall, T. G., and J.R.C. Wheeler. 1979. The effect of income on use of preventive care: An evaluation of alternative explanations. *J. Health Soc. Behav.* 20:397–406.

Rutter, M., B. Maughan, P. Mortimore, J. Ouston, and A. Smith. 1979. *Fifteen Thousand Hours.* Cambridge, MA: Harvard University Press.

Sandler, I. N. 1980. Social support resources, stress, and maladjustment of poor children. *Am. J. Community Psychol.* 8:41–52.

Sarason, B. R., I. G. Sarason, and G. R. Pierce. 1990. *Social Support: An Interactional View.* New York: Wiley-Interscience.

Scarr, S., D. Phillips, and K. McCartney. 1988. *Facts, Fantasies, and the Future of Child Care in America.* Charlottesville, VA: University of Virginia.

Schor, E. L. 1987. Unintentional injuries: Patterns within families. *Am. J. Dis. Child* 141:1280–1284.

Schor, E. L., B. Starfield, C. Stidley, and J. Hankin. 1987. Family health: Utilization and effects of family membership. *Med. Care* 25:616–626.

Seybold, J., J. Fritz, and D. MacPhee. 1991. Relation of social support to the self-perceptions of mothers with delayed children. *J. Community Psychol.* 19:29–36.

Shonkoff, J. P. 1984. Social support and the development of vulnerable children. *Am. J. Public Health* 74:310–312.

South, S. J., and G. Spitze. 1986. Determinants of divorce over the marital life course. *Am. Soc. Rev.* 51:583–590.

South, S. J., and K. M. Lloyd. 1992. Marriage opportunities and family formation: Further implications of imbalanced sex ratios. *J. Marriage Fam.* 54:440–451.

Spivak, H., and M. Weitzman. 1987. Social barriers faced by adolescent parents and their children. *JAMA* 258:1500–1504.

Suchman, E. A. 1965. Social patterns of illness and medical care. *J. Health Hum. Behav.* 6:2–16.

Tessler, R. 1980. Birth order, family size, and children's use of physician services. *Health Serv. Res.* 15:55–62.

Thoits, P. A. 1985. Social support and psychological well-being: Theoretical possibilities. In I. G. Sarason and B. R. Sarason (eds.), *Social Support: Theory, Research, and Application,* pp. 51–72. The Hague: Martinus Nijhoff.

Thomson, E., S. S. McLanahan, and R. B. Curtin. 1992. Family structure, gender, and parental socialization. *J. Marriage Fam.* 54:368–378.

Tinsley, B. J., and D. R. Holtgrave. 1989. Maternal health locus of control beliefs, utilization of childhood preventive health services, and infant health. *J. Dev. Behav. Pediatr.* 10:236–241.

Tyroler, H. A., A. L. Johnson, and J. T. Fulton. 1965. Patterns of preventive health behavior in populations. *J. Health Hum. Behav.* 6:128–140.

U.S. Bureau of the Census. 1967. Household and family characteristics: March 1966. Series P-20, No. 164, p. 3, Table D, April 12. *Current Population Reports.* Washington, DC: U.S. Government Printing Office.

U.S. Bureau of the Census. 1971. Marital status and living arrangements: March 1971. Series P-20, No. 225, November. *Current Population Reports.* Washington, DC: U.S. Government Printing Office.

U.S. Bureau of the Census. 1976. Household and family characteristics: March 1975. Series P-20, No. 291, p. 51, Table 7. *Current Population Reports.* Washington, DC: U.S. Government Printing Office.

U.S. Bureau of the Census. 1990. Marital status and living arrangements: March 1989. Series P-20, No. 445. *Current Population Reports.* Washington, DC: U.S. Government Printing Office.

U.S. Bureau of the Census. 1990. Household and family characteristics: March 1990 and 1989. Series P-20, No. 447. *Current Population Reports.* Washington, DC, U.S. Government Printing Office.

U.S. Department of Labor. 1988. Childcare: A work force issue. *Report of the Secretary's Task Force*, pp. 7–8. Washington, DC, U.S. Government Printing Office.

Wacquant, L. D., and W. J. Wilson. 1989. Poverty, joblessness, and the social transformation of the inner city. In P.H. Cottingham and D.T. Ellwood (eds.), *Welfare Policy for the 1990s*, pp. 70–102. Cambridge, MA: Harvard University Press.

Waller, D., M. Agass, D. Mant, A. Coulter, A. Fuller, and L. Jones. 1990. Health checks in general practice: Another example of inverse care. *Br. Med. J.* 300:1115–1118.

Werner, E. E., and R. S. Smith. 1982. *Vulnerable But Not Invincible: A Study of Resiliant Children and Youth.* New York: McGraw-Hill

Williams, D. R. 1990. Socioeconomic differentials in health: A review and redirection. *Soc. Psychol. Q.* 53:81–99.

Wilson, W. J., and K. Neckerman. 1987. Poverty and family structure: The widening gap between evidence and public policy issues. In W. J. Wilson (ed.), *The Truly Disadvantaged: The Inner City, the Underclass, and Public Policy*, pp. 63–92. Chicago, IL: University of Chicago Press.

Wingert, W. A., W. Larson, and D. B. Friedman. 1968. The influence of family organization on the utilization of pediatric emergency services. *Pediatrics* 42:743–751.

Wise, P. H., M. Kotelchuck, M. L. Wilson, and M. Mills. 1985. Racial and socioeconomic disparities in childhood mortality in Boston. *N. Engl. J. Med.* 313:360–366.

Zigler, E., and K. B. Black. 1989. America's family support movement: Strengths and limitations. *Am. J. Orthopsychiatry* 59:6–19.

Zigler, E., and N. W. Hall. 1988. Day care and its effects on children: An overview for pediatric professionals. *J. Dev. Behav. Pediatr.* 9:38–46.

Zill, N., II. 1985. Family structure and changes in the use of mental health services by U.S. adolescents. *Workshop on Demographic Change and the Well-Being of Children and the Elderly.* Woods Hole, MA: National Academy of Science.

Zill, N., II, and A. Rhoads. 1991. *Assessing Family Strengths in a National Sample of Families with Adolescent Children: Progress Report*, No. 91-04. Washington, DC: Child Trends.

Zill, N., II, H. Sigal, and O.G. Brim, Jr. 1983. Development of childhood social indicators. In E. F. Zigler, S. L. Kagan, and E. Klugman (eds.), *Children, Families, and Government: Perspectives on American Social Policy*, pp. 188–222. New York: Cambridge University Press.

3

Community and Health

DONALD L. PATRICK
and THOMAS M. WICKIZER

Social determinants of health and quality of life—such as social class, gender inequalities, and racism—influence how long people live, how well people live, and the trade-offs made between quantity and quality of life (Patrick and Erickson, 1993). These determinants operate simultaneously at the level of individual and group behavior and at the level of "community." Investigators routinely observe differences in mortality, disease prevalence, and other measures of health status between and within nations, and smaller subdivisions such as states, regions, counties, metropolitan or rural areas, cities, and neighborhoods. The importance of community as a determinant of health is confirmed by observations that geographic variations in health behaviors and outcomes do not disappear when controlling for individual sociodemographic characteristics, availability of health services, and other individual-level variables (Dayal et al., 1984).

That community can affect health behavior and health outcomes provides the rationale for community-based public health interventions in which entire geographic areas are targeted for educational campaigns (Farquhar et al., 1985) and for epidemiologic surveillance and intervention, such as the prevention of AIDS. It also justifies efforts to develop and activate community organizations for health (Lefebvre et al., 1987; Wickizer et al., 1993), environmental measures such as pesticide control and toxic-waste disposal (Ritter and Curry, 1988), and legislative measures regulating individual behaviors, such as speed limits, no-smoking ordinances, and the sale of alcohol (Lestina et al., 1991). If we can understand the association between community and health more fully, we can improve the design and evaluation of community interventions. Too often, well-intentioned public health personnel initiate community-level interventions without a theory of community change, and prolong interventions without thorough understanding of their effectiveness or lack of it.

This chapter will review the prerequisites for identifying and implementing effective

46

community-level interventions. The design of effective community interventions—those that produce optimal outcomes—calls for five kinds of knowledge:

1. A conceptualization of community at different levels. How should *community* be defined in contemporary America?
2. An adequate theory of *how* community affects health. Both the social and the physical environment undoubtedly affect health, but the mechanisms by which this happens are not well understood. How do communities' structural characteristics and processes modify behavior, cause ill health, protect and enhance good health, or promote happiness?
3. A conceptual framework for measuring and comparing widely different communities using a standardized set of domains and measures. What characteristics and processes of a community should be included in an empirical test of the community determinants of health?
4. Evidence from intervention studies of the relationship among community variables, intervening variables such as attitudes and behaviors, and quality-of-life outcomes. Once particular community environments have been identified as harmful or beneficial to health, what are the most effective means of changing such environments?
5. Diffusion of the most effective community interventions. What intervention strategies should be reproduced and financed?

Analyzing how the environment influences health is at least a lifetime undertaking; its scope is encompassing, and the task daunting. This chapter will review selected literature to address the link between community and health, identify conceptual and methodological issues that need to be resolved, and offer suggestions for future research and directions for developing and testing community interventions.

What Is Community?

Agreement has not been reached on a unified definition of community. Indeed, as Hillery (1955, p. 118) observed 50 years ago, there are almost as many definitions of community as there are community theorists. Setting out to identify "areas of agreement" among the many definitions of community, he uncovered 94 definitions. All definitions concerned human beings; beyond this commonality, no agreement emerged from Hillery's analysis. Definitions of community vary according to the discipline of the theorist—sociology, anthropology, health services research, epidemiology, and human or social ecology—and the purpose of the inquiry. This state of affairs is not surprising given that everyone experiences community with their own lens and purpose. Warren (1978) has categorized the various approaches to community as involving space, people, shared institutions and values, social interaction, distribution of power, and a social system. He also noted great changes in American communities in the twentieth century, with increasing orientation of local community units toward extracommunity systems and a corresponding decline in community cohesion and autonomy. These changes are manifested in the division of labor into specialized goods and services, erosion of interests based on locality, stronger ties to the larger society, bureaucratization, a grouping of important functions by commercial enterprises and government, urbanization and suburbanization, and changing values. At the same time there is no single overarching community shared by all, due to the changes that have occurred over the last century in modes of production, in residence patterns, and the global market. The changing situation of the family, gender roles, and generational conflict and/or cooperation, also play a role, as do relationships among social groups defined by race, ethnic identity, property ownership, education, and class.

We begin with the thesis that the nature of contemporary American society is affected by broad social changes, many of them global. These changes continually redefine the different kinds of community in our lives, their relative importance, and their relationship to health and well-being. A single review chapter cannot "update" the observations of the many distinguished analysts who have written volumes on the definition of community. It is tempting to suggest, however, that as the political pendulum swings, definitions vary. When disenchantment with central government and the larger society dominates, there is renewed emphasis on local responsibility and local autonomy. When political leaders sound the clarion call for a national community response, such as that for economic, legislative or health reform, the larger society becomes the focus.

We will group the definitions of community most relevant to our purposes into three broad categories: community as *place*, community as *social interaction*, and community as *social and political responsibility*. Our ranking of relative importance of these definitions of community, and our suggestions about how to investigate or modify their characteristics, emerge from a synthesis of the literature that is influenced by our own professional interests, political ideology, and personal experience.

Community as Place

There has been a trend over the past 25 years to question whether geography is a necessary or even a desirable element in any definition of community. Early theoretical treatment of the notion of community, by contrast, focused heavily on locality. Warren (1978, p. 21) provides a useful articulation of this viewpoint: "The systematic study of the community has developed around the general focus of shared living based on common locality. In a sense, the community is the meeting place of the individual and the larger society and culture."

The "father" of community theory—nineteenth-century German sociologist Ferdinand Toennies—began with just such a geographical definition. Toennies (1887), in his influential *Community and Society*, defined a community as: (a) a group sharing a defined space, and (b) a group sharing common traits. Toennies proposed his two conceptualizations of community as *gemeinschaft* (human association rooted in traditions and emotional attachment, with a focus on solidarity expressed in shared values and joint rituals) and *gesellschaft*, (specialized, formalized and impersonal relationships, with a focus on moral and economic self-interest). These two characterizations do not describe sequential movement from gemeinschaft to gesellschaft through the industrial revolution, nor the contrast between villages and cities. Both concepts are coexisting ideal dimensions relevant to today's communities, in which both economic progress and social solidarity are compelling social goals (Keller, 1988).

Some theorists flatly reject any geographical definition. Robert Nisbet (1970) declared the notion of community dead or dying. In his view, the mobility of modern household units and the decreasing dependence on local areas for the necessities of life have undermined the validity of a geographical definition. Scherer (1972) argued that a "global village" has emerged with the advent of new media that enable people to accept or reject place.

Since the nineteenth century, the geographic definition of community has been expanded by the field of human ecology, which draws analogies between plant ecology and the urban community. The essential characteristics of community as defined by human ecology are a population, territorially organized and more or less rooted in the soil it occupies, whose individual units live in a relationship of mutual interdependence (Park, 1977). What has happened in the modern community is a change in the "soil." The city, large and small, has become the dominant form of community organization, as illustrated by the Lynd and Lynd's *Middletown* (1929), a famous study of social stratification in a small city in midwestern United States. Community "soil" is also influenced by the global economy and mass communication, to the point that there can be more input from outside the locale than inside. The human-ecology movement, moving with the times, has expanded the spatial delimitations of community to encompass both a localized population and ecological boundaries enlarged by transportation and communication.

Community as Social Interaction

A number of theorists have defined community in terms of social interaction, including social support and shared perceptions, beliefs, knowledge, goals, and the like. Durkheim (1897), analyzing geographical variation in rates of suicide, identified the importance of social bonds in counteracting anomie, or social disintegration. Kaufman (1959) proposed an interactional model, in which the community consists of a set of actions carried out by persons working through various associations or groups. Wilkinson (1970), building on Kaufman's work, viewed community as both collective action on the part of organizations and a phenomenological experience on the part of the individual. These definitions stress the dynamic aspects of community as an outgrowth of social interaction that is continually changing. An exact definition of the scope of community, however, is problematic in contemporary society, in which social communication is national and international in scope rather than merely local.

Studies of social networks and social support define community as social interaction. Wellman (1982), describing the concept of "personal communities," declares that location or geography has little or no importance. Network analysts argue that community should be viewed in terms of types of social relations—networks of ties—and not as locality containing sets of potential relations. A vast literature has established a theoretical basis and empirical evidence for a causal connection between social relationships and health (House et al., 1988). Social networks and social support can affect mortality, psychological and physical functioning, health perceptions, how individuals and families manage disease and illness, and many other intermediate health outcomes. Little of this important work has been grounded in a community context, however, and the relationship between geographic community and social relationships remains poorly understood.

Most Americans live in a defined geographic community, and also participate in many personal networks consisting of other equally important associations. Expanding the definition of community to include personal networks, however, distracts attention from an analysis of the social interaction most proximal to the individual. The community *around the person* may have large, unobservable boundaries; the community *next to the person* is bounded, visible and potentially amenable to intervention through social action.

Community as Political and Social Responsibility

From the perspective of health and social services, community can be defined in terms of political boundaries. In fact, Weber (1921–1922), who analyzed past communities seeking to identify how a community came into being and continued to exist, emphasized the importance of political and social motives in the formation of communal groups. Weber's question remains relevant. The National Commission on Community Health Services, for example, has proposed a concept known as "community of solution" to suggest that the most efficient solution to health problems should determine the size and shape of communities (Gray, 1978). Similarly, Patrick (1989) invoked the need for defined boundaries of political responsibility when designing public policy for people with disability. He concluded that achievement of equal opportunity and inclusion in public life for people with disabilities requires that everyone in the community be involved directly or indirectly.

Angell (1951) drew attention to social responsibilities as a definition of community in a series of intercommunity studies conducted from 1935 to 1946. He set out to measure the "moral integration" of American cities from available statistics; moral integration was defined as "cohesiveness that comes from common orientation to the problems of life." (Angell, 1951, p. 2). Angell developed two indexes, one positive and one negative, to measure moral integration: the welfare effort index, created with data on community welfare initiatives from the Department of Labor, and the crime index created with data from the FBI. Angell found a causal relationship between moral integration and ethnic heterogeneity and mobility: the greater the heterogeneity and mobility of a community, the lower the moral integration. Angell viewed racial heterogeneity as detrimental in that "the dominant element in our society—native, white, and Protestant—relies more on segregation as a solution than any other measure." (Angell, 1951, p. 98). In later analyses, Angell added rate of city growth, percentage of married women working, and percentage of rental units in a community as determinants of moral integration. Other hypothesized influences, including city size, income level, church membership, and small-business ownership, were not highly correlated with his indexes of moral integration.

Defining community in terms of shared concerns or responsibilities may either expand or shrink the physical boundaries of community. A community may be geographically proximal to a concern (such as the local community of persons who provide necessary support services to persons with chronic illness) or more distal (such as a national advocacy group for persons with disabilities). The boundaries shift with the nature of the need and the varying involvement of individuals and collectives. Keller (1988, p. 169) defines the essential aspects of community in such a way as to encompass both a specific locale or social concern and the larger political community: "Community, in my view, must include something larger and grander—a collective framework, participation in a common enterprise, a sense of social solidarity that transcends individuals and private networks; and most especially a sense of mutual obligation and responsibility for social survival." Community defined by social welfare is firmly rooted in the tradition of analyses by Plato, Aristotle, Hobbes, and Rousseau on the social contract: community is the extent to which one is willing to give up a part of the self in order to gain a larger benefit. National leaders constantly invoke such a definition of community in asking the nation to support their social goals.

Our own working definition of community integrates the tradition of human ecology to include a spatial or geographic aspect, and the tradition of social responsibility that informs contemporary health policy by promoting health through community organization activities. Community concerns the entire complex of social relationships in a given locale, and their dynamic interaction and evolution in working toward this solution of health problems. the physical boundaries of the locale should be determined by the pattern of relationships; it will be influenced by outlying areas whose extent will vary depending on the activity under consideration. Therefore we agree with Hawley that a community is "that area the resident population of which is interrelated and integrated with reference to its daily requirements whether contacts be direct or indirect" (Hawley, 1950, pp. 257–258). From the standpoint of the social contract, community is the public forum in which individual interests compete with the social good, the *moi humain* and the *moi commun*.

Two types of community studies are included in this review: studies of community as a determinant of health, and studies of community interventions and their effectiveness. Exactly what constitutes a community-level study is often unclear. Studies of health determinants typically focus on a given geographical area and define community as the area within its boundaries. These studies are conducted at the level of the *community* and not the *individual*. In intervention studies, however, confusion persists over what constitutes a community-level intervention, that is, an intervention organized to modify the entire community through community organization and activation, as distinct from interventions that are simply community-based, which may attempt to modify individual health behaviors, such as smoking, diet, or physical activity. These interventions may be located in the community, but they are directed toward individuals and do not necessarily attempt to modify the social or power structure of the community or to reallocate resources within subgroups of the population based on race, gender or class. We use the term community-level to signify interventions that *attempt* to modify the sociocultural context of a community, rather than change individual behaviors or characteristics. However, both types of studies (community-based and community-level) are included in this review.

How Does Community Affect Health?

A conceptual framework specifying the determinants of health and the functions of community within this framework would help in the design, implementation, and evaluation of community-based interventions. Several attempts have been made to design a comprehensive model of the determinants of health for purposes of health services research and community health promotion (Puska et al., 1985; Patrick et al., 1988; Evans and Stoddart, 1990; Green and Kreuter, 1991; Wagner et al., 1991). These models classify the determinants of health status differently, and place different emphasis on health care. All distinguish, however, among the environment, individual behavior, and health status outcomes.

The Canadian Government's (1974) analytic framework, published as *A New Perspective on the Health of Canadians*, offered a useful means of classifying the major determinants of health, using the categories of lifestyle, environment, human biology, and health-care organization. Building on this framework, Evans and Stoddart (1990) developed the more detailed model shown in Figure 3–1.

This model distinguishes the physical and social environment from the individual behaviors and biology that constitute the "host" response. Determinants of health-related outcomes thus include genetic endowment, the physical environment, the social environment, and individual response, both behavioral and biological. Both health outcomes and the physical and social environment are influenced by prosperity, in that there are inevitable economic trade-offs in the investment in health, most notably between health care itself and such other health-promoting activities as income-redistribution programs and subsidy of education.

This causal model provides a sound conceptual basis for considering the influence of community on health. As a determinant of health, community interacts with broader determinants, notably the social and physical environment. Communities contain the social environment, including worksites, schools, families, friends, and a range of organizations and social institutions. These social units are sources of reciprocal social influence that affect the health and well-being of individuals. Individuals and groups

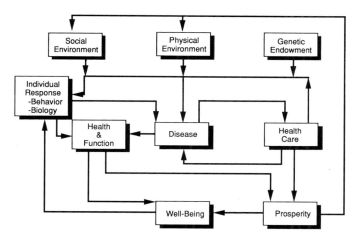

Figure 3-1 A causal model of the determinants of disease, health and function, and well-being (Evans and Stoddart, 1990).

are both agents and recipients of social influence. Community also incorporates the physical environment, and for this reason alone its definition must include a geographic component: the physical environment of a locale, influenced by the larger global environment, affects the health of its residents. For example, the poisonous properties of excessive lead have long been recognized as a serious hazard to mental development, particularly in children (Beasley et al., 1973). Air and water quality are also associated with disease incidence (Bang et al., 1975).

Our task is therefore "unbundling" the social and physical environment as depicted in Figure 3–1. We reviewed the literature on studies whose primary goal was to investigate the effects of social and physical environmental processes on the health of communities. Our main aim is to illustrate the approaches used by these investigations and the scope of their inquiry; the reporting of detailed findings is of less concern. When studies had both social and physical environmental aspects, we categorized them arbitrarily on the basis of their dominant emphasis. We have undoubtedly "disturbed" the intentions of some investigators and overlooked important works on how community affects health.

This review includes studies of multiple geographic communities, e.g., neighborhoods, postal code areas, villages, cities, counties, and countries. In each case, analyses were conducted at the level of community, even if community was only a dummy variable in a regression model. We have excluded studies in which analyses were conducted solely at the individual level, even if several communities were sampled, as well as studies of such poor quality as to prevent adequate description.

This focus on multiple-community studies should not detract attention from case studies that can provide valuable insight into the process of activating and mobilizing communities. Koos' classic, *The Health of Regionville* (1967), offers in-depth understanding of how communities relate to families, how different classes of people interact, how health concerns arise out of unemployment and perceptions of need, and how communities mobilize their health resources. Ethnographic case studies can also capture varying perceptions of the community and of health and illness. Although they have serious limitations, including problems of generalizability and replicability, case studies can help improve practice methods and advance theory about community and health.

A recent case that illustrates the value of the case-study approach is the analysis of one community's response to toxic-waste contamination of its water supply (Brown and Mikkelsen, 1990). In the mid-1970s, residents of Woburn, Massachusetts, an industrial town 15 miles north of Boston, realized that children in the community were contracting leukemia at an alarmingly high rate. On their own initiative, families in Woburn discovered a leukemia cluster, which they attributed to carcinogens that had leached into the drinking-water supply from industrial waste. Citizens of Woburn enlisted the help of "outside" public-health experts and gathered evidence to document the nature and scope of the contamination problem. This effort resulted in the filing of a civil suit against two large corporations on behalf of the families whose children died from leukemia allegedly as a result of the contaminated water supply.

This case traces the development of community activism around the issue of toxic-waste contamination and the important roles that a few key individuals, such as the mother of one of the leukemia victims, played in initiating action. Community mobilization in Woburn, however, encountered problems. Those most affected were lower-middle-class or lower-class families living near the polluted areas. A small group of woman, mothers of the affected children, were outside the power structure; they faced strong opposition. The authors draw attention to the gender and class bias that hindered mobilization of the Woburn community. Even so, the case study reveals the power and influence that a small group of committed citizens exercised on an entire community. Their actions stimulated public debate and, ultimately, public health decisions. Case studies of this type offer insight into complex community mobilization processes and the roles of the various participants. Such insights rarely emerge from multi-community studies using quantitative analyses.

The Social Environment

A community's social environment encompasses characteristics and processes ranging from ethnic composition and occupational and demographic characteristics to the dynamics of community interaction. Forty-eight community studies focusing on social-environmental factors are described in Appendix A. Most of these multi-community studies were published between 1970 and 1991; about half describe communities outside the United States. The outcome measures used are primarily mortality and disease incidence, although several studies focus on mental-health outcomes (Kasl and Harburg, 1975; Gore, 1978; Neil and Jones, 1988; Linn et al., 1989). Most data were collected from population surveys, and both primary and secondary data were used in analyses with similar frequency. We will divide this review of studies of socio-environmental factors into four major groups: socioeconomic status, social stress, social support, and community character.

Socioeconomic Status and Social Class

In general, socioeconomic status has been defined and measured in community-based health studies in much the same ways as in studies of individuals. Individually aggregated data on occupation, education, and income are analyzed as contributors to the health of communities. Other indicators include neighborhood composition (Brooks, 1975), quality of housing (Duvall and Booth, 1978), and unemployment (Black and Laughlin, 1986). The results of these studies support the foregone conclusion that lower socioeconomic status is associated with lower health status.

Brooks (1975) investigated the relationships among low family income, low education, poor housing, percentage of African-Americans, and neonatal and postneonatal mortality rates in 2,237 counties in the United States. Low education and percentage of African-Americans were shown to have direct effects on both components of infant mortality and to account for the associations between income, housing, and rates of infant loss. This analysis reinforces the often-observed independence of socioeconomic variables in relation to health outcomes: how education works is different from how income and/or occupation work. The finding concerning the African-American composition of communities also suggests that family relationships, gender roles, and broad cultural influences not easily measured in community studies may explain the impact of socioeconomic factors on health.

Studies of social environment that incorporate area-based measures of socioeconomic status are susceptible to the ecological fallacy, whereby ecologic correlations are explained in individual terms (Morgenstern, 1982). For example, poverty levels of different geographic areas may be compared and interpreted as though they were accurate measures of the income level of residents in those areas. Area-based studies can be misleading, especially in cities where socioeconomic status can vary greatly within a small area, e.g., within a single block in the United States. Correlations between a community-level characteristic and a given health outcome, i.e., geographical area and mortality, do not always coincide with correlations between individual-level characteristics and health measures. In studies of endometrial cancer, for example, area-based measures of social class such as mean income and educational level did not show the same strong positive association as did measures of the social class of individuals (Liberatos et al., 1988). Kasl and Harburg (1975) question the usefulness of aggregating the characteristics of individuals and of describing environments in the same way as other variables. Even if analyzed identically, variables have different levels of credibility or susceptibility to the ecological fallacy.

Social Stress

Social stress, in community studies, is a conglomerate of two or more variables or processes representing the concepts of economic deprivation, crowding, family insta-

bility, and crime. Stress, which ranges in its manifestations from broad social disorganization to individual psychoendocrine changes, is hypothesized to result when these
social factors cause decrements in health. The evidence for this hypothesis is less consistent than that for socioeconomic status, although studies increasingly implicate
stressful social conditions in mortality, morbidity, and sense of insecurity arising from
increasing urban violence.

Investigators have begun to use socioeconomic data that are available on a consistent and comparable basis to describe areas of residence. Measurement of deprivation
has been one product of this methodological innovation. Carstairs and Morris (1991)
measured deprivation in England, Wales, and Scotland "on a dimension which reflects
the access people have to material resources which . . . permit individuals to play the
roles, participate in the relationships and follow the customary behavior which is expected of them by virtue of their membership in society." These studies defined community using postcode sectors, local government jurisdictions, and health boards. After
considering several different sets of indicators formulated by other investigators, they
decided on overcrowding, male unemployment, low social class, and lack of a car as
indicators of deprivation. All four variables were applied to individuals, not to households. The influence of deprivation on health is strongest in young adults, although
health-status differences are associated with deprivation in older age groups as well.
Area-wide deprivation was shown to have an influence on mortality differentials by
social class, and it is suggested that Scotland's greater mortality differentials by social class is due in part to its adverse socioeconomic circumstances. This study and
others highlight the important influence of economic factors, particularly unemployment, on the well-being of people in affected areas. Social class inequalities exert influence within the political and economic structure of communities. The economic environment of certain communities is thus a target for interventions such as income
maintenance or mixed-income housing in order to promote individual and social well-
being.

Evidence of the deleterious effects of crowded household conditions—constant and
intense interaction, which presumably causes social stress—is mixed. Some community studies using aggregate units of analysis found little evidence that crowding is
damaging to health (Cassel, 1973; Factor and Waldron, 1973). Other studies obtained
positive associations between some form of crowding and infant mortality (Schmitt
1966), mortality (Galle et al., 1972), and admissions to mental hospitals (Galle et al.,
1972). Booth and Cowell (1976), using family-level data from intact families to test
the effects of crowding, found that crowded households and neighborhood conditions
had little or no effect on people's health. Gove and colleagues (1979, 1980) concluded
from a similar study that overcrowding had substantial effects. Differing units of
analysis and methods of study may explain the lack of consistent results across investigators and studies. Alternatively, crowding may have a negative effect on health in
some communities and not others.

In a recent community study of depression in a southern black community, Dressler

(1991) analyzed the role of socially patterned stress in depression. Using a brief measure of depressive symptoms, Dressler and colleagues compared a community in Alabama in which 90 percent of residents are black with data from similar studies in Alameda County, California, and Kansas City, Missouri. The crude prevalence of high depressive symptoms was lower in the Alabama community (20 percent) than in Kansas City (26 percent) or Alameda County (22 percent). Data from Alabama yielded a portrait of a community struggling to keep its head above water economically, where access to jobs and educational opportunities were severely limited. In the face of this adversity, the investigators found that household and family structure and the church were important sources of economic and social support. Households, as opposed to individuals, provided the bulk of the "resistance resources" used to cope with social stress. Just as stress itself is socially patterned, placing a greater burden on disadvantaged groups, responses to stress are undoubtedly conditioned by the social relationships and culture of communities.

Urban Violence

Another component of social stress deserving of particular attention is urban violence. Viewed from a public health perspective, deaths and injuries from assaultive violence have reached epidemic proportions in some U.S. cities (U.S. Department of Health and Human Services, 1986). Urban violence takes several forms, including homicide, assaultive violence, domestic violence, child abuse, sexual assault, and firearm injury. Homicide is of greatest concern for the toll it exacts on urban communities and on minority groups in particular.

In 1987, homicide was the 11th leading cause of death overall in the United States, accounting for nearly 20,812 deaths (U.S. Department of Health and Human Services, 1990). But the risk of homicide varied greatly by race and across communities. In 1983, homicide was the 5th leading cause of death among blacks, 14th among whites, and 9th among persons of other races (Centers for Disease Control, 1987). Meanwhile, homicide was the leading cause of death among black males aged 15 to 34. Because it strikes disproportionately among the young, homicide takes a large toll in terms of years of potential life lost: for blacks, homicide was the 3rd leading cause of years of potential life lost (Centers for Disease Control, 1987).

Though the effects of violence and homicide are exhaustively noted and analyzed, the root causes remain inadequately understood. Unsurprisingly, repeated studies have found the homicide rate to be related to poverty measured in absolute terms (the poverty level) as well as to social inequality measured in relative terms (income dispersion) (Flango and Sherbenou, 1976; Swigert and Farrell, 1976; Muscat, 1988). The violence-inducing consequences of poverty and social inequalities stem from their adverse effects on social relations and social organization (Blau, 1977; Messner, 1982). The high levels of homicide observed among blacks and in certain regions of the country (the South) have given rise to a culture-of-violence theory (Wolfgang and Ferracuti, 1967; Curtis, 1975; Silberman, 1980). The notion that violence may be culturally related has received some support in empirical studies (Blau and Blau, 1982; Messner, 1982; Williams, 1984). Blaming the culture of a community for violence, however, focuses only on proximal determinants.

Williams (1984) points out that the statistical relationship between ethnic membership (black) and homicide rates observed in some studies can be attributed to unmeasured economic factors, and perhaps such other factors as the chronic stress, developmental issues, and mental-health problems experienced by many low-income urban blacks, especially black youth (Baker, 1985; Tardiff, 1985; Brunswick and Merzel, 1988). Limited coping resources and low frustration tolerance in the face of overwhelming emotional, developmental, sociocultural, and environmental stressors may account for the high levels of violence and homicide observed in low-income minority urban areas.

Epidemiologists and other investigators also stress the link between the *availability* of guns in many communities and the homicide rate (Baker, 1985; Hebedoe et al., 1985). Sloan and colleagues (1988), for example, found virtually all of the adjusted excess risk of death from homicide in Seattle, Washington, versus Vancouver, Canada—two geographically proximate cities in the Pacific Northwest that share many social and economic characteristics—to result from the 4.8-fold higher risk of being murdered with a handgun. Handguns are not readily available in Vancouver. For some subgroups of the population, urban violence is not an acute episodic event but a recurrent chronic condition that affects entire communities (Sims et al., 1989).

Social Cohesion

Social cohesion can be viewed as the flip side of social breakdown. A series of studies on "the Roseto Effect" is widely cited as evidence for the positive effects of social cohesion on longevity (Stout et al., 1964; Bruhn et al., 1966; Bruhn and Wolf, 1979; Egoff et al., 1992). Roseto, Pennsylvania, an Italian-American town in eastern Pennsylvania, has been studied intensively since 1962 because of its strikingly low mortality rate from myocardial infarction, as compared to the adjacent town of Bangor and three other nearby control communities. Between 1955 and the early 1960s, Roseto was characterized by ethnic and social homogeneity, close family ties, and cohesive community relationships; it was the kind of town Jimmy Stewart lived in in Frank Capra's *It's a Wonderful Life*. Investigators postulated that Roseto's low rate of myocardial infarction could be attributed to the town's stability, family cohesion, and supportiveness. They also predicted that the loosening of family ties and community cohesion would be accompanied by loss of this protective effect.

In a 50-year comparison of mortality rates, Egoff and colleagues (1992) found a progressive rise in the mortality rate from myocardial infarction among Roseto men and women over the 30-year period between 1935 and 1964. After this period, a sharp increase occurred between 1965 and 1974, accompanying a decrease in social cohesion (Wolf and Bruhn, 1992), as did a similar increase in total mortality. This important study supports the original hypothesis that a decline in social solidarity and homogeneity would lead to more deaths from myocardial infarction. It also suggests that the dynamics of social cohesion need to be investigated more closely in order to understand exactly what was lost in Roseto, and presumably in many other communities, when strong ethnic and family ties disintegrate.

Challenges to social and family cohesion in America have been described powerfully in novels by Amy Tan and Bette Bau Lord on the experience of second-generation Chinese women in San Francisco (Lord, 1981; Tan, 1989). Social mobility, intermarriage, changes in gender roles, the mixing of cultural traditions, and geographical mobility all contribute to a sense of loss of community that profoundly affects identity and stability with multigenerational consequences.

Social cohesion may have other important benefits. Recent research in community psychology has advanced understanding of the phenomenon of "sense of community" and its effects. Sense of community is a complex concept, difficult to define and elusive to measure. McMillan and Chavis (1986) propose a definition with four elements: *membership*, the feeling of belonging and personal relatedness; *influence*, the feeling that one makes a difference to a group and vice versa; *integration and fulfillment of needs*, the expectation that one's needs will be met through membership in the group; and *shared emotional connection*, the belief that members have shared and will continue to share a history. In short, sense of community is a feeling of belonging, and of mattering to one another and to the group, and a shared faith that one's own and others' needs will be met through the commitment to be together (McMillan, 1976). The importance of sense of community stems from its effect on people's behavior and perceptions about their environment, which may increase their willingness to participate in activities and associations that often play a central role in community organization and development. Recent research points to an association between sense of community and participation in voluntary organizations and associations that address local problems (Chavis and Wandersman, 1990).

Sense of community may have a catalytic effect on community action by affecting people's perceptions of their environment, social relations, and perceived control. The stronger the sense of community, the more influence people will feel they have on their immediate environment (McMillan and Chavis, 1986). Thus a sense of community can contribute to individual and community development in a reciprocal fashion: sense of community may stimulate participation in community-action groups and improve their chances for success, which in turn may over time enhance the sense of community.

The potential role of community organizations in addressing social and health problems at the local level (Naparstek et al., 1982; Green, 1986; Moynihan, 1986), and the importance of citizen participation in these organizations (Perlman, 1976; Mayer, 1984; Florin, 1989), has received increased attention in recent years. Chavis and Wandersman (1990) argue that sense of community serves as an important catalytic force, increasing the likelihood of participation in voluntary associations. More generally, sense of community may help further community development by giving people a sense of individual and collective power and a conviction that they can influence events through collective action.

The impact of sense of community on health remains to be investigated. However, direct measures of social relationships provide persuasive evidence that the lack of social relationships is a major risk factor for mortality (Berkman and Syme, 1979; Broadhead et al., 1983; Schoenbach et al., 1986; House et al., 1988). House et al. (1988), after reviewing studies using these measures, suggested that small communities may provide a particularly broad context of social integration and support that benefits most people. However, the relationship between low social integration and mortality may be less valid, or have less variance, in rural and small-town environments, where the social context may provide a moderate level of social integration for everyone except very isolated individuals.

How community promotes social relationships—the essence of Durkheim's inquiry—is not well understood. Community institutions—churchs, professional organizations, political and economic structures—undoubtedly influence social relationships. Americans today are less likely to be married, more likely to be living alone, less likely to belong to voluntary organizations, and less likely to visit informally with others than in previous eras (Veroff et al., 1981). These changes reflect and promote changes in the community that may enhance or inhibit the effects of social ties and their impact on health and well-being.

Community Character

Social ecologists sometimes analyze communities as though they had personalities that could be classified with accuracy and detail: warm and supportive or cold and controlling (Insel and Moos, 1974). The social climate of an environment, in the view of ecologists, shapes the behaviors of its inhabitants, who in turn influence their environment (Insel, 1980). "The person-environment fit," a concept developed by French and colleagues (1972), describes aspects of an environment as either demands or resources. The individual brings his or her own demands and resources to this environment and the environment-person interaction determines the outcomes.

Several studies have measured the social environment in terms of its "personality" and potential influence on the person-environment fit. Notable among them are those by Levine and colleagues (Levine and Bartlett, 1984; Levine et al., 1989), who investigated the relationship between the pace of life, punctuality, and coronary heart disease (CHD) in different communities. Indicators of pace included walking speed and talking speed, the speed with which postal and bank workers respond to requests, and the proportion of individuals wearing watches (concern with clock time). These studies are based on one premise in the controversial theory of the Type-A individual (Friedman and Rosenman, 1974): that time urgency—the chronic struggle to achieve many goals in a short period of time—is detrimental if not toxic to health, and a fundamental feature of coronary-prone behavior.

Extending these notions, Levine and others hypothesize that communities too can be characterized by tempo—some faster-paced and others slower-paced. In a series of studies in Japan, Taiwan, Indonesia, Italy, England, and the United States, it was found that public clocks were most accurate in the most economically developed countries (Japan and the United States), and least accurate in the least-developed country (Indonesia). Pace of life was strongly related to death rates from coronary heart disease across both cities and regions of the country. A possible explanatory factor is that individuals living in fast-paced communities may be more prone to unhealthy behaviors such as cigarette smoking, placing them at greater risk for CHD.

The ecological fallacy is as pertinent to these studies of community character as it is to area-based studies of socioeconomic environments. You can remove the Type-A person from the Type-A environment, in other words, and still find the Type-A person. The notion that communities vary in terms of time urgency has intuitive appeal, however, and matches the observations of people who travel between big cities and slower-paced communities. Depending on the individual's fit with environment, some communities may be more healthful than others.

The Physical Environment

Physical environmental characteristics and processes exert an important influence on a community and the health of its population. These factors include air and water pollution as well as geographic location (urban or rural), climate, noise level, housing, transportation patterns, and other physical forces such as geoseismic activity and fires. The health effects of physical environmental factors have been subjects of epidemiological investigation for over a century. Generally speaking, these studies have identified a population believed to be exposed to some environmental agent and compared its rates of disease with those of an unexposed comparison population. Such investigations do not qualify as community studies as defined here, because the community itself is not the unit of analysis; nor do they systematically examine physical environmental factors with the primary intent of improving understanding of community health.

The physical environmental studies reviewed here are listed in Appendix B. We have grouped these studies into two categories: (1) those examining the effects of pollution, and (2) those aimed at exploring geographical variations in health, particularly urban-rural differences. It should be noted that most studies used multiple sets of measures and often combined social and physical factors.

Pollution

The quality of a community's air and water resources are among the most visible aspects of the physical environment. Over the last several decades, numerous scientific studies have been conducted throughout the world to assess the health effects of exposure to toxic agents and pollutants. Studies have documented adverse health effects of occupational exposure to a variety of industrial agents, such as PCBs (polychlorinated biphenyls) (Landrigan and Markowitz, 1989). Others have documented the adverse effects of exposure to elevated levels of atmospheric pollutants as a result of specific episodes, such as the elevated levels of air pollution that occurred sporadically in New York City during the mid-1960s (Glasser et al., 1967). Knowledge of the health hazards of toxic agents and pollutants has improved over time but remains limited, particularly with regard to the effects of chronic exposure to low levels of pollutants (Doll, 1992).

The air and water pollution studies listed in Appendix B produced mixed findings, some presenting evidence of adverse effects (Blot and Fraumeni, 1976; Bourke et al., 1979; Lloyd et al., 1985; Ong et al., 1991) and others finding little effect (Lan and Shy, 1981; Schechter et al., 1990; Beasley et al., 1973; Lipfert, 1980). These studies examine diverse health outcomes, including acute and chronic respiratory diseases, respiratory cancer mortality, enteric infections and blood-lead levels. They also vary considerably in rigor of design and analysis. Analyzing county-level data for the United States from 1950 to 1969, Blot and Fraumeni (1976) found age-adjusted lung cancer mortality to be associated with proximity to manufacturing industries, based on a multiple regression model that controlled for a number of population and geographic characteristics. High concentrations of manufacturing plants appeared to explain the elevated mortality levels observed in southern coastal communities. This study's success in controlling for possible confounding factors, and the fact that the data base included all U.S. counties over a 20-year period, strengthen the credibility of the findings. Studies that are more local in scope are often less able to control for the effects of factors, such as race and social class, that may confound relationships between measures of pollution and health outcomes (Bourke et al., 1979; Lloyd et al., 1985).

The lack of consistency in findings suggests a need for caution in considering the potential health effects of pollution. Even in communities located near highly visible sources of pollution, such as natural gas refineries, citizen concern about health effects may be difficult to support on scientific grounds (Schecter et al., 1990). Cost and data limitations preclude controlling for confounding factors such as smoking. When studies are able to control for confounding factors, the predicted effects of pollution on health are often attenuated (Lan and Shy, 1981).

Geographic Location and Urban-Rural Differences

A community's geographic location, and in particular its degree of urbanization, may affect health indirectly as well as directly. Certain population subgroups, particularly disadvantaged people, may experience increased mortality due to diseases associated with pollution (Hexter and Goldsmith, 1971). Also, people's health values and attitudes may differ in urban and rural areas, leading to differences in behavior (diet, exercise, smoking, care-seeking) and ultimately health status (Greenberg, 1983).

Observed differences in mortality rates across geographic areas prompted Campbell and Beets (1979) to examine climatological influences. They analyzed mortality data for eight conditions in 143 large U.S. metropolitan areas classified by mean temperature at different times of year. Climate was associated with mortality rates for two of the eight conditions: heart attacks and injuries. The correlations were strongest in the case of heart attacks, with mortality increasing during severe winter weather. Another study, investigating the role of climate in sudden infant death syndrome (SIDS) in eight U.S. communities, showed that infants in cold-wet climates, such as that of Seattle, were more likely to die from SIDS than infants in cities with different climates (Deacon and Williams, 1982). The researchers speculated that weather conditions had an indirect effect on infants at risk through increased prevalence of respiratory infections in the general population.

An observed association between cancer mortality and population density led Connelly (1982) to the hypothesis that environmental differences between urban and rural areas could affect health. Analysis of detailed data on cancer incidence in Colorado and Iowa, examining differences in risk, found the incidence of several types of common cancer, including lung, colon, and bladder cancer, to be significantly higher in the urban areas. These findings were consistent with those of other analyses (Blot and Fraumeni, 1976; Nasca et al., 1980; Mackenbach et al., 1988), though interpretation was problematic because the study was unable to control for smoking status and differential access to medical care. Another study found mortality rates correlated positively with urban location for some diseases but negatively for other diseases, suggesting that mortality rates might be associated with a dimension of socioeconomic status that was not measured (Haynes, 1983). In a study conducted in the Netherlands, researchers found a variable pattern in declines in mortality associated with urban location across different disease conditions (Mackenbach et al., 1988). The researchers attributed the relatively fast decline in mortality from heart disease in urban areas to diffusion of medical technology and of new "healthy" lifestyles. Another study, analyzing the effects of population size on health status (both mortality and morbidity), showed a possible association between community size and mortality measures, including potential years of life lost.

The mixed findings of these regional and/or community variation studies illustrate the complex nature of relationships among factors analyzed by this approach. Again, a major obstacle is the inability or inadequacy of such analyses to take into account other variables that affect health. As Moens (1984) puts it: "Many variables, known and unknown, vary with geography and make the interpretation of geographical difference a complex and confounding matter."

Studies of the physical environment indicate that community characteristics, such as pollution and climate, can influence health. How strong an effect these factors exert, however, is still a matter of considerable debate. As Hart (1991, p. 152) points out, "Tokyo, among the world's largest, most polluted, and congested cities, records the lowest infant mortality and the longest life expectancy of any place on earth. This paradox is testimony to the power of the social and economic environment as a determinant of health." In other words, the social and economic environment can buffer the physical stresses of the environment. Conducting studies that have sufficient control over potentially confounding variables, obtaining accurate and reliable measures of environmental characteristics, and the long latency periods associated with exposure to environmental agents create vexing research problems. Nonetheless, considerable theoretical and empirical support exists for including the physical environment in the examination of community determinants of population health.

Modifying the Physical and Social Environment of a Community

Community efforts to modify the social and physical environment, such as health promotion programs that activate communities or change community power structures, help to identify the characteristics of communities that promote health. By no means do all community health promotion programs seek to change *community*-level characteristics, such as the sense of community or social cohesion. Many aim to change individuals' health behaviors through dissemination of information in the mass media, without modifying community structures or processes. We will concentrate on interventions that have, as an important goal, community organization or the reallocation of community resources across groups of residents.

The Healthy Cities and Healthy Communities Movement

The Healthy Cities Project is a series of global and national networks initially developed by the World Health Organization (Europe) in response to *Global Strategy for Health for All by the Year 2000* (World Health Organization, 1981; Ashton et al., 1986; Ashton and Seymour, 1988). The movement has spawned activity in North America, particularly Canada, whose Healthy Communities Project involves a growing number of cities. The Healthy Cities movement is based on the premise that a city is a place "which shapes human possibility and experience [and] has a crucial role to play in determining the health of those living in it" (Ashton and Seymour, 1988, p. 156). Efforts to promote the health of cities are founded on the principle that such efforts should not be externally administered. Instead, communities should be empowered to: (1) formulate a definition of health for themselves, and (2) decide how best to achieve this aim. The Project thus consists of the growing network of cities using this approach. Hancock and Duhl (1986) who describe the Project as "family therapy for cities," offer a blueprint for implementation that consists of: (1) encouraging and building social networks, (2) encouraging participation in democratic process, e.g., voting and participation in community groups, (3) decentralizing decision-making, and (4) building competence among the population by enhancing coping skills and self-esteem.

Freedom to act in one's own best interests is the paramount principle of the Healthy Cities movement. According to this principle, empowerment cannot be bestowed on a community by a professional organization. "Power" is the ability to choose; thus groups and individuals can only empower themselves (Labonte, 1989). The health challenges of reducing inequities, promoting prevention, and enhancing ability, are achieved though healthy environments that promote self-care and mutual aid. Three implementation strategies have been articulated to achieve these aims: fostering public participation, strengthening community health services, and coordinating healthy public policy.

According to the Healthy Cities and Healthy Communities approach, the extent to which communities are empowered determines how healthy the community will be. No evidence has yet been published on the link between community empowerment and health outcomes, but the appealing messages of community involvement and healthy environments have inspired enthusiasm and energy.

Community-level Health Promotion Programs

Community-level prevention programs focus on social and environmental determinants of health (Kottke et al., 1985; Thompson and Kinne, 1990; Wagner et al., 1991). This approach assumes that permanent, large-scale behavior change is best achieved by changing community norms about health-related behavior and by developing positive role models that support healthful behavior and discourage unhealthful behaviors (Thompson and Kinne, 1990; Wagner et al., 1991). It also seeks changes in the physical, regulatory, and socioeconomic environments to make them more supportive of healthful behavior.

Unlike the high-risk approach to prevention, which seeks to identify people at risk through screening and to provide these high-risk individuals with health care services (Multiple Risk Factor Intervention Trial, 1990), the community approach targets whole populations or broad segments of the community for intervention. This approach to prevention gives emphasis to the role of social and environmental factors as key determinants of health (Kottke et al., 1985; Thompson and Kinne, 1990; Wagner et al., 1991). The community-based approach assumes that permanent, large-scale behavior change is best achieved by changing community norms about health-related behavior and by developing positive role models that support healthful behavior and discourage unhealthful behaviors (Thompson and Kinne, 1990; Wagner et al., 1991). It also seeks changes in the physical, regulatory, and socioeconomic environments to make them more supportive of healthful behavior.

A widely used implementation strategy relies on community organization techniques to mobilize leadership and resources, and to build citizen support for community health interventions (Rothman et al., 1981; Mittelmark et al., 1986; Lefebvre et al., 1987; Kinne et al., 1989; Bracht, 1990). Bracht defines community organization as follows:

> Community organization is a planned process to activate a community to use its own social structures and any available resources (internal or external) to accomplish community goals, decided primarily by community representatives and consistent with local values.

Purposive social change interventions are organized by individuals, groups, or organizations from within the community to attain and then sustain community improvements
and/or new opportunities. (Bracht, 1990, p. 67)

As the above spells out, central to community organization is community involvement
in the design and implementation of interventions (Wandersman, 1981).

Several large-scale community prevention trials have used community organization
strategies to design and implement interventions. The Minnesota Heart Health Program (Mittelmark et al., 1986) used community analysis in communities participating
in cardiovascular risk-reduction interventions to identify organizations and citizen
groups that could help plan interventions and support their implementations. The A Su
Sulud prevention program in Texas (Amezcua et al., 1990) used an approach to community prevention that relied on grassroots community organization methods to stimulate citizen participation and support for health interventions. Other community prevention programs and trials that have used community organization techniques to
develop and implement interventions include the North Karelia Project in Finland
(Kottke et al., 1985), and the National Cancer Institute's Community Intervention Trial
for Smoking Cessation (COMMITT) project (Bracht, 1990).

The effectiveness of these implementation approaches remains unclear, primarily
because evaluation focuses on program impact, most often behavioral change, rather
than the implementation process. One ongoing evaluation that focuses on process is
that of the Western Community Health Promotion Grant Program (CHPGP) (Wagner
et al., 1991), sponsored by the Henry J. Kaiser Family Foundation (Tarlov et al., 1987).
The CHPGP supported community prevention projects directed at cardiovascular disease, cancer, injuries, adolescent pregnancy and substance abuse in 11 western sites of
the United States.

CHPGP projects used a particular "community activation" to develop and implement community health interventions. Rooted in community organization theory, this
approach emphasizes the involvement and coordination of major community institutions in mobilizing community leadership to allocate resources to health promotion
and to improve public awareness of health issues (Wickizer et al., 1993). Community
activation consists of organized efforts to promote community awareness and consensus about health problems, coordinated planning of prevention and environmental
change programs, and interorganizational allocation of resources; it also emphasizes
citizen involvement in these processes. In terms of Rothman's typology of community
organization (Rothman, 1970), community activation is most closely associated with
the social planning model, which emphasizes organizational change and rational planning strategies to achieve change.

Analysis of cross-sectional data indicates that community activation is correlated
with positive health behaviors in both adults and adolescents (Wickizer et al., 1992).
More activated communities had, on average, a lower prevalence of smoking, a higher
percentage of individuals drinking low-fat milk, and a lower percentage of adolescents

engaging in unprotected sex or using marijuana. While the direction of causality cannot be inferred from cross-sectional comparisons, these findings suggest a potential beneficial effect on health stemming from community organization processes.

A Framework for Studying Community and Health

The foregoing review of the literature suggests that substantial evidence is available that community characteristics and community processes affect both health behaviors and health outcomes. Scant evidence exists, however, to illuminate the pathways and processes by which community operates as a direct influence on health or as a mediator between community risk factors and health outcomes. A systematic framework is needed to guide future research examining the relationships between community characteristics and health outcomes. Figure 3–2 represents an attempt to integrate existing knowledge about community and health into such a framework, and to identify the characteristics and processes most in need of future study. The two global realms iden-

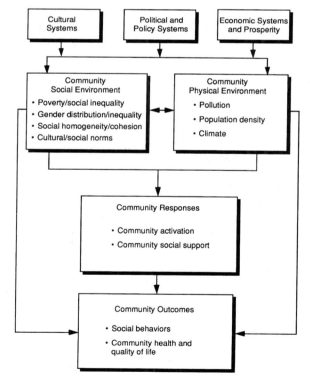

Figure 3-2 An organizing framework for studying community and health. The components of factors listed under Community Social Environment and Community Physical Environment are illustrative. They are not intended to be comprehensive.

tified in the causal model of determinants of health shown in Figure 3–1—the social and physical environment—are influenced by cultural systems (including values, beliefs and rituals, and their meanings in a particular community), the political system that drives health policy and community organization, and economic systems and prosperity (which influence income distribution, housing, employment, and other important determinants of health).

The social and physical environment have many different components; those listed in Figure 3–2 are illustrative, not definitive. We hypothesize that the most important social characteristics of communities are poverty (particularly social inequality), gender distinction or inequalities, and social cohesion. Major physical factors include pollution, population density, and climate; such other factors as food supply and transportation, could also be included. The process of sorting out the best set of operational constructs for measuring community risk characteristics and processes is a challenge for future research.

Figure 3–2 modifies the causal model shown in Figure 3–1 by adding community-level responses (also known as community modifiers)—defined as community activation and community social support; and community-level outcomes—defined as social behaviors and community-level health and quality of life. Thus this model provides for both direct and indirect effects of community: the social and physical environment may affect community outcomes directly, or indirectly through modification of the environment. For example, poverty and inequalities of social class, in addition to their direct effects on the health of a community, may also have an indirect effect through community response. Organizing to provide medical care to poor people is an example of community response, as is provision of income, housing, or educational programs.

Conceptual and Methodological Problems in Future Research

Well-conceptualized and well-conducted observational and intervention-based studies are needed to further understanding of the relationship between community and health. Community studies are not simply aggregated observations of the properties of individuals; community is more than the sum of individuals or even of its component parts such as church groups, political organizations, or civic groups. Studies may find no significant community effect either because it is negligible or because community is not measured adequately. Thus, more systematic approaches are needed to guide community-level investigations.

Conceptualization of Community

Our review indicates considerable variation in the conceptualization of community, even in geographically based studies. It is a genuine challenge to study communities that are defined as local places with distal influences. People undoubtedly derive support in ways that are less localized than in previous eras, when transportation and media were more limited. Many people have meaningful supports at the office, in other cities, and even in other countries. With greater geographic mobility and communication, it is increasingly possible to create personal communities that are temporary, such as the spontaneous intimacy of the bus, airline cabin, or cruise ship. People demonstrate considerable ingenuity in pulling social resources together on the spur of the moment.

Yet locale is still a fundamental concept in the study of communities. Despite increasing or increasingly visible homelessness, most Americans still have homes and view them as a base from which to act. The immediate physical environment clearly affects health and well-being. Of less certainty is the impact of the cultural, social, and psychological environment of the locale on health and well-being. Depending on the level of community interaction and organization, locale can have varied meanings. The meaning of place may differ by social class: for instance, the power to move at will is associated with prosperity and the necessity of moving is associated with poverty. This social variation in the meaning of place should be investigated.

Innovative conceptualizations of communities, particularly the intentional community, the temporary community, and the personal community, deserve to be tested. What accounts for the success or failure of intentional communities, such as ecological communities, long-lasting communities based on spiritual beliefs, or other residential communities that are created with special purpose? Are personal communities, such as health club memberships or volunteer networks, activated for social support once the immediate context in which they sprang up has dissolved? Are individuals able to build community in the welter of transitory experiences available to moderately well-off people? It is likely that transitory communities not rooted in the soil cannot and do not offer the long-term support needed to sustain people through crises or to provide help when illness or social threat strikes. Yet families and individuals show remarkable resilience in putting together communities of support through a combination of informal and formal caring networks. Observational or ethnographic studies of the formation of personal communities in natural settings would help to explain how they form, how they operate, and how they succeed or fail under stressful circumstances.

From the perspective of social and political responsibility, community necessarily involves commitment to others. Informational, emotional, and instrumental support can be provided from a distance, but direct and continuous contact is usually necessary to support vulnerable people. It is a particular challenge to organize informal and formal supports across wide distances, particularly in rural settings. With sufficient resources and attention, almost any community can be activated. But to sustain community involvement and participation requires at least a few dedicated individuals *staying in place* to provide continuity and to hand over the leadership baton to others, often newly arrived in the community.

Thus it is important not only to inquire how important place is to persons, but also whether the importance of place varies with an individual's length of time there and commitment to it. Many Americans suffer from a sense of "lost community" due to physical relocation and/or social mobility, either upward through education and occupation, or downward through unemployment and loss of income. Is this sense of loss of community only nostalgic, or does the Roseto effect generalize to less ethnically based communities and to smaller locales such as neighborhoods? How do individuals and families adapt to the frequent moves, and do such changes affect health? How does sense of community vary by gender, social class, sexual orientation, ethnic identity, housing arrangement, and other social and physical characteristics? Most importantly, how does sense of community translate into high-level well-being?

The studies by Levine and colleagues of the Type-A city are intriguing. Further research is warranted into community as character, the social-psychological community. As influential as the character of a community might be, however, it would be difficult to modify such diffuse cultural processes as speed of walking and level of activity. It might prove more useful to examine the person-environment fit in these communities. Can people be trapped in a social environment that is deleterious to their well-being because they cannot or do not wish to adapt or move?

The links between community and health are sometimes more vividly illuminated in the humanities and in ethnographic and other qualitative studies than in quantitative analyses of primary or secondary data. Close attention should be paid to personal stories about community, and to its meaning to individuals and groups. Such stories help us grasp how community does or does not affect well-being, and what directions we might take in designing and interpreting the results of multi-community studies.

Causal Modeling of Community Determinants of Health

To more fully understand the link between community and health calls for attention to the causal ordering of determinants of community health outcomes. Epidemiological and social science studies of the physical and social environment need to start with a clear causal model, including hypothesized relationships between geography and the concepts pertaining to the physical and social environment. The list of potential determinants of health operating or having an influence at the community level is long: gender, age, marital status, race, education, job opportunities, housing, wage, rates, religion, and numerous characteristics of individuals and communities. Developing causal models of determinants and applying them to particular places requires both a theoretical perspective and empirical tests of that perspective.

The literature suggests increased concentration on relative deprivation and social inequalities as a means of exploring community determinants of health. Community life is patterned by the social and economic structures operating within it, as well as by its physical location: housing stock, property ownership, consumption of goods and services, child care and education, care of people with severe chronic illness and disabilities, and gender roles. Occupation probably has a more tenuous link to community of residence, although working at home is increasing in many different occupations and communities. Systematic inequalities within the community among groups influence the life chances of residents, such as life expectancy, opportunities for education, and mobility. The extent to which these inequalities influence community, or community influences the shape and degree of inequality, is unknown. Rather than studying individual characteristics, future research would benefit from a concentration on social inequalities within communities.

Observational studies are the prime method of investigating community and health. To date these studies have yielded inconsistent results, primarily because they lack uniformity in conceptualization, measurement, and analysis. To develop cumulative knowledge will require repeated assessments of communities using a common set of indicators and health outcomes, including both health behaviors and health status.

Studies of the relationship between environment and health should control for confounding factors, such as smoking habits, in analyses of health outcomes. Too often studies omit such factors, making interpretation of results difficult if not impossible. Measures of socioeconomic status or gender inequality should be included in all studies to control for these important modifying variables. As in the literature on social support, investigators often observe that community has both a direct and an indirect effect on changes in health behavior and health outcomes. These direct and indirect effects, though small, can be studied using multivariate regression analysis. Sociological studies using structural equation modeling will help to pinpoint when and where community effects operate. The most appropriate analyses relate aggregate community characteristics to measures of health, with appropriate adjustments for individual-level variables such as income and ethnic composition. Clearly organized modelling will separate community effects from individual or compositional effects; once individual characteristics enter into the model, community-level effects often disappear.

A related methodological issue concerns inferences about individuals based on aggregate characteristics. The validity of results in community studies is often threatened by the ecological fallacy. One direction for future research might be to sample individual behaviors and outcomes in community studies in order to test the relationship between community variables and individual variation. Such studies suggest that adverse circumstances can have profound effects on households and entire communities, as well as individuals. Though costly, sampling individual characteristics and behaviors will be necessary to validate community-level measures.

Adverse experiences differ in their impact, depending on duration and type. For example, natural disasters such as hurricanes and earthquakes often mobilize communities to provide aid and mutual support to victims; such temporary aid ends once the effects of the disaster have lessened. Continuing economic deprivation and social disorganization, however, may stimulate a more lasting community response, such as community-based social-welfare programs and self-help movements. Though such responses to continuing social stressors may be effective, studies such as those by Angell (1951) and Dressler (1991) suggest that homogeneity is an important determinant of how the community responds and the nature of the social support it provides.

These studies suggest that greater attention should be paid to the homogeneity or heterogeneity of community residents as a determinant of well-being. The accumulated evidence suggests that individuals who live near other people like themselves—with similar culturally based beliefs, values, and behaviors—enjoy the benefits of community more than those whose neighbors are unlike them, particularly if residents are unwilling to mix or no institutionalized arrangements exist for inclusion of differentness. This evidence of the benefits of homogeneity is at odds with liberal or politically correct valuation of cultural diversity. Diversity has benefits that have not been recognized in previous community health studies. Community diversity should be studied in association with sense of community to examine their relationship and potential effects on health and well-being.

Developing Environmental Indicators

Community-level indicators are those that characterize a community as a whole, as opposed to individuals or subgroups within it (Cheadle et al., 1992). Most community-level measures are based on information about individuals for whom individual-level covariate data, such as demographic characteristics, are available. Cheadle and colleagues (1992) refer to such measures as *individual-disaggregated*. These data are then analyzed and interpreted in community summary statistics; no community-level data are collected. Interview surveys are the most frequently used methods for gathering individually disaggregated data.

A second level of data consists of *individual-aggregated* measures, derived from individual-level information but available only in aggregated form, such as census data, mortality rates, accident and injury rates, and most economic data. These data are most commonly used to measure the physical and social environment. Nonetheless, aggregation may not always make sense; nor can the result readily indicate supraindividual phenomena.

The third level of data consists of environmental indicators aggregated at the level of community. Examples of environmental indicators of health behaviors include the number, type, and visibility of no-smoking signs in a workplace, the proportion of communities with no-smoking ordinances, the amount of no-smoking space in a restaurant, and proportion of space in a grocery store devoted to low-fat foods. Other environmental indicators, as illustrated by the studies of Type-A cities, are unobtrusive measures such as the number of public clocks set on the correct time or the observed walking speed of people on the street.

The notion of "healthy communities" suggests a need for more attention to environmental indicators that can be used to characterize whole communities. Such indicators would be a community analogue to health-risk appraisal for individuals. Although environmental indicators offer the advantages of being unobtrusive and not subject to response bias, few efforts have been made to assess and improve their validity and reliability (Koepsell et al., 1992). Creative attempts to design and test environmental indicators in community settings would be welcome.

Approaches to Community Intervention

Generalized approaches to community intervention have yet to be tested thoroughly. It is often difficult to derive tangible objectives for such approaches that can be assessed with measurable indicators. Funders of community interventions must recognize the importance of obtaining evidence to support the concept of community activation. As attractive as this concept is, more evidence is required to know when and how organizing communities promotes well-being.

Collectively, the findings of community-based prevention trials and broader community interventions suggest that these programs can achieve positive results. We know little, however, about whether or how different implementation strategies affect outcomes and ultimate success. Until we know more about this critical question, it will be difficult to advance theory or refine practice methods. This dilemma represents a significant challenge to both organizers and evaluators of change.

Increased attention to how communities affect health and well-being is well deserved. We live in an era rife with reminders that individual behaviors and choices, such as increasing exercise, following a low-fat high-fiber diet, and refusing addictive substances, dictate health. Most people recognize that individual behavior does not arise in isolation from social and cultural influences. Yet it is difficult to place clear blame on the community or the society for the ills experienced as individuals. More often we are grateful for the influence of community, experienced most intensely in times of need such as impending death or physical disaster. If community is important to well-being, it behooves community organizers and researchers to work together for a better understanding of the people among whom we live, the places in which we live, and how we organize both place and people to promote health and well-being.

Appendix A: Selected Community Studies on Social Environmental Characteristics and Processes

Reference	Type and Number of Communities	Dependent/Independent Variable	Summary of Results
Angell 1951	4 U.S. cities	"Moral integration"/crime index, welfare effort index	The greater the heterogeneity and morbidity, the worse the crime index and welfare effort index. City growth, percent of married women working, and percent of rental units also important determinants.
Beiser 1980	5 West African villages	Mental and physical health measures; 29 variables including modernity, exposure, stability, rural-urban, social change, age, gender	Rural and urban groups affected equally by social change. Equal correlation between psychological measures and acculturation scores among both groups.
Blattner, Blair & Mason 1981	3,056 counties in the contiguous U.S.	Mortality-multiple myeloma/geographical-regional, ethnicity, occupation, rural-urban, socioeconomic environment	Increases in mortality rates for multiple myeloma uniform in all geographic regions, urban and rural. Positive correlation with mortality in economic areas w/high Scandinavian population, percent urbanization for white and nonwhite; between whites and number of years of school completed. High correlation w/ white males in petroleum, paper production; lower correlation in glass, printing, leather, stone and clay. Rates highest in far west and mid-central regions for whites and in the northeast for non-whites.
Blot et al. 1976	3,056 U.S. counties	Mortality-large bowel cancer/gender, ethnicity, socioeconomic status, dietary habits, alcohol sales	Ethnic, socioeconomic and urban factors linked to risk of large-bowel cancer only partly explain predominance of this tumor in northern U.S.; geographic peculiarities may identify dietary and other environmental determinants. Mortality consistently elevated in counties with large populations, high incomes and educational levels, and many residents of Irish, Czechoslovak, and German ancestry.
Brooks 1975	3,000 U.S. counties parishes and independent cities	Infant mortality/income, education, housing, race	Percentage of blacks and low educational level two variables with appreciable direct effects on both components of infant mortality. Socioeconomic factors better predictors of postnatal than neonatal mortality rates. Post-neonatal mortality has slightly larger direct effect on infant mortality than does neonatal mortality.

Reference	Disease/variables	Sample	Findings
Bulterys 1990	Sudden infant death syndrome (SIDS)/smoking habits, ethnicity, socioeconomic status	12 U.S. Indian populations	Differences in socioeconomic status, maternal age, birth weight, and prenatal care did not explain higher incidence of SIDS among Northern Indians than among Southwestern Indians. Prevalence of maternal cigarette smoking exceptionally high among Northern Indians and Alaskan Natives, low among Southwestern Indians. Smoking may explain part of the excess of SIDS among Indians in Northern regions.
Burnley 1980	Mortality-ischemic heart disease and cancer/social isolation, housing class, crowding, density, socioeconomic status	3 local government areas and cities in Australia	Crowding, social isolation, housing class, socioeconomic status interrelated. Inner-city mortality level higher than nonmetropolitan. Mortality rates in higher-income, lower-density suburbs with family-centered lifestyle below those of many rural areas and small towns. Inner suburbs and some outer lower-income suburbs have increased mortality rate.
Duxbury 1983	Morbidity/socioeconomic status, socio-cultural environment, living conditions	24 Native Canadian communities	Community factors, including degree of social integration, economic conditions and educational opportunities, strongly related to community health.
Egoff et al. 1992	Mortality-myocardial infarction, congestive heart failure/social cohesion, social support	5 towns in Pennsylvania	Correlation between mortality from heart attack and differences in culture and social cohesion. Decreased mortality in populations characterized by family-centered social life, absence of ostentation, nearly exclusive patronage of local business, and predominance of intra-ethnic marriages.
Engs et al. 1990	Alcohol consumption/religion	Students from 2 colleges in U.S. and Canada	Religious norms more influential in cohesive religious groups, cultural norms more influential among less cohesive groups. Results support Canadian "mosaic" and American "melting-pot" assumption.
Farquhar et al. 1985	Cardiovascular disease/change in health behavior (smoking), change in physiological risk indicators	5 cities in California	Stanford Five-City Project: Examines design and methods to evaluate community-health-education program for prevention of cardiovascular disease; will also test ability of a potentially cost-effective program to prevent cardiovascular disease at the community level.
Farquhar et al. 1977	Coronary heart disease/health behavior, physiological indicators of risk	3 towns in California	Mass-media educational campaigns directed at entire communities possibly very effective in reducing risk of cardiovascular disease.

Reference	Type and Number of Communities	Dependent/Independent Variable	Summary of Results
Foley 1977	274 U.S. counties with a hospital	Health-care differentiation/social structure	Local health system differentiation explains 66% of variance in health care between counties. Variables were community resource level, population base, and support facilities. Differentiation proceeds in a stepwise progression. Change in one or more structural variables necessary to develop a more differentiated system unless extraordinary efforts made to circumvent structural relationships.
Fox, Jones & Goldblatt 1984	4 geographic regions in England	Mortality/environment, social class, socioeconomic status	Geographic areas clustered according to sociodemographic characteristics. Marked differences found between clusters. When clusters disaggregated according to individual characteristics, little homogeneity retained. Individual characteristics (circumstances) better measures of mortality risk than measures derived from geographic areas.
Gore 1978	2 U.S. city and rural communities	Depression and illness/social support, employment, urban-rural	Health differences exist between populations with community support versus nonsupport. Life stress exacerbated by low sense of social support, as evidenced by changes in cholesterol, illness symptoms, and affective response.
Haenszel et al. 1976	2 prefectures in Japan	Stomach cancer/diet, occupation	Supportive evidence of possible protective food effects. Lettuce and celery negatively associated with stomach cancer.
Harburg et al. 1973	4 Detroit neighborhoods	Blood pressure/ethnicity, environment	Blood pressure varies with socio-ecological niches; or combinations of sex, race, and residence, that reflect class position as well as degree of social stressor conditions.
Hume & Womersley 1985	112 postcode sectors in Glasgow, Scotland	Mortality/age, social class, socioeconomic status	Death-rate variability in greater Glasgow correlates with postcode sectors. Highest death rates in more disadvantaged areas of the city and suburbs.
Janes & Pawson 1986	Samoan Communities in California	Chronic and degenerative disease/ethnicity and social support	Samoan social structure acts as buffer for risk factors related to obesity and high blood pressure. Less awareness of Samoan values of family and social structure among children may weaken existing social buffers.
Jenkins 1983	39 mental-health catchment areas, Massachusetts	Mortality-cancer/130 socioeconomic status indicators including socioeconomic status, gender	Social and demographic factors strongly related to mortality from cancer in men, virtually not at all in women.

Reference	Sample	Variables	Findings
Jenkins et al. 1977	39 mental-health catchment areas, Massachusetts	Mortality/demographic, socioeconomic status, housing, unemployment	Mortality excessive in areas with low median income, high percent of families in poverty, unemployment, high percent of nonwhite residents. "Zones of death" suggest additional medical care resources not adequate to address problem.
Kasl & Harburg 1975	4 Detroit census tracts	Mental health and well-being/ethnicity, socioeconomic status	Clear difference in perceptions of environment among high- and low-stress residents, but no consistent association with mental health.
Kushi et al. 1985	3 ethnic groups in Boston and Ireland	Mortality-coronary heart disease/diet	Diet related weakly to development of coronary heart disease.
Laurell et al. 1977	2 villages in Mexico	Morbidity-acute illness/physical environment, socioeconomic status, access to medical services	Impact of rural development on morbidity depends on its particular form in developing countries. Socioeconomic characteristics define groups of high and low morbidity more clearly than do sanitary conditions and access to professional medical care. Success of public health activities depends on capacity to plan the process of change.
Levine & Bartlett 1984	12 cities in various countries	Incidence of coronary heart disease/ punctuality, pace of life	When a variety of cultures are considered, behavior may not be directly related to psychological stress and the coronary-prone personality pattern as in the U.S.
Levine et al. 1989	36 U.S. metropolitan areas	Coronary heart disease/walking speed, talking speed, concern with clock time	People in fast-paced cities more prone to coronary heart disease. Sociological approach to personality processes may suggest answers. On individual level, interaction of personality with temporal norms may be better predictor of well-being than norms alone.
Lilienfeld, Levin & Kessler 1972	U.S. counties	Morbidity and mortality-cancer/ urbanization, socioeconomic status, ethnicity, gender, urban-rural	Inverse relationship of cancer mortality to education in both sexes except males 65 and over, for all forms of cancer combined. Observed differences among patterns of urbanization and cancer. Degrees of urbanization ratios generally higher for nonwhites and males than for whites and females. Increased mortality in urban areas for most neoplasms.
Linn et al. 1989	3 metropolitan counties in Tennessee	Psychological depression/community satisfaction/dissatisfaction	Depression higher for women, low-income families, and individuals with few friends. Low community satisfaction associated with depressive symptoms in both rural and urban southern black communities. Life events unrelated to depression in rural group. In urban group, life events both significant and more important predictor of depressive symptoms than measure of community contentment.

Reference	Type and Number of Communities	Dependent/Independent Variable	Summary of Results
Loudon 1991	Countries	Maternal and child mortality/socioeconomic status	Link between maternal mortality and all components of infant mortality very slight. Causes of mortality differ. Mortality rates insensitive measure of economic deprivation
Mackenbach, Kunst & Looman 1991	39 districts (COROP District)	Mortality/geographical-regional, gender, socioeconomic status, religion, urbanization	Both cultural and economic factors important in geographic mortality patterns in the Netherlands.
Mahaffey et al. 1982	Unspecified U.S. urban/ rural areas	Blood-lead levels/ethnicity, age, urban and rural, geographical, regional, socioeconomic status, urbanization	Racial difference in blood-lead levels may reflect different exposure or absorption or both. In both races there was an increase in the level previously predicted. Significant higher prevalence of elevated lead levels in young children, black and white, in families with income under $6,000.
Marmot & McDowall 1986	Regions of Great Britain	Coronary heart-disease mortality/region occupation, gender, smoking, social class	Mortality from CHD higher in manual than nonmanual occupational classes, and higher in Scotland, Wales, and north of England than in South.
Milliard 1985	2 rural areas in Mexico	Child mortality/quality of farm land, socioeconomic status, housing, marital status	Better housing quality, higher quality farm land, and marriage associated with lower child mortality.
Neff & Husaini 1985	2 Nashville cities and surrounding rural areas	Response to stress/stress, urban/rural, ethnicity, age, socioeconomic status, religion	Moderate alcohol use acts as stress buffer among urban whites. Life events positively related to depressive symptoms in all drinking categories among urban blacks. Protestant identification isolates no differences in consumption.
Neil & Jones 1988	13 remote resource-boom communities in Australia	Mental health/environment, gender, work site, social support	Resident's perception of their environment as stressful had little influence on whether they were classified as probable psychiatric cases. No differences across towns despite different variables.
Pick 1975	29 U.S. Standard Metropolitan Statistical Areas with low migration	Mortality/ethnicity, socioeconomic status, religion, environment	Consistent geographical trends in fertility or life expectancy not apparent.
Pooling Project Research Group 1978	Unspecified U.S. population groups	Coronary heart disease/physiological indicators of health	Risk of first heart attack over next decade in middle-aged white males can be reasonably predicted with measurement of serum cholesterol, blood pressure, and cigarette use.
Puska, Nissinen & Tuomilehto 1985	2 counties in Finland	Cardiovascular disease/health behavior (smoking, diet), gender, change in physiological risk indicators	Well-conceived community-based programs can have important impact on lifestyle and risk-factor levels in the population.

Study	Variables	Findings
Ramachandran & Shastri 1983	Morbidity/socioeconomic status	No significant differences in distance traveled by different socioeconomic groups to medical centers. Different socioeconomic groups may visit different sites due to "status-consciousness." Middle-level centers under utilized.
Sembajwe 1983	Mortality/socioeconomic status, environment	Socioeconomic development more important in lowering mortality in rural Tanzania than provision of health facilities and services.
Singh 1981	Drug and alcohol use and related problems/socioeconomic status, ethnicity, crime and law enforcement, social disorganization, quality of life, population size and density	Global measures such as quality of life of a community not clearly related to outcomes of methadone-maintenance programs. Property-crime rates not related during treatment program to outcomes of drug use and criminality.
Wechsler & Pugh 1967	Morbidity-psychiatric/age, worksite	Findings support the "fit" hypothesis that people with a particular characteristic who live in a community where that characteristic is less common have a higher rate of psychiatric hospitalization than people in communities where it is more common.
Wnuk-Lipinski 1990	Life expectancy/social class, urbanization, gender, region	Inequalities result from economic failure, differences in living conditions, and lifestyles rather than from inefficiencies in the health-care system. Significant inequalities in access to care and quality of care.
Yeracaris & Kim 1978	Mortality/socioeconomic status	Increased socioeconomic differentials between 1960 and 1970, especially for males in central cities and for suburban rings, in spite of reductions in mortality during this period. Mortality rates from heart diseases, malignant neoplasms, and all other causes of death inversely related to socioeconomic status in both central cities and suburban communities.
Young & Garro 1982	Morbidity/health attitudes, access to health care	Variation in use of physicians' services between two areas a consequence of differential access to such treatment, without corresponding degrees of variation in residents' illness beliefs.

Appendix B: Selected Community Studies on Physical Environmental Characteristics and Processes

Reference	Type and Number of	Dependent/Independent Variable	Summary of Results
Bang et al. 1975	3 villages in West Bengal	Morbidity-respiratory infection in children/environment, socioeconomic status, culture, urban-rural	Intensity of infection highest in crowded urban sample. Crowded sleeping quarters and use of contaminated water for sanitary/household needs common to all.
Beasley et al. 1973	3 population groups in Aberystwyth, Wales	Blood-lead level/age, gender, residence	Increasing blood-lead levels with length of residence. Significant increase with age. Gender not significant.
Blot, Fraumeni & Stone 1978	3,056 U.S. counties	Mortality/geographical/regional ethnicity, gender, human behavior	Higher mortality rates associated with urban areas, highly correlated with lung cancer in males and diabetes mellitus in females. No associations with socioeconomic, industrial, or alcohol-consumption indices.
Blot et al. 1979	49 U.S. counties with shipyards	Mortality/occupation, ethnicity, gender	Elevated rates of lung and laryngeal cancer and excess mortality in shipyard counties.
Bourke, Giggs & Ebdon 1979	6 geographic areas near Nottingham, England	Morbidity/gender, social class, water supplies	One water-supply area found to have significantly greater incidence of disease, although no property of the water supply was identified as an important etiological factor.
Byarugaba 1991	Urban, rural and peri-urban areas, Republic of Transkei	Pediatric/urbanization, socioeconomic status	Factors of health status, including diarrhea (and understanding of home treatment), income, breastfeeding, and nutritional status of children, lower in rural area.
Campbell & Beets 1979	143 U.S. Metropolitan Statistical Areas	Mortality rates/environment and climatological variables	Of eight categories of death, climatological variables possibly causal only in heart attacks and accidents.
Chambers et al. 1989	2 towns in Ontario, Canada	Morbidity/water supply, sewage disposal in households, socioeconomic status, geographical location	High frequency of diarrhea and stomach cramps attributed to microbial contamination resulting from area's poor water supply and sewage disposal.
Chapman & Coulson 1972	142 U.S. communities	Infant mortality/geographic location, ethnicity, socioeconomic status	Infant mortality, low birthweights, accident and cirrhosis mortality correlated with high proportion of blacks and low income. High hospitalization rates corresponded with low family income and inner-city location.

Citation	Variables	Findings
Chase 1963	Mortality/geographic location, gender	Average number of physicians, urban percentage of population, population density, and non-white percentage of population all positively correlated with heart disease among males and females.
Cheng 1989	Morbidity/geographic location, urbanization, gender	No significant rural/urban difference in overall minor psychiatric morbidity; however, depression lower in urban women.
Connelly 1982	Cancer incidence/geographic location	Differences in smoking habits and alcohol consumption, occupational exposure to carcinogens, and air pollution possible causes for increased risks for cancer in urban residents.
Deacon & Williams 1982	Sudden infant death/geographic location, climate	Strong dependence of SIDS incidence on cold-wet weather frequency attributed indirectly to amount of respiratory infection in general population.
El-Shaarawi et al. 1976	Mortality/gender, geographic location	County differences in mortality greater for deaths from accidents, violence, and cardiovascular diseases.
Ghosh, Datta & Lamba 1969	Illness/socioeconomic status, environmental measures, sanitation	Morbidity and sickness rates lower in modern community. Environmental sanitation facilities influence difference more than improved socioeconomic conditions.
Gillum et al. 1984	Mortality-heart disease/geographic location	Coronary heart disease trends not explained by incidence of influenza or pneumonia, stroke mortality, hypertension, or cancer mortality. Lifestyle and medical care changes due to general affluence.
Greenberg et al. 1983	Female cancer/geographic location	Rates of respiratory cancer in white females increase at same rate or faster in urban areas than in suburban and rural areas, in contrast to the trend in white male respiratory cancer.
Harmi 1975	Morbidity/socioeconomic status, other social variables, geographic location	Regional differences in chronic morbidity explained by regional variations in illnesses related to availability and use of ambulatory medical care and to local socioeconomic development.

Reference	Type and Number of	Dependent/Independent	Summary of Results
Haynes 1983	35 provinces in Chile	Mortality/geographic location	Geographical patterns in morbidity rates documented: tuberculosis in the north, digestive diseases in the north and central, accidents and violence in the south, and lung cancer in the extreme north.
Johnson 1987	8 U.S. cities/towns	Health-status indices/population size, geographic location	Community size not related to health status. Other factors affecting health were housing, crime, and drug problems.
Kendrick 1980	24 hospital board districts in New Zealand	Cancer incidence/drinking water, socioeconomic status, urbanization, ethnicity, population change, gender	Correlations found between cancer incidence and chemical composition of drinking water, median male income, percentage Maori, population increase, and distribution of doctors.
Klebba 1975	U.S. Standard Metropolitan Statistical Areas, states, regions	Homicides/region, age, gender	Greatest increases in homicides in men other than white, ages 25–29, in South and central cities.
Lan & Shy 1981	5 metropolitan areas in New York	Respiratory disease/air pollution	Significant prevalence of chronic respiratory symptoms associated with area differences in pollution levels found among nonsmokers but not among smokers. Many confounding factors.
Lindtjorn 1990	24 food-distribution sites in southern Ethiopia	Child mortality/environment, drought, malnutrition	Mortality among children highest in relief shelter areas (due to crowding and poor sanitation), in the most arid regions, and during the dry season.
Lipfert 1980	U.S. cities, counties, states	Mortality-cancers/air pollution, socioeconomic status, smoking	Most air-pollution variables not significantly related to mortality (all causes). Cigarette smoking highly significant.
Lloyd et al. 1985	3 census districts in Scotland	Mortality/geographic location, industrial air pollution	Mortality from respiratory cancer and sex ratios of birth significantly related to exposure to air pollution from steel foundry.
Mackenbach et al. 1988	39 regions in the Netherlands	Mortality/geographic location, urbanization, socioeconomic status	Causes of death more amenable to intervention declined faster in less-urbanized lower income areas. For heart disease, mortality declined faster in more urban higher-income areas.

Reference	Location/sample	Variables	Findings
Moens 1984	19 municipalities in Brussels	Mortality/socioeconomic status, gender, environment	Geographic differences in mortality patterns consistent between sexes, but only descriptive determinants of the pattern suggested.
Nasca et al. 1980	140–209 New York cities	Mortality/population density	Increasing incidence of many forms of cancer observed in both sexes with increasing population density. Data on other explanatory variables not considered.
Rogot et al. 1978	473 U.S. cities	Mortality/fluoridation	No consistent relation found between fluoridation and changes in mortality rates, heart disease, or cancer deaths.
Schechter et al. 1990	3 Canadian regions	Mortality/environmental location	No excess mortality found in a population living downwind from a gas refinery.
Sommerfelt et al. 1985	35 villages and field areas in India	Leprosy/socioeconomic status, nutrition, environmental measures	Prevalence of leprosy not correlated with nutritional level, poverty, or illiteracy, and greater in villages than in open fields.
Sullivan-Bolyai et al. 1980	156 Standard Metropolitan Statistical Areas urban and rural areas, Ohio	Reyes syndrome/geographic location, socioeconomic status	Reyes syndrome attack rates higher in urban noncentral areas, among middle and upper socioeconomic groups, and among black children less than 1 year old.
Van Poppel 1981	260 regions in western Europe	Life expectancy/work site variables, geographic location	Male life expectancy higher in agricultural regions, lower in highly urbanized areas and those where mining, heavy industry, or dock yards are located.

Acknowledgments

We are grateful for the assistance in locating and abstracting published documents provided by Margaret Beck, Todd Wagner, Janet Liang, Anneliese Schleyer, Leslie Francis and Adam Atherly. We also thank Michelle Bugge who prepared tables and figures. James House, Ph.D., provided thoughtful comments on an earlier draft of the manuscript.

References

Amezcua, C., A. McAlister, A. Ramirez, R. Espinoza. 1990. A Su Salud: Health promotion in Mexican-American border community. In Bracht, N. (ed.), Health Promotion at the Community Level, pp. 257–276. Newbury Park, CA: Sage.

Angell, R. C. 1951. *The Moral Integration of American Cities*. Chicago, IL: University of Chicago Press.

Ashton, J., P. Grey, and K. Barnard. 1986. Healthy cities—WHO's new public health initiative. *Health Promotion* 1:319–323.

Ashton, J., and H. Seymour. 1988. *The New Public Health*. Philadelphia: Open University Press.

Baker, S. P. 1985. Without guns, do people kill people? *Am. J. Public Health* 75:587–588.

Bang, F., M. Bang, and B. Bang. 1975. Ecology of respiratory virus transmission: A comparison of three communities in West Bengal. *Am. J. Med. Hygiene* 24:326–346.

Beasley, W. H., D. D. Jones, A. Megit, and S. G. Lutkins. 1973. Blood lead levels in a Welsh rural community. *Br. Med. J.* 4:267–270.

Beiser, M. 1980. Coping with past and future: A study of adaptation to social change in West Africa. *J. Operational Psychiatry* 11:140–155.

Berkman, L. F., and L. Syme. 1979. Social networks, host resistance, and mortality: A nine-year follow-up study of Alameda County residents. *Am. J. Epidemiol.* 109:186–204.

Black, D., and S. Laughlin. 1986. *Unemployment and Health*. Glasgow, Scotland: Health Education Dept., Greater Glasgow Health Board.

Blattner, W. A., A. Blair, and T. J. Mason. 1981. Multiple myeloma in the United States, 1950–1975. *Cancer* 48:2547–2554.

Blau, J. R., and P. M. Blau. 1982. The cost of inequality: Metropolitan structure and violent crime. *Am. Soc. Rev.* 47:114–129.

Blau, P. M. 1977. *Inequality and Heterogeneity*. New York: Free Press.

Blot, W. J., and J. F. Fraumeni, Jr. 1976. Geographic patterns of lung cancer: Industrial correlates. *Am. J. Epidemiol.* 103:539–550.

Blot, W. J., J. F. Fraumeni, B. J. Stone, and F. W. McKay. 1976. Geographic patterns of large bowel cancer in the United States. *J. Natl. Cancer Inst.* 57:1225–1231.

Blot, W. J., J. F. Fraumeni, and B. J. Stone. 1978. Geographic correlates of pancreas cancer in the United States. *Cancer* 42:373–380.

Blot, W. J., B. J. Stone, J. F. Fraumeni, Jr., F. Joseph, and L. E. Morris. 1979. Cancer mortality in U.S. counties with shipyard industries during World War II. *Environ. Res.* 18:281–290.

Booth, A., and J. Cowell. 1976. Crowding and health. *J. Health Soc. Behav.* 17:204–220.

Bourke, J. B., J. A. Giggs, and D. S. Ebdon. 1979. Variations in the incidence and the spatial distribution of patients with primary acute pancreatitis in Nottingham 1969–76. *Gut* 20:366–371.

Bracht, N. 1990. *Health Promotion at the Community Level*. Newbury Park, CA: Sage.

Broadhead, W. E., B. H. Kaplan, S. A. James, V. J. Schoenbach, E. H. Wagner, R. Grimson, S. Heyden, G. Tibblin, and S.H. Gehlbach. 1983. The epidemiologic evidence for a relationship between social support and health. *Am. J. Epidemiol.* 117:521–537.

Brooks, C. H. 1975. Path analysis of socioeconomic correlates of county infant mortality rates. *Int. J. Health Serv.* 5:499–514.

Brown, P., and E. J. Mikkelsen. 1990. *No Safe Place.* Berkeley, CA: University of California Press.

Bruhn, J. G., B. Chandler, C. Miller, and S. Wolf. 1966. Social aspects of coronary heart disease in two adjacent ethnically different communities. *Am. J. Public Health* 56:1493–1506.

Bruhn, J. G., and S. Wolf. 1979. *The Roseto Story: An Anatomy of Health.* Norman, OK: University of Oklahoma Press.

Brunswick, A. F., and C. R. Merzel. 1988. Health through three life stages: A longitudinal study of urban black adolescents. *Soc. Sci. Med.* 27:1203–1214.

Bulterys, M. 1990. High incidence of sudden infant death syndrome among northern Indians and Alaska natives compared with southwestern Indians: Possible role of smoking. *J. Community Health* 15:185–194.

Burnley, I. H. 1980. Social ecology of premature mortality in three Australian cities. *Aust. J. Social Issues* 15:305–320.

Byarugaba, J. 1991. The impact of urbanization on the health of black pre-school children in the Umtata District, Transkei, 1990. *S. Afr. Med. J.* 79:444–448.

Campbell, D. E., and J. L. Beets. 1979. The relationship of climatological variables to selected vital statistics. *Int. J. Biometeorol.* 23:107–114.

Canadian Government. 1974. *A New Perspective of Health of Canadians.* (*Lalonde Report*). Ottawa: Department of National Health and Welfare.

Carstairs, V., and R. Morris. 1991. *Deprivation and Health in Scotland,* chaps. 1–6. Aberdeen: Aberdeen University Press.

Cassel, J. 1973. The relation of the urban environment to health: Implications for prevention. *Mt. Sinai J. Med.* 40:539–550.

Centers for Disease Control. 1987. Homicide Surveillance, High Risk Racial and Ethnic Groups—blacks and Hispanics, 1970 to 1983. *MMWR*; 36:634–636.

Chambers, L. W., F. Shimoda, S.D. Walter, L. Pickard, B. Hunter, J. Ford, N. Deivanayagam, and I. Cunningham. 1989. Estimating the burden of illness in an Ontario community with untreated drinking water and sewage disposal problems. *Can. J. Public Health* 80:142–148.

Chapman, J. M., and A. Coulson. 1972. Community diagnosis: An analysis of indicators of health and disease in a metropolitan area. *Int. J. Epidemiol.* 1:75–81.

Chase, H. C. 1963. Variations in heart disease mortality among counties of New York State. *Public Health Rep.* 78:525–534.

Chavis, D. M., and Wandersman A. 1990. Sense of community in the urban environment: A catalyst for participation and community development. *Am. J. Community Psychol.* 18:55–81.

Cheadle, A., E. W. Wagner, T. D. Koepsell, A. Kristal, and D. Patrick. 1992. Environmental indicators: A tool for evaluating community-based health promotion programs. *Am. J. Prev. Med.* 8:345–350.

Cheng, T. A. 1989. Urbanization and minor psychiatric morbidity: A community study in Taiwan. *Soc. Psychiatry Psychiatr. Epidemiol.* 24:309–316.

Connelly, R. R. 1982. Patterns in urban and rural cancer incidence. *Basic Life Sci.* 21:61–91.

Curtis, L. A. 1975. *Violence, Race and Culture.* Lexington, MA: Lexington Books.

Dayal, H., C. Y. Chiu, R. Sharrar, J. Mangan, I. Rosenwaike, S. Shapiro, A. J. Henley, R. Goldberg-Alberts, and J. Kinman. 1984. Ecological correlates of cancer mortality patterns in an industrialized urban population. *J. Nat. Cancer Inst.* 73:565–574.

Deacon, E. L., and A. L. Williams. 1982. The incidence of the sudden infant death syndrome in relation to climate. *Int. J. Biometeorol.* 26:207–218.

Doll, R. 1992. Health and the environment in the 1990s. *Am. J. Public Health* 82:933–940.

Dressler, W. W. 1991. *Stress and Adaptation in the Context of Culture: Depression in a Southern Black Community*. Albany, NY: State University of New York Press.

Durkheim, E. 1897. *Suicide*. (Translated by J. A. Spaulding and G. Simpson and reprinted in 1951). New York: Free Press.

Duvall, D., and A. Booth. 1978. The housing environment and women's health. *J. Health Soc. Behav.* 19:410–417.

Duxbury, L. E. 1983. The relative effects of community characteristics and health care environment on Indian health and use of health care facilities in the Sioux Lookout Zone. Waterloo, Ontario: University of Waterloo.

Egoff, B., J. Lasker, S. Wolf, and L. Potvin. 1992. The Roseto effect: A 50-year comparison of mortality rates. *Am. J. Public Health* 82:1089–1092.

El-Shaarawi, A. H., W. H. Cherry, W. F. Forbes, and R. L. Prentice. 1976. A statistical model for studying regional differences in observed mortality rates, and its application to Ontario during 1964–1968. *J. Chron. Dis.* 29:311–330.

Engs, R. C., D. J. Hanson, L. Gliksman, and C. Smythe. 1990. Influence of religion and culture on drinking behaviors: A test of hypotheses between Canada and the USA. *Br. J. Addict.* 85:1475–1482.

Evans, R. G., and G. L. Stoddart. 1990. Producing health, consuming health care. *Soc. Sci. Med.* 31:1347–1363.

Factor, R., and I. Waldron. 1973. Contemporary population densities and human health. *Nature* 243:381–384.

Farquhar, J. W., N. Maccoby, P. D. Wood, J. K. Alexander, H. Breitrose, B. W. Brown, Jr., W. L. Haskell, A. L. McAlister, A. J. Meyer, J. D. Nash, and M. P. Stern. 1977. Community education for cardiovascular health. *Lancet.* 1:1192–1195.

Farquhar, J. W., S. P. Fortmann, N. Maccoby, W. L. Haskell, P. T. Williams, J. A. Flora, C. B. Taylor, B. W. Brown Jr., D. S. Solomon, and S. B. Hulley. 1985. The Stanford Five-City Project: Design and methods. *Am. J. Epidemiol.* 122:323–334.

Flango, V. E., and E. L. Sherbenou. 1976. Poverty, urbanization and crime. *Criminology* 14:331–346.

Florin, P. 1989. *Nurturing the Grassroots: Neighborhood Volunteer Organizations and America's Cities*. New York: New York Citizens Committee for New York City.

Foley, J. W. 1977. Community structure and the determinants of local health care differentiation: A research report. *Soc. Forces* 56:654–660.

Fox, A. J., D. R. Jones, and P. O. Goldblatt. 1984. Approaches to studying the effect of socioeconomic circumstances on geographic differences in mortality in England and Wales. *Br. Med. Bulletin* 40:309–314.

Freidman, M. P., and R. H. Rosenman. 1974. *Type A Behavior and Your Heart*. New York: Knopf.

French, J.R.P., W. Rodgers, and S. Cobb. 1972. Adjustment as person–environment fit. In G. Coelho and J. E. Adams (eds.), *Coping and Adaptation*, pp. 316–334. New York: Basic Books.

Galle, O. R., W. R. Gove, and J. M. McPherson. 1972. Population density and pathology: What are the relations for man? *Science* 176:23–30.

Ghosh, R. N., S. P. Datta, and K. Lamba. 1969. A study on environment and morbidity in an urban area. *Indian J. Public Health* 13:166–171.

Gillum, R. F., D. R. Jacobs, R. V. Luepker, R. J. Prineas, P. Hannan, J. Baxter, O. Gomez-Marin, T. E. Kohke, H. Blackburn. 1984. Cardiovascular mortality trends in Minnesota, 1960–1978. The Minnesota Heart Survey. *J. Chron. Dis.* 37:301–309.

Glasser, M., L. Greenberg, and F. Field. 1967. Mortality and morbidity during a period of high levels of air pollution, New York, November 23–25, 1966. *Arch. Environ. Health* 15:684–694.

Gore, S. 1978. The effect of social support in moderating the health consequences of unemployment. *J. Health Soc. Behav.* 19:157–165.

Gove, W., M. Hughes, and O. Galle. 1979. Overcrowding in the home: An empirical investigation of its possible pathological consequences. *Am. Soc. Rev.* 44:59–80.

Gove, W. R., and M. Hughes. 1980. The effects of crowding found in the Toronto Study: Some methodological and empirical Questions (A comment on Booth and Edwards, ASR 1976). *Am. Soc. Rev.* 45:864–870.

Gray, S. 1978. *Community Health Today.* New York: Macmillan.

Green, L. W. 1986. The theory of participation: A qualitative analysis of its expression in national and international health policies. *Advances in Health Education and Health Promotion* 1(a):211–236.

Green, L. W., and Kreuter M. W. 1991. *Health Promotion Planning: An Educational and Environmental Approach.* Mountain View, CA: Mayfield.

Greenberg, M., D. Barrows, P. Clark, S. Grohs, S. Kaplan, and N. Newton. 1983. White female respiratory cancer mortality. A geographic anomaly. *Lung* 161:235–243.

Greenberg, M. R. 1983. *Urbanization and Cancer Mortality*, chaps. 4–6. New York: Oxford University Press.

Haenszel, W., M. Kurihara, F. B. Locke, K. Shimuzu, and M. Segi. 1976. Stomach cancer in Japan. *J. Natl. Cancer Inst.* 56:265–274.

Hancock, T., and L. J. Duhl. 1986. *Healthy Cities: Promoting Health in the Urban Context.* A background working paper for the Healthy Cities Symposium Portugal, 1986. Copenhagen: WHO.

Harburg, E., J. C. Erfurt, C. Chape, L. S. Hauenstein, W. J. Schull, and M. A. Schork. 1973. Socioecological stressor areas and black-white blood pressure: Detroit. *J. Chron. Dis.* 26:595–611.

Harni, A. 1975. Regional variations in the development of illness in Finland. *Br. J. Prev. Soc. Med.* 29:249–257.

Hart, N. 1991. The social and economic environment and human health. In W. W. Holland, R. Detels, G. Knox (eds.), *Oxford Textbook of Public Health*, Vol. 1, 2nd Edition, pp. 152–180. New York: Oxford University Press.

Hawley, A. H. 1950. *Human Ecology: A Theory of Community Structure.* New York: The Ronald Press.

Haynes, R. 1983. The geographical distribution of mortality by cause in Chile. *Soc. Sci. Med.* 17:355–364.

Hebedoe, J., A.V. Charles, J. Neilsen, F. Grymer, B. N. Moller, B. Moller-Madson, and S.E.T. Jensen. 1985. Interpersonal violence: Patterns in a Danish community. *Am. J. Public Health* 75:651–653.

Hexter, A. C., and J. R. Goldsmith. 1971. Carbon monoxide: Association of community air pollution with mortality. *Science* 172:265–267.

Hillery, G. A. 1955. Definitions of community: Areas of agreement. *Rural Society* 20:111–125.

House, J. S., K. R. Landis, and D. Umberson. 1988. Social relationships and health. *Science* 241:540–545.

Hume, D., and J. Womersley. 1985. Analysis of death rates in the population aged 60 years and over of greater Glasgow by postcode sector of residence. *J. Epidemiol. Community Health* 39:357–363.

Insel, P. M. 1980. Task force report: The social climate of mental health. *Community Ment. Health J.* 16:62–78.

Insel, P. M., and R. H. Moos. 1974. Psychological environments: Expanding the scope of human ecology. *Am. Psychol.* 29:179–188.

Janes, C. R., and I. G. Pawson. 1986. Migration and biocultural adaptation: Samoans in California. *Soc. Sci. Med.* 22:821–834.

Jenkins, C. D. 1983. Social environment and cancer mortality in men. *Massachusetts Department of Public Health* 308:395–398.

Jenkins, C. D., R. W. Tuthill, S. I. Tannenbaum, and C. R. Kirby. 1977. Zones of excess mortality in Massachusetts. *Massachusetts Department of Public Health* 296:1354–1356.

Johnson, K. S. 1987. Health status and community size: Is there a relationship? Fort Collins, Colorado, Colorado State University.

Kasl, S. V., and E. Harburg. 1975. Mental health and the urban environment: Some doubts and second thoughts. *J. Health Soc. Behav.* 16:268–282.

Kaufman, H. F. 1959. Toward an interaction conception of community. *Soc. Forces* 38:8–17.

Keller, S. 1988. The American dream of community: An unfinished agenda. *Sociol. Forum* 3:167–183.

Kendrick, B. L. 1980. A spatial, environmental and socioeconomic appraisal of cancer in New Zealand. *Soc. Sci. Med.* 14D:205–214.

Kinne, S., B. Thompson, N. J. Chrisman, and J. R. Hanley. 1989. Community organization to enhance delivery of preventive health services. *Am. J. Prev. Med.* 5:225–229.

Klebba, A. J. 1975. Homicide trends in the United States, 1900–1974. *Public Health Rep.* 90:195–204.

Koepsell T. D., E. H. Wagner, A. C. Cheadle, D. L. Patrick, D. C. Martin, P. H. Diehr, E. P. Perrin, A. R. Kristal, C. H. Allan-Anrilla, and L. J. Dey. 1992. Selected methodological issues in evaluating community-based health promotion and disease prevention programs. *Annu. Rev. Public Health* 13:31–57.

Koos, E. L. 1967. *The Health of Regionville*. New York: Hafner Publishing.

Kottke, T. E., P. Puska, J. T. Salonen, J. Tuomilehto, A. Nissinen. 1985. Projected effects of high-risk versus population-based prevention strategies in coronary heart disease. *Am. J. Epidemiol.* 121:697–704.

Kushi, L. H., R. A. Lew, F. J. Stare, C. R. Ellison, M. el Lozy, G. Bourke, L. Daly, I. Graham, N. Hickey, R. Mulcahy, and J. Keraney. 1985. Diet and 20-year mortality from coronary heart disease. The Ireland-Boston Diet-Heart Study. *N. Engl. J. Med.* 312:811–818.

Labonte, R. 1989. Community and professional empowerment. *Can. Nurse* 85:23–28.

Lan, S., and C. Shy. 1981. Effect of air pollution on chronic respiratory disease in the New York City metropolitan area, 1972. *Environ. Health Perspect.* 42:203–214.

Landrigan, P. J., and S. Markowitz. 1989. Current magnitude of occupational disease in the United States: Estimates from New York State. *Ann. N. Y. Acad. Sci.* 72:27–45.

Laurell, A. C., J. B. Gil, T. Mchetto, J. Paloma, C. P. Rulfo, M. R. de Chavez, M. Urbino, and N. Velazquez. 1977. Disease and rural development: A sociological analysis of morbidity in two Mexican villages. *Int. J. Health Serv.* 7:401–423.

Lefebvre, R. C., T. M. Lasater, R. A. Carleton, and G. Peterson. 1987. Theory and delivery of health programming in the community: The Pawtucket Heart Health Program. *Prev. Med.* 16:80–95.

Lestina, D. C., A. F. Williams, A. K. Lund, P. Zador, and T. P. Kuhlmann. 1991. Motor vehicle crash injury patterns and the Virginia seat belt law. *JAMA* 265:1409–1413.

Levine, R. V., and K. Bartlett. 1984. Pace of life, punctuality, and coronary heart disease in six counties. *J. Cross-Cultural Psychol.* 15:233–255.

Levine, R. V., K. Lynch, K. Miyake, and M. Lucia. 1989. The type A city: Coronary heart disease and the pace of life. *J. Behav. Med.* 12:509–524.

Liberatos, P., B. G. Link, and J. L. Kelsey. 1988. The measurement of social class in epidemiology. *Epidemiol. Rev.* 10:87–121.

Lilienfeld, A. M., M. L. Levin, and I. I. Kessler. 1972. Mortality, urbanization, and socioeconomic status. In *Cancer in the United States*, pp. 215–232. Cambridge, MA: Harvard University Press.

Lindtjorn, B. 1990. Famine in Southern Ethiopia 1985–1986: Population structure, nutritional state, and incidence of death among children. *Br. Med. J.* 301:1123–1127.

Linn, J. G., B. A. Husaini, R. Whitten-Stovall, L. R. Broomes. 1989. Community satisfaction, life stress, social support, and mental health in rural and urban southern black communities. *J. Community Psychol.* 17:78–88.

Lipfert, F. W. 1980. Statistical studies of mortality and air pollution: Multiple regression analyses by cause of death. *Sci. Total Environ.* 16:165–183.

Lloyd, O. L., G. Smith, M. M. Lloyd, Y. Holland, and F. Gailey. 1985. Raised mortality from lung cancer and high sex ratios of births associated with industrial pollution. *Br. J. Ind. Med.* 42:475–480.

Lord, B. B. 1981. *Spring Moon: A Novel of China.* New York: Harper & Row.

Loudon, I. 1991. On maternal and infant mortality 1900–1960. *Soc. Social Hist. Med.* 4:29–73.

Lynd, R. S., and H. M. Lynd. 1929. *Middletown.* New York: Harcourt, Brace & World.

Mackenbach, J. P., C.W.N. Looman, A. E. Kunst, J.D.F. Habbema, and P. J. van der Maas. 1988. Regional differences in decline of mortality from selected conditions: The Netherlands, 1969–1984. *Int. J. Epidemiol.* 17:821–829.

Mackenbach, J. P., A. E. Kunst, and C.W.N. Looman. 1991. Cultural and economic determinants of geographical mortality patterns in The Netherlands. *J. Epidemiol. Community Health* 45:231–237.

Mahaffy, K. R., J. L. Annest, J. Roberts, and R. S. Murphy. 1982. National estimates of blood lead levels: United States, 1976–1980. *N. Engl. J. Med.* 307:573–579.

Marmot, M. G., and M. E. McDowall. 1986. Mortality decline and widening social inequities. *Lancet* 2:274–276.

Mayer, S. E. 1984. *Neighborhood Organizations and Community Development.* Washington DC: Urban Institute Press.

McMillan D. W. 1976. Sense of community: An attempt at definition. Unpublished manuscript, Nashville, TN: George Peabody College for Teachers.

McMillan D. W., and D. M. Chavis. 1986. Sense of community: A definition and theory. *J. Community Psychol.* 14:6–23.

Messner, S. F. 1982. Poverty, inequality, and the urban homicide rate. *Criminology* 20:103–114.

Millard, A. V. 1985. Child mortality and economic variation among rural Mexican households. *Soc. Sci. Med.* 20:589–599.

Mittelmark, M. B., R. V. Luepker, D. R. Jacobs, N. F. Bracht, R. W. Carlaw, R. S. Crow, J. Finnegan, R. H. Grimm, R. W. Jeffery, F. G. Kline, R. M. Mullis, D. M. Murray, T. F. Pechacek, C. L. Perry, P .L. Pirie, and H. Blackburn. 1986. Community-wide prevention of cardiovascular disease: Education strategies of the Minnesota Heart Health Program. *Prev. Med.* 15:1–17.

Moens, G.F.G. 1984. Some aspects of the geographical mortality pattern of the Brussels population in 1970. *Soc. Sci. Med.* 18:59–62.

Morgenstern, H. 1982. Uses of ecologic analyses in epidemiologic research. *Am. J. Public Health* 72:1336–1344.

Moynihan, D. P. 1986. *Family and Nation.* San Diego: Harcourt, Brace, Jovanovich.

Multiple Risk Factor Intervention Trial. 1990. Mortality rates after 10.5 years for participants in the Multiple Risk Factor Intervention Trial. *JAMA* 263:1795–1801.

Muscat, J. E. 1988. Characteristics of childhood homicide in Ohio, 1974–1984. *Am. J. Public Health* 78:822–824.

Naparstek, A. J., D. E. Biegall, and H. R. Spiro. 1982. *Neighborhoods Networks for Humane Mental Health Care*. New York: Plenum Press.

Nasca, P. C., W. S. Burnett, P. Greenwald, K. Brennan, P. Wolfgang, and K. Carlton. 1980. Population density as an indicator of urban-rural differences in cancer incidence, upstate New York, 1968–1972. *Am. J. Epidemiol.* 112:362–375.

Neff, J. A., and B. A. Husaini. 1985. Stress-buffer properties of alcohol consumption: The role of urbanicity and religious identification. *J. Health Soc. Behav.* 26:207–222.

Neil, C. C., and J. A. Jones. 1988. Environmental stressors and mental health in remote resource boom communities. *Australian and New Zealand Journal of Sociology* 24:435–458.

Nisbet, R. 1970. *The Quest for Community*. New York: Oxford University Press.

Ong, S. G., J. Liu, C. M. Wong, T. H. Lam, A.Y.C. Tam, D. Hedley, and A. J. Hedley. 1991. Studies on the respiratory health of primary school children in urban communities of Hong Kong. *Sci. Total Environ.* 106:121–135.

Park, R. E. 1977. Human Ecology. In R. L. Warren (ed.), *New Perspectives on the American Community: A Book of Readings*, pp. 45–57. Chicago: Rand McNally College Publishing.

Patrick, D., and P. Erickson. 1993. *Health Status and Health Policy: Quality of Life in Evaluation and Resource Allocation*. New York: Oxford University Press.

Patrick, D. L., J. Stein, M. Porta, C. Q. Porter, and T. C. Ricketts. 1988. Poverty, health services, and health status: Lessons from rural America. *Milbank Q.* 66:105–136.

Patrick, D. 1989. A sociomedical approach to disablement in the community. In D. Patrick and H. Peach (eds.), *Disablement in the Community*, pp. 1–18. Oxford: Oxford University Press.

Perlman, J. E. 1976. Grassrooting the system. *Social Policy* 7:4–20.

Pick, J. B. 1975. Correlates of fertility and mortality in low-migration standard metropolitan statistical areas. *Soc. Biol.* 24:69–83.

The Pooling Project Research Group. 1978. Relationship of blood pressure, serum cholesterol, smoking habit, relative weight and ECG abnormalities to incidence of major coronary events: Final Report of the Pooling Project. *J. Chron. Dis.* 31:201–306.

Puska, P., A. Nissinen, and J. Tuomilehto. 1985. The community-based strategy to prevent coronary heart disease: Conclusions from the ten years of the North Karelia Project. *Ann. Rev. Public Health* 6:147–193.

Ramachandran, H., and G. S. Shastri. 1983. Movement for medical treatment: A study in contact patterns of a rural population. *Soc. Sci. Med.* 17:177–187.

Ritter, L., and P. B. Curry. 1988. Regulation of pesticides in Canada. *Toxicol. Ind. Health* 4:331–340.

Rogot, E., A. R. Sharrett, M. Feinleib, and R. R. Fabsitz. 1978. Trends in urban mortality in relation to fluoridation status. *Am. J. Epidemiol.* 107:104–112.

Rothman, J. 1970. Three models of community organization practice. In F. M. Cox, J. L. Erlich, and J. Teresa, *Strategies of Community Organization*, pp. 25–45. Itasca, ILL: Peacock.

Rothman, J., J. Erlich, and J. Teresa. 1981. *Changing Organizations and Community Programs*. Beverly Hills, CA: Sage.

Schechter, M. T., W. O. Spitzer, M. E. Hutcheon, R. E. Dales, L. M. Eastridge, C. Hobbs, S. Suissa, P. Tousignant, and N. Steinmetz. 1990. A study of mortality near sour gas refineries in southwest Alberta: An epidemic unrevealed. *Can. J. Public Health* 81:107–113.

Scherer, J. 1972. *Contemporary Community*. London: Tavistock Publications.

Schmitt, R. 1966. Density, health, and social organization. *Am. Inst. Planners J.* 32:38–39.

Schoenbach, V. J., B. H. Kaplan, L. Fredman, and D. G. Kleinbaum. 1986. Social ties and mortality in Evans County, Georgia. *Am. J. Epidemiol.* 123:577–591.

Sembajwe, I. S. 1983. Socioeconomic factors affecting mortality in rural Tanzania. *J. Biosoc. Sci.* 15:487–500.

Silberman, C. E. 1980. *Criminal Violence, Criminal Justice.* New York: Vintage.

Sims D. W., B. A. Bivins, F. N. Obeid, H. M. Horst, V. J. Sorensen, and J. J. Faith. 1989. Urban trauma: A chronic recurrent disease. *J. Trauma* 29:940–946.

Singh, B. K. 1981. The effects of community structure on during-treatment outcomes of methadone maintenance programs. *Int. J. Addict.* 16:1183–1196.

Sloan, J. H., A. L. Kellerman, D. T. Reay, J. A. Ferris, T. Koepsell, F. P. Rivara, C. Rioz, L. Gray, J. LoGero. 1988. Handgun regulations, crime, assaults, and homicide. *N. Engl. J. Med.* 319:1256–1262.

Sommerfelt, H. H., L. M. Irgens, and M. Christian. 1985. Geographic variations in the occurrence of leprosy: Possible roles played by nutrition and some other environmental factors. *Int. J. Lepr. Other Mycobact. Dis.* 53:524–532.

Stout, C., J. Morrow, E. N. Brandt, and S. Wolf. 1964. Study of an Italian-American community in PA; Unusually low incidence of death from myocardial infarction. *JAMA* 188:845–849.

Sullivan-Bolyai, J. Z., J. S. Marks, D. Johnson, D. B. Nelson, F. Holtzhauer, F. Bright, T. Kramer, and T. J. Halpin. 1980. Reye syndrome in Ohio, 1973–1977. *Am. J. Epidemiol.* 112:629–638.

Swigert, V. L., and R. A. Farrell. 1976. *Murder, Inequality, and the Law: Differential Treatment in the Legal Process.* Lexington, MA: Lexington Books.

Tan, A. 1989. *The Joy Luck Club.* New York: Putnam.

Tardiff, K. 1985. Patterns and determinants of homicide in the United States. *Hosp. Community Psychiatry* 36:632–639.

Tarlov, A. R., B. H. Kehrer, D. P. Hall, S. E. Samuels, G. S. Brown, M.R.J. Felix, and J. A. Ross. 1987. Foundation work: The health promotion program of the Henry J. Kaiser Family Foundation. *Am J. Health Promotion* 2:74–80.

Thompson, B., and S. Kinne. 1990. Social change theory: Applications to community health. In N. Bracht (ed.), *Health Promotion at the Community Level*, pp. 45–66. Newbury Park, CA: Sage.

Toennies, F. 1887. *Community and Society.* Translated by Charles P. Loomis, 1957. East Lansing, MI: Michigan State University Press.

U.S. Department of Health and Human Services. 1986. *Report of the Surgeon General's Workshop on Violence and Public Health.* Leesburg, VA: Health Resources and Services Administration.

U.S. Department of Health and Human Services. 1990. *Healthy People 2000: National Promotion and Disease Prevention Objectives.* Washington, D.C.: Government Printing Office.

van Poppel, E.W.A. 1981. Regional mortality differences in western Europe: A review of the situation in the seventies. *Soc. Sci. Med.* 15D:341–352.

Veroff, J., E. Douvan, and R. A. Kulka. 1981. *The Inner American: A Self-Portrait from 1957 to 1976.* New York: Basic Books.

Wagner, E. J., T. D. Koepsell, C. Anderman, et al. 1991. The evaluation of the Henry J. Kaiser Family Foundation's Community Health Promotion Grant Program: Design. *J. Clin. Epidemiol.* 44:685–699.

Wandersman, A. 1981. A framework of participation in community organizations. *J. Appl. Behav. Sci.* 17:27–58.

Warren, R. L. 1978. *The Community in America.* Boston: Houghton Mifflin.

Weber, M. 1921–1922. *Economy and Society*. (Edited by G. Roth and C. Wittich, translated by E. Fischhoff, 1968.) New York: Bedminster Press.

Wechsler, H., T. F. Pugh. 1967. Fit of individual and community characteristics and rates of psychiatric hospitalization. *Am. J. Soc.* 73:331–338.

Wellman, B. 1982. Studying personal communities. In P.V. Marsden, and N. Lin (eds.), *Social Structure and Network Analysis*, pp. 61–80. Beverly Hills, CA: Sage.

Wickizer, T. M., E. H. Wagner, M. Vonkorff, A. Cheadle, D. Pearson, W. Beery, and J. Maesar. 1992. *An Approach to Assessing Community Activation for Health Promotion: Methods and Preliminary Findings* Department of Health Services, University of Washington. (Unpublished Report.)

Wickizer, T. M., M. Vonkorff, A. Cheadle, J. Maeser, E. H. Wagner, D. Pearson, W. Beery, and B. M. Psaty. 1993. Activating communities for health promotion: A process evaluation method. *Am. J. Public Health* 83:561–567.

Wilkinson, K. P. 1970. The community as a social field. *Soc. Forces* 48:311–322.

Williams, K. R. 1984. Economic sources of homicide: Reestimating the effects of poverty and inequality. *Am. Soc. Rev.* 49:283–289.

Wnuk-Lipinski, E. 1990. The Polish country profile: Economic crisis and inequalities in health. *Soc. Sci. Med.* 31:859–866.

Wolf, S., and J. G. Bruhn. 1992. *The Power of a Clan: The Influence of Human Relationship on Heart Disease*. New Brunswick, NJ: Transaction.

Wolfgang, M. E., and F. Ferracuti. 1967. *The Subculture of Violence*. London: Tavistock.

World Health Organization. 1981. *Global Health for All By the Year 2000*. Geneva: WHO.

Yeracaris, C. A., and J. H. Kim. 1978. Socioeconomic differentials in selected causes of death. *Am. J. Public Health* 68:342–351.

Young, J. C., and L. Y. Garro. 1982. Variation in the choice of treatment in two Mexican communities. *Soc. Sci. Med.* 16:1453–1465.

4

Race and Health: A Multidimensional Approach to African-American Health

GARY KING and DAVID R. WILLIAMS

At the turn of the century, W. E. B. Du Bois (1903), the distinguished American sociologist, declared that the problem of the twentieth century is the color line. The issues of race and racism have plagued this country since its very beginning, and remain a disturbing and volatile component of the American dilemma. The roots of the problem, as historians (Franklin, 1980; Stampp, 1956; Davis, 1966; Bennett, 1966; Jordan, 1968), sociologists (Silberman, 1964; van den Berghe, 1967; Blauner, 1972; Wilson, 1980) and other observers (de Tocqueville, 1835; Myrdal, 1944) have determined, lie in the nature of the relationships established by Europeans in their contacts with and conquests of, physically distinct and culturally disparate peoples throughout the world.

Jordan (1968) explains that sixteenth and seventeenth century Europeans viewed their production systems and technology, social institutions, and culture (specifically their religion, moral codes, and sexual practices) as superior to those of darker peoples, particularly "uncivilized" Africans. Consequently, the concept of color acquired value-laden meanings that expressed and reinforced the "superiority" of whiteness over blackness. For example, "white and black connoted purity and filthiness, virginity and sin, virtue and baseness, beauty and ugliness, beneficence and evil, god and the Devil" (Jordan, 1968). Underlying and propelling this belief and value system was the imperative for a cheap and bountiful supply of labor to exploit the promise of the New World. In the Western hemisphere, this belief system helped to justify the introduction and development of the African slave trade and to absolve the European conscience. What resulted was an institutionalized social system and ideology of racial subjugation and oppression.

93

The social history of Africans in this country since 1619 has been the dominant theme in the study of American race and ethnic relations. Owing to the peculiar debt and inheritance of the African diaspora, the differences in social status, human and civil rights and life chances of African-Americans[1] have been well documented (Blackwell, 1985; Wilson, 1980, 1987; Jaynes and Williams, 1989). Disparities between blacks and whites in income, education, occupation, community development, criminal activity, housing, and social indicators confirm the continuing legacy of the American past and the present dangers. Each era in American history reflects the "original sin" of Western civilization and the uniquely American contradictions between racial subjugation and the ethos of freedom, justice, and equality.

Sociologists have rightly taken credit for developing theoretical frameworks for analyzing and conducting most of the research on this form of intergroup relations. The central sociological paradigm that will inform this discussion is the majority-minority model of racial group dominance and subordination (Wirth, 1945; Frazier, 1949; van den Berghe, 1967; Vander Zanden, 1972). A *majority group* is defined as a group that uses its power to control vital social institutions and processes and to maintain the status quo (Blauner, 1972). In American society, whites collectively constitute the majority or dominant group.

A *minority group* (Wirth, 1945; Burkey, 1978) refers to a collective that, regardless of size, is distinguishable on the basis of color, language, culture, sex, religion, or other recognizable features. Moreover, a minority group exerts less power than the majority group over societal decision-making processes, controls fewer vital social resources, and is unequal in access to opportunity structures, social rewards, and status (economic, political, and health status) as a result of discrimination, intentional or unintentional. Accordingly, African-Americans are appropriately defined as a minority group. In practically all spheres of life, interaction between minority and majority group members reflects individual and group status in society. Thus, relations between blacks and whites in American society are products of individual and institutional racism as well as other expressions of social stratification (e.g., social class differences, sexism).

Thus health care issues ranging from health belief systems, through the epidemiology of disease, to prevention and treatment cannot be approached in a social vacuum— that is, they cannot be viewed as unaffected by racial inequality in American society.

Our aim in this chapter is to examine "the race factor" and the health of African-Americans from different perspectives. Following a brief overview of the health status of African-Americans and a review of work on African-American health, we will address the conceptual meaning and empirical application of the race variable in public health research, including a critical discussion of race and racism in epidemiological research. The limitations of socioeconomic status as a theoretical and empirical variable in health research will be examined, as well as the current debate about race ver-

---

1. Although some argue for a substantive distinction between the terms black and African-American, we use the terms interchangeably.

sus social class as the key predictor of health beliefs, behavior, and status (Navarro, 1989, 1991; Freeman 1989). Finally, we will look critically at the epidemiological and social science research on blacks and the challenges facing black community-based health initiatives and intervention research. By way of caveat, this discussion is applicable to other minorities and other multiracial societies, but refers specifically to African-Americans.

The Epidemiology of Disease Among African-Americans

A major effort was launched by the U.S. government in 1984 to document the extent of health inequalities experienced by racial and ethnic minority groups. It focused on four groups: blacks, native Americans, Hispanics, and Asian/Pacific Islanders. The resulting multivolume report, published in 1985 (U.S. Department of Health and Human Services, 1985), estimated that there were 60,000 excess annual deaths in the African-American population. That is, about 60,000 fewer annual deaths would have occurred among blacks if their death rate had been the same as whites. Though comparative data of this kind masks the heterogeneity of the black population, it nonetheless highlights the health problems of blacks.

The report identified six causes of death that are responsible for 80 percent of the excess deaths: cancer; cardiovascular and cerebrovascular disease; chemical dependency; diabetes; homicide, suicide, and unintentional injuries; and infant mortality and low birth weight. The health status of the black population, as measured by a broad range of indicators, has declined every year since 1984, while that of the general population has improved (Sullivan, 1991). Among some subgroups of the African-American population, health problems have reached crisis proportions. For example, a study of mortality rates for African-Americans in the central Harlem health district of New York City found that black males between the ages of 25 and 44 are six times more likely to die than white males, and that the life expectancy of adult males in Harlem is lower than that of males in Bangladesh (McCord and Freeman, 1990). Interestingly, Du Bois (1906) made a similar observation almost 100 years ago in *The Health and Physique of the Negro American*.

What follows is a concise summary of certain health status differences between African-Americans and whites (U.S. Department of Health and Human Services, 1985, 1991).

1. *Infant mortality*. Though the infant mortality rate for both blacks and whites has declined throughout this century, the ratio of black to white infant mortality rates increased between 1975 and 1987 (Rice, 1991). The increase in the ratio of black to white infant mortality rates reflected a higher decline in infant mortality among whites than among blacks. Data from the 1983–1985 birth cohorts, based on linked birth and death records, reveal that the infant mortality rate for blacks continues to be more than twice that of whites (18.7 versus 9.0 deaths per 1,000 live births).

2. *Low birth weight.* Weight of less than 2,500 grams at birth, (i.e., low birth weight) is a major risk factor for infant morbidity and mortality. In 1988, the percent of low-birth-weight infants born to black mothers was more than twice that of their white peers (13.3 percent and 5.7 percent respectively). Moreover, the approximately 1 percent annual decline in low birth weight evident among both racial groups in the 1970s did not continue into the 1980s.

3. *Homicide.* Among young black men, homicide was the leading cause of death (59 per 100,000) in 1988. This rate was more than 7 times that of white males (8 per 100,000); the rate for the nation as a whole that year was 9 per 100,000. Native American and Hispanic youth had homicide rates 3 to 4 times that of whites, while the rate among Asian youth was slightly lower than for whites. About half of white, black, and Asian murder victims between the ages of 15 and 34 were killed with handguns.

4. *AIDS.* Initially most prevalent in the white middle-class homosexual community, AIDS (acquired immunodeficiency syndrome) is increasing most quickly among black and Hispanic residents of central city areas, as a result of intravenous drug abuse. The number of AIDS cases among blacks, Hispanics, and native Americans aged 13 and older increased respectively by 123%, 114%, and 123% between 1992 and 1993 (CDC, 1994a). Cumulatively between 4 and 11 percent of white, Asian, and native American males with AIDS contracted the disease through intravenous drug abuse, compared to 38 percent of Hispanics and 37 percent of blacks. Black and Hispanic women, who comprise only 19 percent of all women in the United States, represented 75 percent of reported cumulative AIDS cases among women, as of June 1994. Equally alarming is the fact that 80 percent of all children with AIDS are either black or Hispanic (CDC, 1994b).

5. *Cancer.* African-Americans have higher cancer incidence and mortality rates than do whites, and they survive fewer years with the disease. The American Cancer Society estimates (Boring et al., 1992) that cancer incidence rates are about twice as high for blacks as they are for whites. Mortality rates, over a 30-year period have increased 66 percent for black men (compared to 21 percent for white men) and 10 percent for black women (compared to a nonmeaningful change in the rates for white women). Examined by specific sites, data from the National Cancer Institute (U.S. Department of Health and Human Services, 1986) reveal that incidence rates are higher among blacks for carcinomas of the breast (women under 40), esophagus, lung (males), pancreas, prostate, stomach, and for multiple myeloma. Mortality rates are higher for cancers of the cervix, esophagus, larynx, lung, pancreas, prostate, and for multiple myeloma. While 54 percent of whites survived 5 years or more after diagnosis (1983–1988), only 38 percent of blacks lived this long with the disease. This disparity in survival status reflects such factors as differences in the quality of medical care and the stage of diagnosis.

6. *Diabetes and cardiovascular disease.* The prevalence of diabetes is 1.5 times higher among blacks than whites. Blacks also have higher rates of cardiovascular

disease (heart disease and stroke) than do whites. The rate for blacks between the ages of 25 and 44 is 2.5 times that for whites in the same age group (44 per 100,000 compared to 17 per 100,000). For stroke, the death rate among blacks in the 45 to 64 age group is three times that of whites (86 per 100,000 compared to 29 per 100,000).

7. *Life expectancy.* Despite striking gains in life expectancy at birth over the course of this century for both blacks and whites (in 1900 life expectancy at birth was 47.3 years for the entire population and 33 years for blacks) the gap between blacks and whites persists, and the gap between black men and white men has recently been widening. In 1988, life expectancy at birth for white males was 72.3 years, compared to 64.9 years for black males. For white women, life expectancy is 78.9 years, compared to 73.4 for their black counterparts. According to a recent report, four causes of death—cardiovascular disease, homicide, cancer, and infant mortality—account for almost three quarters of the differential.

8. *Mental health.* Blacks are disproportionately exposed to social conditions considered to be important antecedents of psychiatric disorder, but they do not have higher rates of mental illness than whites. The latest and best evidence come from two large population-based studies. The first, the National Institute of Mental Health's Epidemiologic Catchment Area (ECA) study found that blacks tend not to have higher rates of discrete psychiatric disorders than whites (Robins and Regier, 1991). The pattern of lower rates of illness in all of the major psychiatric disorder categories for blacks compared to whites, was even more pronounced in the National Comorbidity Study—the first national study of psychiatric disorders in the U.S. (Kessler et al., 1994). The sole exception to this generalization is anxiety disorders (especially phobias) for which blacks' rates exceed those of whites. Historically, blacks have had lower suicide rates than whites. Suicide rates have recently increased among black males, but the age patterns of suicide varies across race (Griffith and Bell, 1989). For white males, the highest suicide rates are among those over age 65; for black males, suicide peaks in the 25–34 age group. The increase in suicide among young black males probably reflects a growing hopelessness about their meager opportunities in this society. The cumulative evidence on black mental health suggests that the resources and strengths of the black community may provide protection against the onslaught of pathogenic stressors.

Historical Factors in the Health of African-Americans

Differences in health status between blacks and whites are not new. The findings reported above reflect a historical pattern in American society of differential treatment, rights, and privileges regarding health and medical care, and unequal social status based on race. In *Medicine and Slavery: The Diseases and Health Care of Blacks in Antebellum Virginia*, for example, Todd Savitt (1978) documents the striking differences in illness patterns and medical care accorded blacks and whites during slavery. The diseases that afflicted African slaves were in most cases directly attributable to lack of proper food, clothing, and shelter and to the occupational hazards and unsanitary conditions that abounded on plantations and in slave quarters. These abject conditions resulted in epidemic contagions of infectious diseases such as respiratory illnesses (tuberculosis, influenza, streptoccal disease, pneumonia, and the like), intestinal diseases (dysentery, typhoid fever) and other maladies, including malaria. This situation presented two major dilemmas for whites. For the slavemaster, a reduction in the number of slaves, or in production due to poor health, resulted in a net economic loss. For whites generally, infectious disease among slaves was ominous since contagion respected no color boundaries. Consequently, Savitt concludes that it was in the direct economic and public health interests of slaveowners and the larger white community to provide medical attention (however meager or crude) to slaves.

Health differences between blacks and whites during the antebellum period served an important purpose other than epidemiological description. These differences were conveniently used to justify the status of blacks as slaves (Savitt, 1978; Kiple and King, 1981; Jones, 1981). Racial differences in disease status were taken as evidence of blacks' inherent biological inferiority: thus no amount of social or medical intervention could be expected to make them equal to whites. Krieger (1987) provides an incisive analysis of how prevailing seventeenth and eighteenth century racist dogma about the genetic constitution and health problems of African-Americans were used to furnish a scientific rationale for slavery. Foremost among the proponents of this early articulation of scientific racism were medical practitioners (Kiple and King, 1981; Jones, 1981). Physicians such as Samuel Cartwright and Josiah Nott published and lectured extensively about differences in the physiology, mental stability, and physical health of blacks and whites. In his zeal, Cartwright even invented diseases unique to blacks: *drapetomania*, peculiar to runaway slaves, literally meant "flight from home madness"; *dyaesthesia Aethiopica* was known as "rascality" or, with greater sophistication, "insensibility of nerves" and "hebetude of mind" (Krieger, 1987; Stampp, 1956). Using "reductionist, biological determinist, and ahistorical assumptions," they attempted to link medical science and spurious statistical data about racial disparities in health status to a belief system ranking blacks as biologically inferior to whites (Krieger, 1987).

Du Bois' *The Philadelphia Negro: A Social Study* (1899), one of the first empirical sociological works published in this country, reports the findings of a descriptive epidemiological comparison of the health status of blacks and whites. As Du Bois notes, data from the 1884–1890 U.S. Census revealed:

> a much higher death rate at present among Negroes than among whites; this is one measure of the difference in social advancement. . . . The Negroes exceed the white death rate largely in consumption, pneumonia, disease of the urinary system, heart disease and dropsy, and in still-births; they exceed moderately in diarrheal diseases, diseases of the

nervous systems, malarial and typhoid fevers. The white death rate exceeds that of Negroes for diphtheria and croup, cancer and tumor, diseases of the liver, and deaths from suicide.

Edward Beardsley (1988) provides a vivid and probing discussion of the health and social problems facing blacks in the South during the twentieth century in *A History of Neglect: Health Care for Blacks and Mill Workers in the Twentieth-Century South.* He demonstrates that the vast majority of deaths among blacks in the South were caused by tuberculosis, heart disease, diseases of infancy, and pneumonia. Beardsley also offers a social history of the institutional structures (specifically, the public health system and the medical profession), political economy (e.g., mill industry and agricultural production), and cultural parameters and infrastructures that affected the health and medical care of African-Americans. Another significant historical work, by historian David McBride's *Integrating the City of Medicine: Blacks in Philadelphia Health Care, 1910–1965* (1989), offers another incisive historical account and a comprehensive review of the roles of black physicians and health care workers, public health movements, institutional racism, and the processes of change.

The aforementioned titles, as well as others (Torchia, 1975), on the history of race and racism and the public health of African-Americans are in the tradition of social science "race scholarship," contributing to an understanding of the significance of race by vividly linking past events to present reality. These historians trace social conditions, ideas, movements, power dynamics, and public policies that led to unequal and discriminatory institutional systems of care, a paucity of black health professionals, community disintegration, diminished life chances and opportunity structures, and eugenic movements and racist ideologies. They have thus laid a foundation for examining the social evolution of the relationship between health and race in American society. In so doing, they make clear that the government reports and epidemiological data presented above simply mirror, in many important ways, the record of the past.

The Meanings of Race

Among the first important contributions of the social sciences were studies of race relations (Du Bois, 1899; Park, 1913; Johnson, 1934), ethnic lifestyles and assimilation. The social milieu that has produced differential opportunity and reward structures as well as supremacist ideologies based primarily on skin color has often required fairly stringent standards for classifying racial group membership. In conducting and analyzing research on race and ethnic relations, social scientists have had to assign conceptual and empirical meaning and clarity to terms that are intrinsically nebulous and interchangeable.

This review of the literature on the concept of race has identified six specific difficulties or topics: (1) the non-existence of so-called "pure" races; (2) the lack of a clear and consistent definition of race; (3) the social genesis and function of racial classifications; (4) the role of racism; (5) methodological problems resulting from the varied meanings of race; and (6) the practical implications of different conceptions of race.

Biologists and physical anthropologists have long debated the meaning and value of race (Montagu, 1942, 1964; Hulse, 1962; Dobzhansky, 1964; Gossett, 1965; Baker, 1967; Damon, 1969; Fortney, 1977). Dobzhansky (1964) argues that the term race exists as a consequence of natural evolution and considers it an important medium whereby scientists can convey their understanding of comparisons between racial groupings. Baker (1967), in his review of the biological concept, argues that the greater the mating isolation and environmental differences, the greater the genetic differences between populations. Racial classifications, which he terms "interim structures for dealing with genotypic and phenotypic distances," will likely persist for the foreseeable future as a useful analytic tool in human biology research and thus in the social sciences as well. In a similar vein, Damon (1969) argues that despite the imperfection of racial classifications and the need to distinguish between "biological homogeneity" (race) and "cultural homogeneity" (ethnic group), the concept has important application as an epidemiological research tool and as a guide for public health strategies. Nevertheless, he maintains that racial disparities in health should not be presumptively ascribed to biologic etiology "unless cultural and environmental factors can be ruled out."

Lasker and Tyzzer (1982), on the other hand, argue strongly that, as a biological concept, race has little practical utility or meaning to the scientific study of behavioral genetics (e.g., mentality and intelligence). In their view, " 'pure' races of Homo sapiens never existed" due to interbreeding and extensive genetic variation within and between races. All human genetic pools have undergone some degree of amalgamation through mutation, natural selection, migration and admixture. There is greater genetic variation within racial groups than between them (Polednak, 1989). Therefore any unqualified empirical or theoretical formulation treating race as a singular pedigree is misleading and fallacious (Hulse, 1962; Fortney, 1977).[2] Consequently, Lasker and Tyzzer prefer the term *social race* as opposed to *biologic race* on the grounds that the significance of race is primarily social, and assert that differences are often emphasized "for the sake of maintaining a superior economic and social position." Specifically mentioned, by the authors, is controversy about race and the nature versus nurture explanations of temperament and intelligence.

With regard to public health research, Cooper (1984) argues against the scientific validity of biologic notions of race. Genetic markers or tests, he asserts, are seldom employed as valid and reliable indicators of biological differences among racial groups.[3] Cooper criticizes epidemiological research for its frequent assumption that "some important proportion of the racial differential may be explained by population

---

2. This point is not at odds with the fact that, because of their genetic composition, certain diseases predominate among particular racial and ethnic groups.

3. The emerging field of genetic epidemiology along with reliable and practical genetic tests may in the near future provide biologic validation for typological categories of race.

genetics." He also poses a number of critical questions about human variation and changing gene frequency, and about the ambiguity and arbitrariness or relative importance attached to particular phenotypic traits. In American society, for example, skin color as a race criterion is considered biologically salient, primary and sufficient for cross-group comparisons regardless of disease category (e.g., sickle cell anemia or cancer) or other phenotypic characteristics (e.g., eye color, hair texture). Cooper rejects this "discordant" argument and promotes the view of race as a social concept whose meaning and relevance are socially defined.

One reason why definitions of race are so inconsistent and unclear is that researchers employ the concept to measure every important indicator associated with racial inequality or difference. Presumably group socioeconomic status, cultural lifestyles and values, genetic predispositions and racism are all being measured by the race variable. Such a categorical or composite approach precludes independent analysis of the separate effects of each implied construct or determinant. It is unrealistic to expect a single variable to measure every aspect of racial oppression or diversity. Moreover, such a variable does not adequately assess (even after controlling for other predictors) intra-group diversity among blacks (Landry, 1987). Not all blacks are poor and genetically similar; nor do they all practice the same cultural traditions, have the same degree of admixture (Polednak, 1989; Keith and Herring, 1991) or experience racism to the same extent (Wilson, 1980, 1987; Kessler and Neighbors, 1986).

A number of observers (Frazier, 1947; Blauner, 1972; Burkey, 1978; Wilson, 1980; Cooper, 1984; Cooper and David, 1986) have pointed out that the established racial classifications or taxonomies in American society evolved from systems of stratification, power and ideology. Others (Montagu, 1964; Lasker and Tyzzer, 1982; Osborne and Feit, 1992) have concluded that current racial and ethnic designations have little relevance to science and are essentially pragmatic or politically expedient categories (Weissman, 1990; Hahn, 1992; Hahn et al., 1992).

In short, we view race as a social construct whose practical utility is determined by a particular society or social system. As Baker (1967, p. 21) asserts:

> Races have no more or less reality than "chairs" since both are human informational constructs which will linguistically and conceptually persist only as long as they serve the purposes of the concept users.

As previously described, social scientists who conduct research on the relationship between race and health in American society are confronted with the powerful historical legacy of social stratification, discrimination, and oppression based on phenotypic characteristics such as skin color. Racial demarcation on the basis of skin color has never been an absolute or definite process. Historically, interracial liaisons between blacks and whites produced a "mulatto class" that developed into recognizable subracial groupings or communities in certain parts of the country, such as New Orleans and Washington, D.C. Frazier (1957) documents the genesis and social advantages of this group. A superb and more recent discussion of this issue appears in the book by Davis (1991), *Who is Black? One Nation's Definition*. His primary contention is that the "one drop" principle has historically defined, both legally and socially, who is black in American society.

Contemporary manifestations of racism have evolved from this historical legacy. In this connection, racial identification should not be equated with racism. The former term may reflect both the acceptance of the prevailing racial taxonomy and an internalized cultural or historical affinity. On the other hand, racism refers expressly to a history and contemporary manifestation of structural inequality (e.g., institutional racism) and discrimination and/or ideology based on color supremacy. It is possible that a person identifying as black may not believe in racial oppression or be more inured, exculpating, or ignorant of racism than other blacks. An important question is to what extent are the life chances or opportunities qualitatively better or different among "believers" and "nonbelievers."

The explanatory power of a unitary indicator of race is likely to be limited because it does not directly or sufficiently capture the effects of racism in American society. Thus while there is ample reason and precedent to collect data about phenotypic identity, the social significance of race is not singularly embodied in or represented by any one variable. Seldom are historical context or theoretical discussions linking the past and the present employed as explanatory constructs or indicators. Further, the residual or unexplained variance is rarely adequately explained by other variables such as gender, psychosocial measures, social class, or socioeconomic status.[4] Indicators of both institutional and individual racism must be developed and included as variables in public health and epidemiological research.

Racism must not only be studied from the perspective of the individual (Krieger, 1990) and the society as a whole; its manifestations in health and medicine must also be empirically confronted. A few recent studies have documented or inferred discriminatory practices in medical technology (Wenneker and Epstein, 1989), access to care (Blendon et al., 1989; Sullivan, 1991) and public policies (Kushnick, 1988; Council on Ethical and Judicial Affairs, 1990; Rice and Winn, 1990; Hutchinson, 1992).

The view that race is immodifiable also promotes an indifference to measuring racism. This viewpoint derives from a particular conception of race. Conventionally, *race* is conceived and employed as a fixed measure (i.e., phenotypically determined by racial identification), and not as something that can be changed or modified.[5] *Racism* on the other hand, whether individual or institutional, could increase or decrease over

---

4. If in fact the significance of race as a empirical variable is declining, one would expect to see an appreciable increase in the amount of variance being explained by nonracial factors or interaction effects.

5. By way of qualification, there are circumstances in which a person's racial identification can change: when a person has been "passing" as a member of one racial group and then decides to change; when the definitions or boundaries of race change, as in the case of a Creole or "mulatto" group that has been "absorbed" by a more encompassing classification (black); or when new categories emerge for official classification purposes, such as "multiracial" or black or white Hispanic. The sociological significance of these circumstances is that race is not "physiologically" constant, but dynamic and subject to change based on social imperatives.

time and be a continuous indicator. Moreover, it could measure structural barriers more precisely than the all inclusive race construct and thus yield clearer interpretations of findings.

A recent article by Osborne and Feit (1992) asks a provocative question, "Is racial research in medicine racist?" The authors assert that an underlying assumption of research using racial comparisons:

> that the results obtained are a manifestation of the biology of racial differences; race as a variable implies that genetic reasons may explain differences in incidence, severity, or outcome of medical conditions. (p. 275)

Scientists and medical researchers, they argue, are not immune to racial bias, conscious or otherwise. Thus racism—as expressed by the "concept that the behavior, social achievements and intellectual capacity of humans are genetically determined by race"—may be accepted or promoted individually or institutionally within the medical profession. They also maintain that a focus or emphasis on "ethnic categorization" minimizes or reduces other possible explanatory variables such as lifestyle factors and socioeconomic status.

Osborne and Feit also express doubt about whether, due to its elusiveness, the concept of race can be defined adequately to be useful in scientific research. They ask, for example, "How white is white?" and "At what point in one's ancestry does race change?" Published research on sexually transmitted diseases is cited to demonstrate the problems that arose when investigators fail to explicate their hypotheses; comparative race results can be interpreted as evidence of biologic risk factors, as opposed to behavioral or social risk factors; and genetic etiology rather than social causation (poverty and racism) can be assumed.

The failure to measure racism reflects generic shortcomings in epidemiology and public health research. Criticism of the field has pointed out its atheoretical approach (Liberatos et al., 1988). The lack of a clearly defined theoretical framework about social phenomena such as race and racism contributes to overquantification at the expense of a scientific or policy-directed approach. The lack of a well developed theory about the association between race and health practically assures problems in defining terms, interpreting data, and replicating findings.

Wilkinson and King (1987) provide a critique of the conceptual, methodological, and policy implications of using race as a variable in health research. Employing a sociological framework, the authors pose various questions about how social scientists apply the term in empirical research and its meaning as a social construct (e.g., cultural or socioeconomic variable). Rarely, they maintain, do researchers specify or operationally define race. This failure, in their view, leads to ambiguity in interpreting research findings, "calls into question the validity and reliability of social science and health research." Moreover, nonspecification or misunderstanding of the intended conceptual application of race as an independent variable does not give a clear and consistent direction for public policy and programmatic initiatives. They also explain the sociological basis for distinguishing between race and ethnicity, and the problems that a lack of specificity may cause in the interpretation of study results.

Another criticism of the use of race in epidemiological research and statistical compilations is offered by Weissman (1990) in his review of the federal government Directive No. 15 (1978) on racial and ethnic classification standards. Under this classification scheme, five basic race and ethnic groups are recognized by the U.S. government for statistical reporting purposes: white non-Hispanic, black non-Hispanic, Hispanic, native American (i.e., American Indians, Eskimos, Aleuts), Asian and Pacific Islander, and unspecified. Weissman points out the ambiguity and confusion resulting from the use of this typology and questions whether race and ethnicity can be considered "a useful marker for genetic variation." He concludes that valid scientific findings will not result from research employing these definitions and implores researchers to define their concepts clearly, to specify the rationale for using these groupings, and, depending on the nature of the investigation, to employ "techniques of modern genetics to define and subdivide populations."

Jones and her colleagues (1991), reviewing the use of the term *race* in the *American Journal of Epidemiology* over a period spanning almost 50 years, produced a quantitative assessment of trends in the uses of race in epidemiological research. Their findings indicate that, despite expanded scientific interest in the effects of race, "there is an increasing trend toward the explicit exclusion of 'nonwhite' subjects and the selection of predominantly 'white' base populations for study." The inclusion of "nonwhite" populations in epidemiological research, regardless of hypothesized race-associated differences, is strongly encouraged. The authors recommend addressing problems in the use of race through a precise definition and measurement of the variable; explication of socioeconomic, cultural, and genetic differences; and devoting subsequent research to race-associated results.

Crews and Bindon (1991) suggest that the concept *ethnicity* is a more valid representation of social, cultural, and biological variability than race. Criticizing previous uses of the term *ethnicity*, they comment on the "multifactorial aspects of ethnicity" and propose an ecological-evolutionary perspective. This approach would entail an analysis of "ethnic differences in physiology, genetics, beliefs, and life-style . . . as a result of biological and cultural adaptations by particular human groups that have maintained some degree of relative cultural or reproductive isolation." This view maintains that ethnic group differences associated with health status are likely to result from sociocultural patterns and ecological systems.

Hahn (1992) reviews the validity of federal health statistics based on prevailing racial and ethnic designations. Approaching the problem from a methodological perspective, he examines four primary assumptions regarding the race and ethnic group taxonomy:

(1) The categories of "race" and "ethnicity" and specific racial and ethnic group designations are consistently defined and ascertained. (2) The categories and designations are un-

derstood by the populations questioned. (3) Survey enumeration, participation, and response rates are high and similar for all populations. (4) The responses of individuals are
consistent in different data sources and at different times. (p. 268)

Addressing the first assumption, Hahn criticizes Directive 15 because of the difficulties (tautology and nonmutual exclusivity of terms) in applying criteria for defining
race and ethnic groups, and incongruities among federal data sources and between the
respondents' and interviewers' labeling of race and ethnicity. With regard to the second assumption, Hahn notes considerable measurement error due to differences between popular understandings of race and ethnicity and survey instrumentation. Con-
testing the accuracy of the third assumption, Hahn identifies four methodological
problems that skew government health data: (1) underregistration of births, although
quite small and mainly limited to older data sets, do differ markedly by race and ethnic
group; (2) misclassification of race at death, leading to "exaggerating white mortality
and minimizing mortality among races other than white"; (3) census miscounts (undercounting of blacks and Hispanics and overcounting of American Indians); and (4) nonresponse. Lastly, Hahn notes the indistinctness of racial and ethnic boundaries that
occur in group identity over time. To rectify such shortcomings, Hahn proposes clearly
defining the terms *race* and *ethnicity* for public health purposes, scientific validation of
the concepts, more vigorous assessment and correction of measurement error incurred
through respondent errors and periodic and systematic evaluation of racial and ethnic
health statistics.

Epidemiologists and other public health researchers have been criticized for emphasizing individual level data, such as lifestyle factors associated with knowledge, beliefs, attitudes, and behavior. Although these factors are relevant to health behavior
and health status, they should not be regarded as surrogates for structural factors
(poverty or medical indigence, institutional racism, unavailability of services) and
other social causes (cultural mores, historical effects, competing priorities). Generally
speaking, researchers have not found that studies of knowledge, attitudes, and practices
(KAP) or the health belief model to have produced adequate explanations of health behavior and outcomes (Williams, 1990). Yet there continues to be an inordinate preoccupation with such indicators.[6] Moreover, conferring primacy to micro-level explanatory variables tends to lead to public policies and programs that minimize or disregard
systemic and other sociological strategies and focus almost exclusively on individual
attribution.

In epidemiology and public health, where the physical and social sciences often converge, there is no clear consensus on the meaning of race (Cooper, 1984; Cooper and

---

6. This orientation may be ascribed to three factors: (1) the large number of behavioral scientists (especially clinical and social psychologists) in public health; (2) the greater methodological
sophistication in measuring individual level variables and in standardized scales and instruments;
and (3) greater receptiveness to individual based interpretations on the part of public policy makers and government bureaucrats.

David, 1986; Wilkinson and King, 1987; Hahn, 1992; Osborne and Feit, 1992). Cooper and David (1986) state that the earliest discussions in the scientific literature about its interpretation and significance were recorded in the mid-eighteenth century.

Definitions and classification schemes also vary depending on the context in which they are used. In health, research focusing on racial differences must address (implicitly or explicitly) the issue of biological or hereditary factors; some genetic attributes and diseases predominate among certain physically distinct groups (Damon, 1969; Polednak, 1989). Thus race, like gender (but unlike social class or socioeconomic status), takes on a different connotation when used in a health or medical context because it reflects the duality of race or gender as both a biological and sociological variable. Rarely, however, do social scientists, except for physical anthropologists, consider biologic and genetic variables in their research. They typically view the role of biology and genetics as either immeasurable and constant across groups, irrelevant, limited to specific disease entities, or outside of their area of expertise.

Opinions diverge about the relative significance of social and biological conceptions of race as determinants of health behavior and health status. In the etiology of major specific chronic diseases such as cerebrovascular disease, certain neoplasms, and cardiovascular disease, the role of genetic differences (and, by implication, racial differences) is widely considered secondary to environmental causation. There is probably greater agreement about the diminished relevance of genetic factors to acute, episodic, and infectious diseases than their importance regarding chronic diseases. Our position is that social and environmental factors are the major reasons why blacks have excess mortality and morbidity rates and experience a poorer quality of life than do whites.

As an alternative, we contend that the key focus should be to measure the primary components of racial inequality or difference. This would require reconstruction and development of specific indicators of race-related behavior. But such an approach would compel researchers to provide definitive formulations of the theoretical premises underlying each specific indicator of race-related behavior.

We also encourage the use of social historical perspectives in public health research. An ahistorical approach—a failure to acknowledge and embody the past—can produce myopic and static theories and research (Mills, 1959; Gouldner, 1970). Moreover, on a larger scale, what results is a tremendous "historical vacuum" in the social sciences, which gives added credence and opportunity for proponents of biological and genetic research to advance intergenerational theories or propositions about health phenomena based on heritability. Ahistorical approaches also enable simplistic and fragmented social theories and explanations (for instance, the culture of poverty) to gain currency and acceptability as intellectual paradigms and policy solutions.

In sum, so-called "pure" races, especially as recognized in the American context, do not exist. If in fact, races ever were "pure," they are not presently so constituted. Furthermore, the notion of "pure" races has historically served to foster group supremacy and other group subjugation. We are convinced that races are fundamentally artificial categories serving a predefined social purpose or outcome. Thus, the nature of the categories can and does shift depending on the historical context, misclassifications (Hahn, 1992; Hahn et al., 1992), migration and admixture (Polednak, 1989), and the social environment.

Understanding Racial Differences in Health

Race has conventionally been employed as an aggregate indicator. Understanding racial disparities in health is contingent on (1) identifying specific factors that may affect health status; and (2) systematically assessing these factors as determinants of differences between the races in health status. This requires more information than is usually collected either by federal health agencies or by most researchers.

Figure 4–1 provides an organizational framework or model for understanding racial differences in health status. It posits an etiological relationship and interaction among the various components of race, and a broad range of intervening variables, as determinants of biological processes and health status. Each component may affect health status directly or indirectly, depending on the biological nature of the disease or illness. The model is dynamic, since the relative contribution of each component is dependent on broader societal influences and changes in life course. For example, increases and decreases in societal racism or SES may affect the impact of these variables on health.

The model illustrates that race is a proxy for biological, cultural, socioeconomic, and sociopolitical factors, as well as for racism. All these components of race are inter-

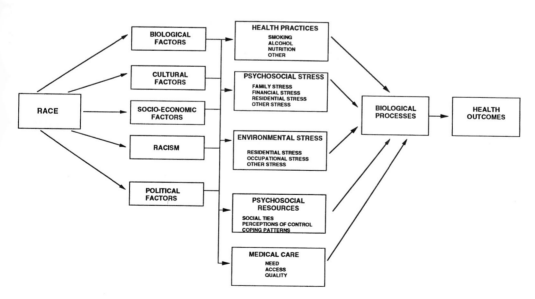

Figure 4-1 A framework for understanding the relationship between race and health.

related and can interact with each other. They exert their effects through more proximal mechanisms or intervening factors, including health practices, psychosocial stress,
environmental stress, psychosocial resources, and medical care. Each component of
race—biology, culture, socioeconomic status, political power and racism—may impact
any of the intermediary factors, which in turn relate to each other in ways that may
produce both additive and interactive effects.

Components of Race

Biological Factors

As we have seen, the biological or genetic contribution of race to health status is likely
to be small. Even so, it is not appropriate to rule out genetics completely without empirical verification. As the model specifies, intervening risk factors and resources ultimately influence health outcomes through biological mechanisms. Thus it is crucial to
make the conceptual distinction between innate and acquired biological factors. Many
researchers view any observed biological difference between the races as *prima facie*
evidence of underlying genetic variation. But since social processes also have physiological effects on organisms (Geronimus, 1992), mere identification of different biological characteristics and/or mechanisms in groups living under different environmental conditions does not necessarily indicate genetic differences. For example, the
hemodynamic profile of hypertension in blacks differs from that of whites. It is possible that socioeconomically linked dietary differences—for instance, blacks consume
less potassium than whites—are responsible for these racial differences (Williams,
1992). Also, exposure to certain occupational hazards (carcinogenic agents) or environmental hazards (radiation, lead poisoning, food contaminants) can alter biological
functions and result in increased risks and altered disease status.

Culture

Culture has traditionally been defined as a socially acquired "way of life" transmitted
from one generation to another (Murdock, 1965). Social scientists have employed the
"way of life" concept as a prism to explain why and how people form belief systems,
establish normative behavior, interact with others, and organize their social existence.
The role of culture is a central topic in the behavioral and social sciences, at least in
part, because of the need to explain social disparities in a culturally diverse society
(Spector, 1979; Zola, 1966).

   Cultural influences on health and medical care involve such basic aspects of human
behavior and belief systems as religious practices, language, folk medicine, diet, dress,
norms and values, and help-seeking behavior. These cultural practices in turn have an
impact on perceptions of symptoms, definitions of illness, delivery of health services,
disease prevention, health promotion, medical practice, and patient adherence (Snow,
1978; Jackson, 1981).

   African-American culture is not monolithic. It is influenced by dominant white

Anglo-Saxon Protestant cultural traditions, behaviors, values and norms. More importantly, it is diverse in matters of geography, religion, ethnicity, and social class. Green (1978) has proposed a comprehensive typology for understanding the heterogeneity of the black population. This framework divides into nine distinctive "cultural-ecological areas" that vary in history, economics, and social and environmental factors, among which are religion, class structure, dominant family type, land ownership, color stratification, and community cohesiveness. The nine cultural-ecological areas are (1) the Tidewater-Piedmont area (eastern Maryland, Virginia, and North Carolina); (2) the coastal southeast or "Gullah" area (South Carolina and eastern Georgia); (3) the Black Belt or lowland southern area (central and western Georgia, Alabama, Mississippi, parts of Tennessee, Kentucky, Arkansas, Missouri, Louisiana, and Texas); (5) areas of Indian influence (Oklahoma and parts of Arkansas and Kansas); (6) the Southwestern area (west Texas, New Mexico, Arizona, and California); (7) the old eastern colonial area (New Jersey, Pennsylvania, New York, Massachusetts); (8) the midwestern and far western area (from Illinois west to Washington state); and (9) post-1920 metropolitan northern and western ghetto areas (large inner cities such as New York, Detroit, Chicago, and San Francisco). Green points out that most of the research on blacks to date has focused on two of these nine areas (the Black Belt and the major inner cities).

Ethnicity is a conventional term sociologists have traditionally employed to refer to cultural phenomena associated with distinct religions, nationalities, or language groups. However, because race as a taxonomic concept continues to have greater sociological import with reference to African-Americans, the model treats culture as a definable and measurable component of race. Ethnicity is in turn a predictor of cultural variation in the black population. The African-American population in the United States includes many twentieth-century immigrants from the Caribbean basin countries and from Africa. The Caribbean or West Indian population includes Hispanics from countries such as Cuba, the Dominican Republic, and Panama; Haitians and other persons from the French-speaking Caribbean; and English-speaking groups. West Indian immigrants to the United States number about 1 million, about half of whom settled in and around New York City (Kasinitz, 1992). According to one estimate (Hill, 1983), West Indians and their descendants constitute as much as 10 percent of the African-American population. Studies in the Northeast have documented that black immigrant populations differ from each other and from the native-born black population in terms of health (Kleinman et al., 1991; Fruchter et al., 1990; Russo et al., 1981), the pattern of variation depending on the health outcome under consideration.

The overreliance of epidemiological studies on a race comparison paradigm, in which the health status of blacks is compared to that of whites, has masked the heterogeneity of the black population in terms of health. Recent studies demonstrate, for instance, that marital status (Williams et al., 1992a) and socioeconomic status (Williams et al., 1992b) predict variations in the distribution of psychiatric disorders within the black population. These studies also indicate that sociodemographic variation in the distribution of illness within the black population resembles—with certain important, striking differences—the observed patterns for whites.

Our viewpoint is that culture is a product of adaptation to the ecological environment and social structure. It does not evolve independently, nor is it unaffected by "external reality" (geography, climate) and broader social forces (e.g., subsistence conditions, economic forces, imperialism).

Socioeconomic Factors

Health status disparities between blacks and whites must be understood within the context of a broader and virtually universal phenomenon: despite general improvements in health status, broad-based social and economic change, and advances in health care technology and the delivery of medical services, socioeconomic status (SES) remains a powerful predictor of health throughout the industrialized world and in poorer Third World countries (Marmot et al., 1987; Williams, 1990). Socioeconomic status is an important correlate of race; and for this reason, it is inadequate to present data by race without controlling for SES. Researchers frequently find that adjusting their results for SES substantially reduces or even eliminates racial disparities in health. Two recent examples will suffice. An analysis of cancer incidence rates in three U.S. metropolitan areas between 1978 and 1982 documented that most of the racial differences disappeared when controls for socioeconomic status were employed (Baquet et al., 1991). And recent analyses of the Charleston Heart Study data found that differences in mortality for blacks versus whites do not remain significant after controlling for SES (Keil et al., 1992).

For several reasons, however, adjusting for or stratifying results according to SES is not enough. First, the prevailing measures of SES (income, education, and occupational status, or some combination of the three) are imperfect proxies for the concept of SES (Liberatos et al., 1988). They do not capture all the dimensions of variations in social stratification that can affect health status. Health care researchers have yet to employ theoretically driven measures of social class (e.g., Wright and Perrone, 1977; Robinson and Kelley, 1979), and have failed to assess all the dimensions of social stratification that may be linked to health status.

Second, the standard SES indicators do not have the same meanings for different races. A given level of occupational status may have different health consequences across race. Employed blacks, for example, are more likely than whites to be exposed to occupational hazards and carcinogens even after controlling for job experience and education (Robinson, 1984). Whites also receive higher income returns on education than blacks (Jaynes and Williams, 1989). A given level of income may provide less purchasing power to blacks than to whites: compared to their white counterparts, low SES blacks pay more for both rent (Cooper, 1984) and food (Alexis et al., 1980). When blacks purchase homes, they also pay higher lending rates for mortgages (Pol et al., 1982).

Racial differences in assets are even more striking. At every income level, whites have more wealth than blacks (Blau and Graham, 1990). At comparable levels of income, for example, blacks have less valuable homes and less housing equity than whites (Parcel, 1982). In general, whites earn one and a half times as much income as blacks, but possess four times as much wealth (Birnbaum and Weston, 1974; Blau and Graham, 1990). These patterns reflect substantial racial differences in the inheritance patterns of wealth and in intergenerational transfers of wealth. Middle-class blacks are more likely than their white counterparts to be first-generation members of the middle class and among the wealthiest persons in their families. They are thus not unlikely to receive assets from other relatives. Among whites, but not among African-Americans, for example, marriage increases the likelihood of an intergenerational transfer of assets to be used in purchasing a home (Parcel, 1982). Middle-class blacks are also likely to be providing material support to poorer family members. Little attention has been given to the health consequences of racial differences in wealth; wealth may prove to be an important component of SES in assessing racial differences in health status.

Third, measures of current SES do not fully capture lifetime exposure to deprived conditions. Observed health risks may be associated with the long-term effects of previous socioeconomic circumstances. Whatever their current SES, adults may be affected by deprivations and deficits experienced during childhood (Williams, 1990). For example, lack of preventive medical care in childhood may set in motion processes that cannot be reversed even with ample access to health care later in life. Low-birth-weight babies have higher risks of morbidity on a broad range of indicators of childhood health status (McCormick, 1985). Given the high prevalence of low-birth-weight infants in the black population, a substantial proportion of African-Americans may experience long-term health consequences linked to problems of infancy and childhood.

These differences suggest that a given level of SES may be more strongly linked to adverse health outcomes for blacks than for whites. Researchers have not explored this possibility in a systematic way, though several studies have documented that SES interacts with race to produce higher levels of morbidity and mortality among blacks. A recent study found that low-birth-weight African-American infants born to college-educated parents had almost twice the risk of death (1.82; adjusted for age, parity, prenatal care, and marital status) as white infants in college-educated families (Schoendorf et al., 1992). Similarly, it has consistently been found in the mental health literature that SES interacts with race to produce markedly higher levels of psychological distress among low SES blacks than among their white peers (Kessler and Neighbors, 1986; Ulbrich et al., 1989). Future research must assess whether interaction effects of this kind reflect true differences between the races in the impact of SES, or merely the limitations of our current SES indicators.

Surprisingly, analyses of data from the five large-probability samples of the ECA study reveal that low-SES white males have higher rates of psychiatric disorder than their black counterparts (Williams et al., 1992b). Could a low-SES position for a white male be so dissonant from societal expectations as to have serious psychological sequelae? Alternatively, the authors of the study suggest the finding may reflect biased estimates of the distribution of disease among African-American males due to the noncoverage of this population in epidemiological studies. In addition to their high rates of nonresponse in community samples, black males also are disproportionately represented among institutional (e.g., prison) and marginal (e.g., homeless) populations, whose rates of illness are likely to be high. The conventional approach to addressing this issue is to use post-stratification weights to make the sample correspond to that of the U.S. Census estimates of the population. Weighting is not an effective solution, however, because nonrespondents are unlikely to be similar to respondents. By the U.S. Census Bureau's own estimates, furthermore, its net undercount for specific age groups of the adult black male population ranges between 10 and 20 percent (National Center for Health Statistics, 1991). Undercounting may be much higher in certain urban areas. At present, the degree to which noncoverage of African-American men biases the findings of epidemiological studies is not known. Since this problem is probably growing more acute with time, health researchers cannot afford to ignore it.

Racism

Racism is explicitly included in the model as a component of race that can have pervasive effects on health status. The experience of racial bias can have pathogenic effects on individuals, and institutionalized racism in the health care sector can lead to deficiencies and inequities in the quality of medical care. Harburg and colleagues (1973b) offered early evidence that the experience of unfair treatment can adversely affect health: they found that people who responded to unfair treatment with suppressed hostility (the combination of stifling anger and feeling guilty if anger is expressed) were more likely to have hypertension. This was found to be true for both black and white males. It is likely that black people who live and work under conditions of acute social and economic deprivation would be exposed to particularly high levels of unfair treatment.

In a small study of black and white women, Krieger (1990) explored the relationship between rates of hypertension and the experience of racial and gender discrimination. Among the black women who experienced unfair treatment, she found those who kept quiet and accepted it were four times as likely to have high blood pressure as those who talked about it or took other action in response. Gender discrimination was unrelated to hypertension for white women. It is instructive that black women were six times more likely than whites to respond passively to unfair treatment, suggesting that they perceived themselves (probably accurately) as having little recourse in such encounters. Moreover, black women who reported that they had experienced no racial or gender discrimination were two to three times as likely to have high blood pressure as those who had reported experiencing unfair treatment. Apparently an internalized denial of racial and gender bias leads to adverse changes in health status.

The experience of racial discrimination is not uniform among blacks. One recent study, documented that darker-skinned blacks in the United States are twice as likely to experience racial discrimination as their lighter-skinned peers (Keith and Herring, 1991). Similarly, research by Dressler (1991) in both the United States and Brazil indicates that the struggle for desirable resources is more acute for darker-skinned blacks than for their lighter-skinned counterparts. Thus, darker skin color may be a social characteristic predictive of reduced access to economic and social resources among lower-SES African-Americans. One recent study consistent with this viewpoint documented that skin color interacts with SES to affect rates of blood pressure among blacks. At low levels of SES, blood pressure is higher in darker-skinned people; at higher levels of SES, skin color is unrelated to blood pressure (Klag et al., 1991). Health researchers who invoke the concept of discrimination must give more systematic attention to measuring such discrimination and to assessing its potential consequences on health status.

Institutionalized racism also affects the receipt of health care. In the words of the former Secretary of Health and Human Services, Dr. Louis Sullivan, "there is clear, demonstrable, undeniable evidence of discrimination and racism in our health care system" (Sullivan, 1991). The Council on Ethical and Judicial Affairs (1990) of the American Medical Association recently reviewed the evidence of persistent and pervasive racial differences in the quality of health care in the United States. Compared to their black counterparts, whites are more likely to receive coronary angiography, bypass surgery, angioplasty, chemodialysis, intensive care for pneumonia, and kidney transplants. These differences persist even after adjustment for the severity of illness, income, and insurance status. Whites are more likely to be on a waiting list for kidney transplants (Council on Ethical and Judicial Affairs, 1990), and they wait only half as long as blacks (Sullivan, 1991). These latter examples provide compelling evidence that discrimination must be at work. Blacks in psychiatric treatment are less likely than whites to receive psychotherapy, and more likely to receive less intensive treatment, for shorter periods of time, with less experienced therapists (Council on Ethical and Judicial Affairs, 1990). Rice (1991) also indicates that blacks are twice as likely as their white peers not to receive prenatal care (40 percent compared to 21 percent). Blacks also spend 3 days more waiting to be placed in a nursing home than their white counterparts (Weissert and Cready, 1988).

Though racism in the health care system is still a neglected topic, the growing body of evidence reviewed above suggests that it is an important individual and structural impediment to seeking health care, as well as to interaction with medical systems and professionals. Ultimately, it is clear, racism adversely affects health status. Understanding its role in health status differences between the races requires researchers to pay more than lip service to the construct. Future research must give more attention to development of theoretically informed measures of racism and to the examination of its role in health.

Political Power

Power is another neglected variable in research on racial differences in health status. LaVeist (1992), in discussing the link between political empowerment and health status, reviews evidence that the political empowerment of blacks may lead to more community-level political participation, increases in black employment, and improvement in overall quality of life. These improvements in social conditions may in turn lead to improvements in health status. In an analysis of neonatal mortality rates in U.S. central cities, LaVeist documented a strong negative association between black political power and postneonatal mortality rates.

Intervening Mechanisms

The intervening mechanisms or proximal factors shown at the center of the model are viewed as the superficial or surface causes of racial disparities in health (Lieberson, 1985; Williams, 1990). This formulation has two implications. First, these variables are dynamic and change over time. In fact, the specific risk factors linked to high rates of morbidity and mortality for African-Americans have changed over time, as the major causes of death have shifted from infectious communicable diseases to chronic degenerative ones. The relative gap in health status between the races, however, has not been substantially altered. Second, because these intervening mechanisms are secondary to the basic causes (racism, political, socioeconomic, cultural, and biological factors), modification of these risk factors alone is unlikely to lead to reductions in racial disparities in health status. As long as the basic societal causes remain operative, interventions directed at superficial influences will likely give rise to new intervening factors without altering the outcome (Williams, 1990).

Health Practices

Health behaviors are measured at the level of the individual, and their distribution is typically regarded as due to personal choice and preference. We will illustrate the role of larger societal factors in affecting their distribution by focusing on cigarette smoking and alcohol abuse. These two behaviors are primary determinants of the heavy burden of disease in the black population. The aforementioned federal government report on black and minority health identified six causes of death as responsible for 80 percent of the 60,000 annual excess deaths in the black population (U.S. Department of Health and Human Services, 1985). As Table 4–1 indicates, cigarette smoking and alcohol abuse are risk factors for five of the six causes of death.

Blacks have higher rates of smoking and are more likely to abuse alcohol than whites. These patterns reflect a noteworthy historical shift in the distribution of these health practices. Prior to the 1950s, rates of smoking and alcohol abuse were higher among whites than blacks (Williams, 1992a). The social distribution of these health behaviors is dependent on cooperative efforts by the state and powerful economic interests. There is a positive association between the availability of alcohol and its consumption. In every state, government policies control the availability of alcohol; these policies have led to the presence of more retail outlets for alcoholic beverages in black and poor neighborhoods than in more affluent areas (Rabow and Watt, 1984). The financial resources that the alcohol and tobacco industries control have led to a symbiotic relationship with the state, and have equipped them to co-opt other influential

Table 4-1 The Leading Causes of Death for Blacks and Their Associated Risk Factors

Causes of Death	Risk Factors
Cardiovascular disease	Smoking, high blood pressure, elevated serum cholesterol, obesity, diabetes, lack of exercise.
Cancers	Smoking, alcohol, solar radiation, worksite hazards, environmental contaminants, diet, infectious agents.
Homicide, suicide, and unintentional injuries	Alcohol or drug misuse, stress, handgun availability.
Diabetes	Obesity.
Infant mortality	Low birth weight, maternal smoking, nutrition, stress, time of prenatal care, age, marital status.
Cirrhosis of the liver	Alcohol.

Source: U.S. Department of Health and Human Services, 1985, Vol. 2.

groups that might otherwise attempt to mobilize the state to act against them. In 1987, Phillip Morris and R. J. R. Nabisco provided over $4.3 million to black, Hispanic, labor and women's groups (Levin, 1988). These groups included the Congressional Black, Hispanic, and Women's Caucuses, the National Urban League and the United Negro College Fund. Moreover, some companies (such as the Adolph Coors Company which agreed to invest $625 million over five years in black and Hispanic areas) explicitly tie their continued economic support to increased consumption of the companies' products (Hacker et al., 1987).

Social and economic stress are important predictors of alcohol and tobacco consumption. Cigarette smoking and alcohol use are socially approved ways to cope with, and temporarily escape from, adverse working and living conditions. People smoke to reduce distress, anger, fear, and nervous tension (Benfari et al., 1982). Smoking rises among women when they enter the labor force and among high-school graduates who are unable to find work (Stark, 1982). Other data reveal that cigarette smoking increases during periods of high stress (Conway et al., 1981). Similarly, sales of alcoholic beverages increase during economic recessions and periods of increasing unemployment (Singer, 1986).

Some populations or groups may also be more vulnerable than others to certain health behaviors because of synergistic effects. Cigarette smoking (Cooper and Simmons, 1985) and alcohol use (Lex, 1987), for example, affect blacks more adversely than whites. It is likely that black smokers are exposed more to toxic working and residential environments than are their white peers. Failure to characterize these environmental exposures in studies of smoking and health may overestimate the effects of smoking (Sterling and Weinkam, 1989).

Psychosocial Stress

The differential distribution of stress is likely to play an important role in accounting for health status differences between the races. A substantial portion of the black population lives in low-income rural or inner-city environments, where they are likely to be exposed to multiple stressors. Low socioeconomic status restricts people to certain types of housing and locales, and compromises the quality of life. Intertwined with low SES is a stressful lifestyle typically characterized by poor nutrition, poor education, crime, traffic hazards, substandard and overcrowded housing, low-paying jobs, unemployment and underemployment, and lack of health insurance and access to basic health services. Low-SES blacks have higher levels of unemployment, underemployment, and marital disruption than their white counterparts (Dohrenwend and Dohrenwend, 1970). They are also more likely to be underemployed.

Current measures of stress that are biased toward the stressors experienced by the middle class do not adequately characterize the stressful conditions faced by the poor in general and the black poor in particular. There may be qualitative differences across the races in the experience of stress. Wilson (1987) indicates that the black poor are increasingly concentrated in depressed inner-city neighborhoods, while the white urban poor are more evenly dispersed, many residing in relatively safe and comfortable neighborhoods. The literature suggests that the stress of life in urban residential areas may significantly impact health status. The classic ecological studies of Harburg and his colleagues (1973a,b) found that residence in stressful urban areas is related to adverse changes in health. Residents of Detroit census tracts characterized by high levels of economic deprivation (low median income and years of formal education), residential instability, marital instability, and crime had higher blood pressure levels than those who lived in census tracts with more favorable conditions. This association was stronger among blacks than whites. In low stress areas, moreover, the blood pressure levels of black and white males did not differ.

Garbarino and colleagues (1992) have examined the impact of community violence as a neglected variable in stress research. They point out that individuals who live in inner-city housing projects are twice as likely to experience violence as other people, and that violence affects not only the victims but also those who witness it and have to live with the consequences. Repeatedly witnessing traumatic events may have an additive effect, especially on children. Children chronically exposed to family and community violence may tend to respond with desensitization, resignation, and addiction. More importantly, they may harbor lifelong vulnerabilities. Violence also depletes the social and material resources available to support the child and family. Living in "urban war zones" where physical safety cannot be assumed, and/or having to maintain a constant psychological vigil to cope with the ubiquitous incidence of racial bias, may lead many African-Americans to live in a state of heightened vigilance that takes toll on the human organism.

Recent studies of racial differences in diurnal blood pressure provide evidence consistent with this viewpoint. Using ambulatory blood pressure measurement procedures, these studies have consistently found that average daytime blood pressure levels were equivalent for blacks and whites. However, blacks experienced a smaller nocturnal decline than whites, such that blacks have higher blood pressure levels while they are asleep (Hashfield et al., 1989; James, 1991; Murphy et al., 1988). This higher baseline level of blood pressure may be partly responsible for the greater organ damage that black hypertensives experience, compared to their white peers (Murphy et al., 1988). Other recent experimental evidence indicates that stress may have more adverse effects on African-Americans than on whites (Light et al., 1987).

Age is a variable routinely employed in epidemiological studies to capture biological processes. Researchers should keep in mind that age may also be a proxy for certain social processes (Geronimus, 1992). For example, racial differences in blood pressure tend to be evident only in adulthood. This finding may indicate a lag in the effect of environmental exposures, or rapid increase of hypertension in young black adults as they confront restricted socioeconomic opportunities and truncated options (Williams, 1992b). Similarly, ratios of black to white neonatal mortality rates increase with the age of the mother from the teens through the twenties. Geronimus (1992) has proposed a "weathering hypothesis" to account for this pattern. She points out that the teenage years may be the optimal years (biologically) for childbearing. Poor mothers have poor health status prior to becoming pregnant; given the chronic and cumulative nature of these adverse conditions, risk will increase with age. The older the mother, the longer her exposure to environmental assaults and the greater her vulnerability to adverse pregnancy outcomes. Thus, the degree of exposure to risk factors (which age sometimes captures) may be an important predictor of their impact. Geronimus' (1988) work also suggests that excess neonatal mortality among blacks is not due simply to high rates of teenage pregnancy.

Environmental Stress

In addition to exposure to high levels of noise, crowding, and other stressors of impoverished inner city environments, African-Americans may also be disproportionately exposed to toxic chemicals. Until recently, researchers have given inadequate attention to environmental toxic exposure in efforts to account for racial differences in health. An analysis of the distribution of hazardous waste sites in the United States revealed that race was the strongest predictor of proximity to hazardous waste facilities, even after adjustment for socioeconomic factors (Commission for Racial Justice, 1987). Central city residents are five times more likely to be exposed to air and water pollution than their suburban peers, and predominantly black poor rural residents are disproportionately likely to be exposed to health-threatening toxic materials from industrial plants (Bullard and Wright, 1987). Lead poisoning is also a serious health problem in inner-city neighborhoods, where large numbers of minority children live and play.

Brajer and Hall (1992) document that, although the highest income families generate 4 to 6 times as much air pollution as do poor families, they are less likely to live in areas where air pollution levels are high. According to their analyses, poor blacks and Hispanic residents experience higher levels of air pollution than do high-income people and Anglos or Asians.

Psychosocial Resources

Research efforts to fully characterize the risk factors and vulnerabilities of the African-American population must be balanced by attempts to identify its strengths and health enhancement resources. An exclusive focus on social pathology distorts the struggles and strengths of a disadvantaged population that continues to survive. Two social institutions frequently nominated for research attention in this regard are the family and the black church.

It is widely believed that strong family ties and the extended black family system buffer the deleterious effects of stress on health. This belief is consistent with the substantial literature suggesting that supportive social relationships are among the most powerful determinants of health (House et al., 1988). However, direct evidence of the health-enhancing role of social ties within the black community is limited. Some of the strongest evidence comes from small qualitative studies, such as Carol Stack's (1975) classic work on mutual support networks among black women. More quantitative studies, however, suggest that levels of social relationships are higher among whites than blacks (Strogatz and James, 1986). Some researchers have attributed an idyllic quality to the social networks of blacks, as if they were a panacea for a broad range of health problems. In reality, though these networks facilitate survival, they are likely to generate stress as well as support (Belle, 1982). Moreover, limited evidence suggests that health status is more strongly linked to the negative aspects of social ties than to the supportive ones (Rook, 1984). Cutbacks in government-provided social services over the last decade have probably increased the burdens and demands on the supportive services provided by black families. How these families are coping with these new demands in the face of economic contraction and decline in socioeconomic position is not known. To examine this question requires a dynamic perspective on social institutions and a recognition that they exist within a larger sociopolitical context and are frequently forced to adapt to the constraints of this environment.

The black church is also a critical source of social integration. Congregation-based friendship networks can function as a type of extended family, offering supportive social relationships to individuals throughout the life cycle (Taylor and Chatters, 1988). The African-American population is arguably the most religious subgroup in the industrialized world (Gallup Report, 1985), and its high level of religious involvement may modify the negative consequences of stress and promote psychological well-being. Griffith and colleagues (Griffith et al., 1980, 1984) have demonstrated that for black congregants, participation in religious services provides therapeutic benefits equivalent to those of formal psychotherapy. The emotional expressiveness and active congregational participation that characterize some African-American church services can promote "collective catharsis" in ways that facilitate the reduction of tension and the release of emotional distress (Gilkes, 1980). We know of no studies, however, that have measured involvement in public religious rituals and its relationship to health status.

The extent to which individual psychological resources, such as perceptions of control and coping strategies, may mitigate the effects on health status of adverse living and working conditions remains to be assessed. It is clear, however, that even these coping strategies need to be understood within their larger social context. This is well illustrated by the ground-breaking studies of "John Henryism" and blood pressure by Sherman James and colleagues (1983, 1987). The John Henryism construct is based on the black American folktale of a strong but uneducated steel driver who died of exhaustion immediately after besting a mechanical steel drill; a high score on a John Henryism scale reflects a predisposition to cope actively with stress and to work toward success against all odds. These researchers found that the effectiveness of this coping strategy depends on the individual's social and economic resources. That is, individuals who scored high on John Henryism but had not finished high school had three times as much hypertension as high school graduates who also scored high on the John Henryism. Interestingly, John Henryism was unrelated to blood pressure in whites.

Medical Care

Recent national surveys indicate the persistence of large variations in both the quantity and the quality of medical care among racial and ethnic groups (Andersen et al., 1986; Blendon et al., 1989). Blendon and colleagues, for example, reveal that blacks are almost twice as likely as whites to receive medical care in hospital clinics, emergency rooms, and similar settings where an individual is likely to see a different provider on each visit and thus lack continuity in care. The same survey found blacks to be more dissatisfied than whites with the quality of care they received, apparently for very good reasons. In addition to spending more time in the waiting room than whites, blacks were also more likely to report inadequacies in explanation of the seriousness of the illness or injury, in the provision of information about medication, in the discussion of tests or examination findings, and in inquiry about the presenting health problem.

In the United States, access to health care is a function of employment status. Most health insurance is made available through employment, but 75 percent of uninsured persons are members of households with at least one working adult (Short et al., 1990). A recent study by the Agency for Health Care Policy Research found that, between 1977 and 1987, the proportion of the black population without health insurance increased from 18 to 25 percent (Short et al., 1990). Overall, the number of uninsured Americans under age 65 rose at four times the rate of population growth over this 10-year period, with blacks and Hispanics accounting for half the increase in the number of people with neither public nor private health insurance. Of poor people under 65, the proportion with no insurance rose from 23 to 38 percent; the proportion with private insurance coverage fell from 34 to 31 percent. The study also documented that a substantial proportion of the uninsured population consists of the working poor. About 40 percent of uninsured blacks, 23 percent of Hispanics, and 19 percent of whites belong to families with no working adult. Thus the overwhelming majority of uninsured persons in the United States are in families with adults who work but either do not have employer provided insurance or cannot afford insurance premiums.

With regard to the health care reform debate and initiatives, access to health care is not solely a matter of having insurance coverage. Many residents in poor and minority communities are less likely to have access to health services because of the paucity of physicians, health care institutions, and other providers in these areas. In addition, the infrastructure (e.g., administrative operations, automation, plant structures) of these fa- cilities will require an infusion of funds to redress longstanding problems related to pa- tient care, transportation, health services research, and cost containment. Another im- portant consideration is the need for health care providers to deal with multicultural issues such as language barriers in written and oral communications with patients; in- creasing knowledge of and promoting sensitivity toward different values and beliefs, norms, and behaviors regarding health; and increasing the representation of racial and ethnic minorities in health care. Lastly, national health care reform is not likely to be effective and sustaining for poor and minority communities if basic structural prob- lems are not adequately addressed.

The Challenges of Health Intervention Research in African-American Communities

Specific public policies and programs have been instituted to enlist community groups, especially the medically indigent and minority groups, in the effort to reduce disease and promote health. A wide array of intervention programs and evaluation research (intervention research) focusing on chronic disease (such as cardiovascular disease and cancer), multiple risk factors (including substance abuse, hypertension, lack of exer- cise, poor diet and nutrition), and infectious diseases (such as AIDS and tuberculosis), have been implemented and targeted to specific population groups. Among the major challenges facing investigators who target black populations are (1) community agita- tion for power or empowerment, (2) change and conflict, and (3) the limitations of health interventions.

Empowerment

This popular and ambiguous buzzword is frequently used as a synonym for community participation in health interventions. One of the earliest discussions of empowerment is Paulo Freire's work (1970) on the impoverished in Brazil. Freire describes empower- ment education as a means of achieving personal and social change, and defines it as a social action process that promotes the participation of people, organizations, and com- munities in gaining control over their lives. The basic process, according to Waller- stein and Bernstein (1988), consists of (1) group efforts to identify problems, (2) criti- cal assessment of the social and historical roots of the problem, and (3) development of strategies to overcome obstacles in achieving goals. For communities or minority groups that enjoy little power or share few societal resources, empowerment is an ef- fort to increase their abilities to participate in and control social and political processes that affect them.

For many public health researchers, empowerment ideas and programs may appear threatening, particularly if they involve nontraditional arrangements for sharing power and project resources. In many urban black communities, researchers will no longer have complete or unilateral control over decisions involving their projects. Community participation and input are the norm. The challenges facing the social science community are to understand and accept the idea and reality of empowerment as a fair means of power sharing and to establish formal and informal mechanisms for resolving problems.

Change and Conflict

The inevitability of change and the dynamic character of health behavior are important processes that need to be examined more fully. In this context, the reference is not to short-term changes as measured by responses to outcome variables in quasi-experimental research designs. This type of change is often temporary, multifaceted, and frequently inexplicable. Studies examining changes in health behavior—regressive or progressive—that are linked to material or structural conditions and racial discrimination would contribute greatly to our understanding of individual behavior (McKinlay, 1975; Williams, 1990). Studies of relapse and regressive health behavior among African-Americans are particularly necessary because of their marginal existence and because of likely fluctuations in socioeconomic status (that is, unemployment and underemployment). One important unanswered question is to what extent acquired health behaviors (smoking cessation, health diets, exercise regimens) are relinquished during times of structural stress (reduced economic productivity, family disruptions, and the like).

There is considerable potential for conflict, overt or subtle, in relations between public health researchers and black communities—especially the urban poor. One source of such conflict is differing perspectives on health as a personal or community priority. In some communities, health competes and sometimes conflicts with other social obligations and priorities, such as economic survival, family roles, and personal preferences. Other sources of conflict are social class, race or ethnicity, religion, folk medicine, culture and language, and community relations with health care institutions.

From a sociological perspective, such conflict may be unavoidable. It is an integral part of the competition for finite resources that characterizes the interaction between majority and minority groups. Researchers and community members or target groups may have different interests, priorities, and motivations for participating in health intervention projects. Many black community residents, organizations and leaders feel that researchers have exploited them—by failing to inform and involve them in key decisions, by taking much but leaving very little, and by misusing study results (Blauner and Wellman, 1973). Moreover, there are compelling historical reasons for such perceptions. The classic example is the Tuskegee Institute syphilis study sponsored by the U.S. Public Health Service (Jones, 1981) of a controlled study of the effects of untreated syphilis on 500 black men in Macon County, Alabama. This incident remains vivid in the collective memories of many-African American communities, and the bitterness it generated may be enduring—especially with regard to the participation of African-Americans in certain public health intervention efforts, such as those aimed at AIDS and cancer.

Intracommunity conflict is exemplified by the previously mentioned ties between the tobacco industry and certain black community organizations and businesses (NAACP, Urban League, United Negro College Fund, the Congressional Black Caucus, *Ebony* and *Essence* magazines), "unhealthy" alliances that conflict with many community efforts to reduce cigarette smoking among blacks (Cooper and Simmons, 1985). Some community organizations, on the other hand, contend that they accept support from the tobacco industry to further "higher priorities" such as racial equality, social justice, and economic opportunities.

These issues are germane to majority-minority relations in American society because they represent different or conflicting perspectives on problems involving unequal social statuses. That is, because of the subordinate group status of African-Americans, civil rights organizations are inclined to view the problem in light of "more pressing" or critical efforts to eliminate racism and bring about fundamental changes in American society. A common assumption underlying this position is that the health status and medical care of black Americans result primarily from basic human rights (social justice and equality). Thus, if such "core dilemmas" or "higher priorities" are addressed, then the health status of blacks will automatically improve.

Civil rights groups argue further that these "higher priorities" will be effective in decreasing cigarette smoking because they will lead to greater upward mobility and economic viability. Improved socioeconomic status, it is assumed, will make people more aware of the negative health effects of smoking and to increase cessation. Another point raised by civil rights organizations is that those who argue against accepting tobacco industry monies offer no substantive options for replacing their support. Were they to refuse it, black communities and the goals for which they are fighting would be the ultimate victims.

Limitations of Health Interventions

Even under the best of circumstances, intervention research and health promotion efforts are often frustrating. Uncontrollable factors influence the success of projects: weather (cold, daylight saving time), bureaucratic red tape, the state of the economy, weak institutional infrastructures, crime, language and cultural barriers, insensitive researchers, and conflicting priorities. Asking racial and ethnic minorities to change health behaviors is often taken to imply inferiority, negativity, and a rejection of their cultural lifestyles and norms. Seldom are they offered positive and relevant alternatives.

Even if these problems were minimized or eliminated, there are still severe limitations regarding how much could be accomplished. In a sobering and perceptive essay on the limits of health promotion, Levin (1987) describes a number of perplexing issues and obstacles confronting health professionals, policy makers, and researchers. His critique, although not focused on African-Americans, is relevant because it address issues related to social structure and diversity. A key point he makes is that health promotion efforts may be inimical to basic American values of individualism. Another is that some communities (notably minorities and the poor) may resist health interventions for fear of losing control. Levin notes that "health promotion itself is not totally reliable" because its messages change. Periodic "health updates" often create considerable confusion about what to believe and how to behave. ("If everything causes cancer, why change one's habits?")

Levin also discusses the shortcomings of approaches that focus on a single disease or risk factor. A single intervention program or health outcome may not reduce morbidity or mortality or improve and extend the life of the poor. This suggests a need to consider multifaceted strategies for dealing with disease or risk factors and to focus on "structural barriers to a health promoting life" (Levin, 1987).

It is suspected that many health promotion programs are pursued in lieu of dealing with racial discrimination, national health care reform, environmental pollutants, drug and food industry exploitation, public policy reform, social justice, education, and employment (Grace, 1991). Until these problems are addressed, black and other poor and disadvantaged populations will continue to have higher morbidity and mortality rates.

As America prepares to enter the twentieth-first century, and as the nation becomes more diverse, Du Bois' prophetic statement about the problem of the color line continues to be accurate, and appears likely to remain so for the foreseeable future. Unequal social status between majority and minority groups, particularly black and white Americans, will continue to permeate all spheres of life. Health is one of many spheres impacted by intergroup relations.

The challenge to the scientific community and to health professionals is to reject obsolete and simplistic intellectual paradigms and empirical methods involving race and health, and to develop new and more powerful tools of analysis. As we have demonstrated, prevailing conceptualizations of race are inadequate and lead to flawed measurement of so-called race effects in health. In addition, the relationship of race to socioeconomic indicators has been obscured and misunderstood because of inadequate conceptualization of both race and socioeconomic status. We have offered a framework for examining the significance of race, in its multiple manifestations in the hope that it will help advance efforts to meet the challenge. We have delineated similar challenges with regard to health intervention and research targeting African-American communities. Improvements in health status, however, will require less innovation and more redirection—specifically, addressing structural determinants of health as opposed to lifestyle factors.

Acknowledgments

We wish to thank Anthony Polednak, Ronald L. Taylor and the participants in the *Authors' Working Conference on Society and Health* for helpful comments on an earlier version of this paper. This research was supported in part by grants NCI-5-PO1CA-42101 from the National

Cancer Institute and AG-07904 from the National Institute of Aging. Please address all correspondence to Gary King, Ph.D., Department of Community Medicine and Health Care, School of Medicine, University of Connecticut Health Center, Farmington, CT 06030-1910.

References

Alexis, M., G. H. Haines, Jr., and L. S. Simon. 1980. *Black Consumer Profiles*. Ann Arbor, MI: Division of Research, Graduate School of Business Administration, University of Michigan.

Anderson, R. M., A. L. Giachello, and L. A. Aday. 1986. Access of Hispanics to health care and cuts in services: A state of the art overview. *Public Health Rep.* 101:238–252.

Baker, P. T. 1967. The biological race concept as a research tool. *J. Physical Anthropol.* 27:21–26.

Baquet, C. R., J. W. Horm, T. Gibbs, and P. Greenwald. 1991. Socioeconomic factors and cancer incidence among blacks and whites. *J. Natl. Cancer Inst.* 83:551–557.

Beardsley, E. H. 1988. *A History of Neglect: Health Care for Blacks and Mill Workers in the Twentieth-Century South*. Knoxville, TN: The University of Tennessee Press.

Belle, D. E. 1982. The impact of poverty on social networks and supports. *Marriage Fam. Rev.* 5:89–103.

Benfari, R., J. Ockene, and K. McIntyre. 1982. Control of cigarette smoking from a psychological perspective. *Annu. Rev. Public Health* 3:101–128.

Bennett, L. 1966. *Before the Mayflower: A History of the Negro in America 1619–1964*. Baltimore: Penguin Books.

Birnbaum, H., and R. Weston. 1974. Home ownership and the wealth position of black and white Americans. *Rev. Income Wealth* 21:103–118.

Blackwell, J. E. 1985. *The Black Community: Diversity and Unity*. New York: Dodd, Mead.

Blau, F. D., and J. W. Graham. 1990. Black-white differences in wealth and asset composition. *Q. J. Eco.* 105:321–339.

Blauner, R. 1972. *Racial Oppression in America*. New York: Harper & Row.

Blauner, R., and D. Wellman. 1973. Toward the decolonization of social research. In J. A. Ladner (ed.), *The Death of White Sociology*, pp. 310–330. New York: Vantage Books.

Blendon, R., L. Aiken, H. Freeman, and C. Corey. 1989. Access to medical care for black and white Americans. *JAMA* 261:278–281.

Brajer, V., and J. V. Hall. 1992. Recent evidence on the distribution of air pollution effects. *Contemp. Policy Issues* 10:63–71.

Bullard, R., and B. H. Wright. 1987. Environmentalism and the politics of equity: Emergent trends in the black community. *Mid-American Rev. Sociology* 12:21–38.

Burkey, R. M. 1978. *Ethnic and Racial Groups: The Dynamics of Dominance*. Menlo Park, CA: Cummings.

Boring, C. C., T. S. Squires, and C. W. Health, Jr. 1992. Cancer statistics for African Americans. *CA Cancer J. Clin.* 42:7–17.

Center for Disease Control. 1994a. Update: Impact of the expanded AIDS surveillance case definition for adolescents and adults on case reporting—United States. *Morbidity and Mortality Weekly Report*, March 11, 1994.

Center for Disease Control. 1994b. *HIV/AIDS Surveillance Report* 6:9–24.

Commission for Racial Justice. 1987. *Toxic Wastes and Race in the United States: A National Report on the Racial and Socioeconomic Characteristics of Communities with Hazardous Waste Sites*. New York: United Church of Christ.

Conway, T., H. Ward, R. Vickers and R. Rahe. 1981. Occupational stress, and variation in cigarette, coffee and alcohol consumption. *J. Health Soc. Behav.* 22:155–165.

Cooper, R. S. 1984. A Note on the biologic concept of race and its application in epidemiologic research. *Am. Heart J.* 108:715–723.

Cooper, R. S., and B. E. Simmons. 1985. Cigarette smoking and ill health among black Americans. *NY State J. Med.* 85:344–349.

Cooper, R. S., and R. David. 1986. The biological concept of race and its application to public health and epidemiology. *J. Health Polit. Policy Law* 11:97–116.

Council on Ethical and Judicial Affairs. 1990. Black-white disparities in health care. *JAMA* 263:2344–2346.

Crews, D. E., and J. R. Bindon. 1991. Ethnicity as a taxonomic category in biomedical and biosocial research. *Ethnicity and Disease* 1:42–49.

Damon, A. 1969. Race, ethnic group, and disease. *Soc. Biol.* 16:69–80.

Davis, D. B. 1966. *The Problem of Slavery in Western Culture.* Ithaca, NY: Cornell University Press.

Davis, F. J. 1991. *Who is Black? One Nation's Definition.* University Park, PA: Pennsylvania State University Press.

de Tocqueville, A. 1835. *Democracy in America.* (Edited by R.D. Heffner and reprinted in 1956.) New York: Mentor Books.

Directive No. 15. 1978. Race and ethnic standards for federal statistics and administrative reporting. *Federal Register* 43:19269–19270.

Dobzhansky, T. 1964. *Heredity and the Nature of Man.* New York: Harcourt, Brace & World.

Dohrenwend, B., and B. Dohrenwend. 1970. Class and race as status-related sources of stress. In S. Levine and N.A. Scotch (eds.), *Social Stress,* pp. 111–140. Chicago: Aldine.

Dressler, W. 1991. Social class, skin color, and arterial blood pressure in two societies. *Ethnicity and Disease* 1:60–71.

Du Bois, W.E.B. 1899. *The Philadelphia Negro: A Social Study.* New York: Schocken Books.

Du Bois, W.E.B. 1903. *The Souls of Black Folks.* Chicago: A.C. McClurg.

Du Bois, W.E.B. 1906. *The Health and Physique of Negro Americans.* Atlanta, GA: Atlanta University Press.

Fortney, N. D. 1977. The anthropological concept of race. *J. Black Studies* 8:35–54.

Franklin, J. H. 1980. *From Slavery to Freedom: A History of Negro Americans,* 5th edn. New York: Alfred A. Knopf.

Frazier, E. F. 1947. Sociological theory and race relations. *Am. Soc. Rev.* 12:265–271.

Frazier, E. F. 1949. Race contacts and the social structure. *Am. Soc. Rev.* 14:1–11.

Frazier, E. F. 1957. *The Black Bourgeoisie.* New York: Free Press.

Freeman, H. P. 1989. Cancer in the socioeconomically disadvantaged. *Cancer* 39:266–288.

Freire, P. 1970. *The Pedagogy of the Oppressed.* New York: The Seabury Press.

Fruchter, R. G., K. Nayeri, J. C. Remy, C. Wright, J. G. Feldman, J. G. Boyce, and W. S. Burnett. 1990. Cervix and breast cancer incidence in immigrant Caribbean women. *Am. J. Public Health* 80:722–724.

Gallup Report. 1985. *Religion in America—50 Years: 1935–1985.* Princeton, NJ: Princeton Religious Research Center.

Garbarino, J., N. Dubrow, K. Kostelny, and C. Pardo. 1992. *Children in Danger: Coping With the Consequences of Community Violence.* San Francisco, CA: Jossey-Bass.

Geronimus, A. T. 1988. On teenage childbearing and infant mortality in the United States. *Popul. Dev. Rev.* 13:246–279.

Geronimus, A .T. 1992. The weathering hypothesis and the health of African-American women and infants: Evidence and speculations. *Ethnicity and Disease* 2:207–221.

Gilkes, C. 1980. The black church as a therapeutic community: Suggested areas for research into the black religious experience. *J. Interdenominational Theological Center* 8:29–44.

Gossett, T. F. 1965. *Race: The History of an Idea in America.* New York: Schocken Books.

Gouldner, A. W. 1970. *The Coming Crisis of Western Sociology.* New York: Basic Books.

Grace, V. M. 1991. The marketing of empowerment and the construction of the health consumer: A critique of health promotion. *Int. J. Health Serv.* 21:329–343.

Green, V. 1978. The black extended family in the United States: Some research suggestions. In D. B. Shimkin, E. M. Shimkin, and D. A. Frate (eds.), *The Extended Family in Black Societies,* pp. 378–387. The Hague: Mouton.

Griffith, E., T. English, and V. Mayfield. 1980. Possession, prayer and testimony: Therapeutic aspects of the Wednesday night meeting in a black church. *Psychiatry* 43:12–128.

Griffith, E., J. Young, and D. Smith. 1984. An analysis of the therapeutic elements in a black church service. *Hosp. Community Psychiatry* 35:464–469.

Griffith, E., and C. Bell. 1989. Recent trends in suicide and homicide among blacks. *JAMA* 262:2265–2269.

Hacker, A. G., R. Collins, and M. Jacobson. 1987. *Marketing Booze to Blacks.* Washington, DC: Center for Science in the Public Interest.

Hahn, R. A. 1992. The state of federal health statistics on racial and ethnic groups. *JAMA* 267:268–271.

Hahn, R. A., J. Mulinare, and S. M. Teutsch. 1992. Inconsistencies in coding of race and ethnicity between birth and death in US infants: A new look at infant mortality, 1983 through 1985. *JAMA* 267:259–263.

Harburg, E., J. Erfurt, C. Chape, L. Havenstein, W. Scholl, and M. A. Schork. 1973a. Socioecological stressor areas and black-white blood pressure: Detroit. *J. Chron. Dis.* 26:595–611.

Harburg, E., J. Erfurt, L. Havenstein, C. Chape, W. Schull, and M. A. Schork. 1973b. Socio-ecological stress, suppressed hostility, skin color, and black-white male blood pressure: Detroit. *Psychosom. Med.* 35:276–296.

Hashfield, G. A., B. S. Alpert, E. S. Willey, G. W. Somes, J. K. Murphy, and L. M. Dupaul. 1989. Race and gender influence ambulatory blood pressure patterns of adolescents. *Am. J. Hypertens.* 14:598–603.

Hill, R. B. 1983. *Comparative Socio-Economic Profiles of Caribbean and Non-Caribbean Blacks in the U.S.* Paper presented at the International Conference on Immigration and the Changing Black Population in the United States, University of Michigan Center for Afro-American and African Studies, Ann Arbor, Michigan, May 18–21.

House, J. S., K. R. Landis, and D. Umberson. 1988. Social relationships and health. *Science* 241:540–545.

Hulse, F. S. 1962. Race as an evolutionary episode. *Am. Anthropol.* 64:929–945.

Hutchinson, J. 1992. AIDS and racism in America. *J. Natl. Med. Assoc.* 84:119–124.

Jackson, J. J. 1981. Urban Black Americans. In A. Hardwood (ed.), *Ethnicity and Medical Care,* pp. 37–129. Cambridge, MA: Harvard University Press.

James, G. D. 1991. Race and perceived stress independently affect the diurnal variation of blood pressure in women. *Am. J. Hypertens.* 4:382–384.

James, S., S. Hartnett, and W. Kalsbeek. 1983. John Henryism and blood pressure differences among black men. *J. Behav. Med.* 6:259–278.

James, S., D. Strogatz, S. Wing, and D. Ramsey. 1987. Socioeconomic status, John Henryism, and hypertension in blacks and whites. *Am. J. Epidemiol.* 126:664–673.

Jaynes, G. D. and R. M. Williams. 1989. *A Common Destiny: Blacks and American Society.* Washington, DC: National Academy Press.

Jones, C. P., T. A. LaVeist, and M. Lillie-Blanton. 1991. Race in the epidemiologic literature: An examination of the American Journal of Epidemiology, 1921–1990. *Am. J. Epidemiol.* 134:1079–1084.

Jones, J. H. 1981. *Bad Blood: The Tuskegee Syphilis Experiment—A Tragedy of Race and Medicine*. New York: Free Press.

Johnson, C. S. 1934. *The Shadow of the Plantation*. Chicago, IL: University of Chicago Press.

Jordan, W. D. 1968. *White Over Black: American Attitudes Toward the Negro, 1550–1812*. Baltimore, MD: Penguin Books.

Kasinitz, P. 1992. *Caribbean New York: Black Immigrants and the Politics of Race*. Ithaca, NY: Cornell University Press.

Keil, J. E., S. E. Sutherland, R. G. Knapp, and H. A. Tyroler. 1992. Does equal socioeconomic status in black and white men mean equal risk of mortality? *Am. J. Public Health* 82:1133–1136.

Keith, V., and C. Herring. 1991. Skin tone and stratification in the black community. *Am. J. Soc.* 97:760–778.

Kessler, R. C., and H. W. Neighbors. 1986. A new perspective on the relationships among race, social class, and psychological distress. *J. Health Soc. Behav.* 27:107–115.

Kessler, R. C., K. A. McGonagle, S. Zhao, C. B. Nelson, M. Hughes, S. Eshleman, H-U. Wittchen, and K.S. Kendler. 1994. Lifetime and 12-month prevalence of *DSM-III-R* psychiatric disorders in the United States. *Arch. Gen. Psychiatry* 51:8–19.

Klag, M. J., P. K. Whelton, J. Coresh, C. E. Grim, and L. H. Kuller. 1991. Association of skin color with blood pressure with low socioeconomic status. *JAMA* 265:599–602.

Kiple, K. F. and V. H. King. 1981. *Another Dimension to the Black Diaspora: Diet, Disease, and Racism*. Cambridge, U.K.: Cambridge University Press.

Kleinman, J. C., L. A. Fingerhut, and K. Prager. 1991. Differences in infant mortality by race, nativity status, and other maternal characteristics. *Am. J. Dis. Child.* 145:194–199.

Krieger, N. 1987. Shades of difference: Theoretical underpinnings of the medical controversy on black/white differences in the United States, 1830–1870. *Int. J. Health Serv.* 17:259–278.

Krieger, N. 1990. Racial and gender discrimination: Risk factors for high blood pressure? *Soc. Sci. Med.* 30:1273–1281.

Kushnick, L. 1988. Racism, the National Health Service, and the health of black people. *Int. J. Health Serv.* 18:457–470.

Landry, B. 1987. *The New Black Middle Class*. Berkeley, CA: University of California Press.

Lasker, G. W., and R. N. Tyzzer. 1982. *Physical Anthropology*. New York: Holt, Rinehart & Winston.

LaVeist, T. A. 1992. The political empowerment and health status of African-Americans: Mapping a new territory. *Am. J. Soc.* 97:1080–1095.

Levin, L. S. 1987. Every silver lining has a cloud: The limits of health promotion. *Soc. Policy* (Summer) 18:57–60.

Levin, M. 1988. The tobacco industry's strange bedfellows. *Bus. Soc. Rev.* 65:11–17.

Lex, B. W. 1987. Review of alcohol problems in ethnic minority groups. *J. Consult. Clin. Psychol.* 55:293–300.

Liberatos, P., B. Link, and J. Kelsey. 1988. The measurement of social class in epidemiology. *Epidemiol. Rev.* 10:87–121.

Lieberson, S. 1985. *Making It Count: The Improvement of Social Research and Theory*. Berkeley, CA: University of California Press.

Light, K., P. Obrist, A. Sherwood, S. James, and D. Stogatz. 1987. Effects of race and marginally elevated blood pressure responses to stress. *J. Hypertens.* 10:555–563.

Marmot, M. G., M. Kogevinas, and M. A. Elston. 1987. Social/economic status and disease. *Annu. Rev. Public Health* 8:111–135.

McBride, D. 1989. *Integrating the City of Medicine: Blacks in Philadelphia Health Care, 1910–1965*. Philadelphia: Temple University Press.

McCord, C., and H. P. Freeman 1990. Excess mortality in Harlem. *N. Engl. J. Med.* 322:173–177.

McCormick, M. 1985. The contribution of low birth weight to infant mortality and childhood morbidity. *N. Engl. J. Med.* 312:82–90.

McKinlay, J. B., and S. J. McKinlay. 1977. The questionable contribution of medical measures to the decline of mortality in the United States in the twentieth century. *Milbank Q.* 55:405–428.

Mills, C. W. 1959. *The Sociological Imagination.* New York: Oxford University Press.

Montagu, A. 1964. *The Concept of Race.* Toronto: Collier-Macmillan.

Murdock, G. P. 1965. *Culture and Society.* Pittsburgh: University of Pittsburgh Press.

Murphy, M. B., K. S. Nelson, and W. J. Elliott. 1988. Racial differences in diurnal blood pressure profile. *Am. J. Hypertens.* 12:55A.

Myrdal, G. 1944. *An American Dilemma.* New York: Harper.

National Center for Health Statistics. 1991. *Vital Statistics of the United States, 1988, Vol. 2., Mortality, Part A.* Washington, D.C.: U.S. Public Health Service.

National Center for Health Statistics. 1991. *Health, United States: 1990.* Hyattsville, MD: U.S. Public Health Service.

Navarro, V. 1989. Race or class, or race and class. *Int. J. Health Serv.* 19:311–314.

Navarro, V. 1991. Race or class or race and class: Growing mortality differentials in the United States. *Int. J. Health Serv.* 21:229–235.

Osborne, N. G., and M. D. Feit. 1992. The use of race in medical research. *JAMA* 267:275–279.

Parcel, T. 1982. Wealth accumulation of black and white men: The case of housing equity. *Soc. Problems* 30:199–211.

Park, R. E. 1913. Racial assimilation in secondary groups. *Publication of the American Sociological Society* 8:75–82.

Polednak, A. P. 1989. *Racial and Ethnic Differences in Disease.* New York: Oxford University Press.

Pol, L. G., R. F. Guy, and A. J. Bush. 1982. Discrimination in the home lending market: A macro perspective. *Soc. Sci. Q.* 63:716–728.

Rabow, J., and R. Watt. 1984. Alcohol availability, alcohol beverage sales, and alcohol related problems. *J. Stud. Alcohol* 43:767–801.

Rice, D. P. 1991. Ethics and equity in U.S. health care: The data. *Int. J. Health Serv.* 21:637–651.

Rice, M., and M. Winn. 1990. Black health care in America: A political perspective. *J. Natl. Med. Assoc.* 82:429–437.

Robins, L., and D. Regier (eds.). 1991. *Psychiatric Disorders in America: Epidemiologic Catchment Area Study.* New York: Free Press.

Robinson, J. 1984. Racial inequality and the probability of occupation-related injury or illness. *Milbank Q.* 62:567–590.

Robinson, R., and J. Kelly. 1979. Class as conceived by Marx and Dahrendorf: Efforts on income inequality and politics in the United States and Great Britain. *Am. Soc. Rev.* 44:38–58.

Rook, K. S. 1984. The negative side of social interaction: Impact on psychological well-being. *J. Pers. Soc. Psychol.* 46:1097–1108.

Russo, R. M., R. Patel, T. A. Laude, S. V. Rajkumar, and V. J. Gururaj. 1981. Infant feeding practices by ethno-cultural grouping. *J. Medi. Soci. NJ* 78:737–740.

Savitt, T. L. 1978. *Medicine and Slavery: The Diseases and Health Care of Blacks in Antebellum Virginia.* Urbana, IL: University of Illinois Press.

Schoendorf, K .C., C.J.R. Hogue, J .C. Kleinman, and D. Rowley. 1992. Mortality among infants of black as compared with white college-educated parents. *N. Engl. J. Med.* 326:1522–1526.

Short, P. F., L .J. Cornelius, and D. E. Goldstone. 1990. Health insurance of minorities in the United States. *J. Health Care Poor Underserved* 1:9–24.

Silberman, C. E. 1964. *Crisis in Black and White*. New York: Random House.

Singer, M. 1986. Toward a political economy of alcoholism. *Soc. Sci. Med.* 23:113–130.

Snow, L. F. 1978. Sorcerers, saints and charlatans: Black folk healers in urban America. *Cult. Med. Psychiatry* 2:69–106.

Spector, R. E. 1979. *Cultural Diversity in Health and Illness*. New York: Appleton-Century-Crofts.

Stack, C. B. 1975. *All Our Kin: Strategies for Survival in a Black Community*. New York: Harper & Row.

Stampp, K. M. 1956. *The Peculiar Institution: Slavery in the Ante-Bellum South*. New York: Random House.

Stark, E. 1982. Doctors in spite of themselves: The limits of radical health criticism. *Int. J. Health Serv.* 12:419–457.

Strogatz, D. S., and S. A. James. 1986. Social support and hypertension among blacks and whites in a rural, southern community. *Am. J. Epidemiol.* 124:949–956.

Sterling, T. H., and J. J. Weinkam. 1989. Comparison of smoking-related risk factors among black and white males. *Am. J. Ind. Med.* 15:319–333.

Sullivan, L. W. 1991. Effects of Discrimination and Racism on Access to Health Care. *JAMA* 266:2674.

Taylor, R. J., and L. M. Chatters. 1988. Church members as a source of informal social support. *Rev. Religious Res.* 30:193–203.

Torchia, M. M. 1975. The tuberculosis movement and the race question, 1890–1950. *Bull. Hist. Med.* 49:152–168.

Ulbrich, P., G. Warheit, and R. Zimmerman. 1989. Race, socioeconomic status, psychological stress: An examination of differential vulnerability. *J. Health Soc. Behav.* 30:131–146.

U.S. Department of Health and Human Services. 1985. *Report of the Secretary's Task Force on Black and Minority Health*. Washington, DC: United States Government Printing Office.

U.S. Department of Health and Human Services. 1986. *Cancer Among Blacks and Other Minorities: Statistical Profiles*. NIH Publication No. 86-2785. Washington, DC.:

U.S. Department of Health and Human Services. 1991. *Health Status of Minorities and Low-Income Groups: 3rd edn*. 1991. Washington, DC: Government Printing Office.

van den Berghe, P. L. 1967. *Race and Racism: A Comparative Perspective*. New York: Wiley.

Vander Zanden, J. W. 1972. *American Minority Relations*. New York: Ronald Press.

Wallerstein, N., and E. Bernstein. 1988. Empowerment education: Freire's ideas adapted to health education. *Health Ed. Q.* 15:379–394.

Weissert, W. G., and C. M. Cready. 1988. Determinants of hospital-to-nursing home placement delays: A pilot study. *Health Serv. Res.* 23:619–647.

Weissman, A. 1990. Race-ethnicity: A dubious scientific concept. *Public Health Rep.* 105:102–103.

Wenneker, M. B., and A. M. Epstein. 1989. Racial inequalities in the use of procedures for patients with ischemic heart disease in Massachusetts. *JAMA* 261:253–257.

Wilkinson, D. and G. King. 1987. Conceptual and methodological issues in the use of race as a variable: Policy implications. *Milbank Q.* (Suppl. 1) 65:56–71.

Williams, D. R. 1990. Socioeconomic differentials in health: A review and redirection. *Soc. Psychol. Q.* 53:81–99.

Williams, D. R. 1992. Social structure and the health behavior of blacks. In K. W. Schaie, J. S. House, and D. Blazer (eds.), *Health Behaviors and Health Outcomes*, pp. 59–64. Hillsdale, NJ: Erlbaum.

Williams, D. R. 1992. Black-white differences in blood pressure: The role of social factors. *Ethnicity and Disease* 2:126–141.

Williams, D. R., D. T. Takeuchi, and R. K. Adair. 1992a. Marital status and psychiatric disorders among blacks and whites. *J. Health Soc. Beha.* 33:140–157.

Williams, D. R., D. T. Takeuchi, and R. K. Adair. 1992b. Socioeconomic status and psychiatric disorder among blacks and whites. *Social Forces* 71:179–194.

Wilson, W. 1980. *The Declining Significance of Race: Blacks and Changing American Institutions*. Chicago: University of Chicago Press.

Wilson, W. 1987. *The Truly Disadvantaged*. Chicago: University of Chicago Press.

Wirth, L. 1945. The problem of minority groups. In Ralph Linton, (ed.), *The Science of Man in the World Crisis*. New York: Columbia University Press.

Wright, E., and L. Perrone. 1977. Marxist class categories and income inequality. *Am. Sociol. Rev.* 42:32–55.

Zola, I. K. 1966. Culture and symptoms—an analysis of patients presenting complaints. *Am. Sociol. Rev.* 31:615–630.

5

Gender, Health, and Cigarette Smoking

DIANA CHAPMAN WALSH, GLORIAN SORENSEN, and LORI LEONARD

The purpose of this book is to look at the ways in which social structures and social processes affect health and the quality of life. We are not asking whether society itself produces preventable risks to health—we know that it does—but more searchingly, we are asking how those risks are generated and felt. The social factor that this chapter examines is gender. Gender offers especially rich material for probing relationships between society and health because it is both a basic biological distinction (labeled *sex*) and a fundamentally social one (labeled *gender*); both of these are deeply enmeshed in historical and political matrices that are clear creations of human agency.

Gender illuminates how potent and obdurate social structure can be. In every known society, whether one emerges as a boy or a girl says as much about one's future options and prospects as does any accident of location at birth. But gender relations also remind us that social structures, even those that originate in the genome, reflect choices that ordinary humans are making, and could be making differently. Announcing the newborn infant's sex to herald its arrival is the first in a series of choices (however unconscious and ritualistic) that transform biology into social destiny.

A Distinctive Lens: Society and Health

We propose to examine whether and how a society-and-health lens brings a distinctive focus to the complex relationships between gender and health. As Hall (1992) suggests, investigations of health can ignore gender, control for gender, or analyze for gender. In the past, most investigators have adopted one of the first two strategies; we opt for and will enlarge on the third. We will seek not only to analyze a health problem "for gender," but to do so in an effort to understand gender as an organizing social force. This means considering gender both as an independent variable that may affect health and as a phenomenon that itself requires explication and analysis.

Analyzing for gender can uncover stereotype and bias. As one example, finely grained studies of depression following widowhood have challenged the assumption that vulnerability to a specific life event varies by sex. New research suggests that loss of a spouse is not the same event for men and for women; the practical impact is different, as is the pathway to mental distress. The strains of household management are the principal mechanism linking depression to widowhood for men, whereas for women the pathway runs through financial strain (Umberson et al., 1992).

Analysis of health outcomes for the effect of gender will, we contend, spotlight unstated assumptions, illuminate large gaps in knowledge, and expand prevailing models of the antecedents and correlates of health. It will also raise new questions about the health-care system and the social construction of knowledge about the health of women and men. The overwhelming emphasis to date when comparing men and women, or considering individuals, assumes static "sex roles" and obscures deeper and more generic, but potentially modifiable, social structures and social processes that compromise health and quality of life for women and men in positions of relative disadvantage.

Our point of departure is a brief survey of research traditions in gender and health. We will identify the questions that have produced the dominant research paradigms, and summarize that research with an eye to whether, and if so how, the underlying models or assumptions are limiting. We will then sketch the contours of a broader, structurally oriented model of gender and society. Next we will use this broader model to reframe questions about associations between gender and one very salient health risk: cigarette smoking. Finally, we will spell out the implications of our analysis for understanding and for research.

Prevailing Research Traditions in Gender and Health

Scholarly and empirical writings on gender and health often begin with or assume two well-established facts that have been fully described, and partially explained, in the literature (Verbrugge 1985a; Waldron 1982, 1983b; Wingard 1984). The first is that women live longer than men, and enjoy a striking mortality advantage at every point along the life span. American women average 7 extra years of life compared to men (male life expectancy at birth is 72.0 years, versus 78.8 years for females; U.S. Bureau of the Census, 1992).

During the first year of life almost one third more male than female infants die, and, by age 75 women outnumber men by nearly a factor of two (Waldron 1976, 1982, 1983a). This pattern holds across racial and socioeconomic lines (black women live longer than black men and longer than white men) and in virtually every industrialized country. Finnish women enjoy the largest advantage over their countrymen and Greek women the smallest (Verbrugge, 1985a).

The second, apparently contradictory, fact is that women are "sicker" than men. They report more illness and mental distress, are less likely to rate themselves in excellent health, are more frequently disabled or confined to bed (they report about 25 percent more days of restricted activities and some 40 percent more days in bed), and use more medical care (twice as much between the ages of 17 and 44) and more prescription drugs, especially psychoactive medications. Even when all aspects of reproductive health are controlled for in careful analyses, women have acute illness rates roughly 20–30 percent higher than men's. Only in the case of injuries do men have substantially higher rates (Verbrugge, 1985a).

A third, more recent trend further complicates the picture: in the past two decades, sex differences in morbidity and mortality have begun to change. From the early 1900s until about 1970, excess male mortality increased steadily. As risks of death declined for both sexes, women gained more than men. But starting around 1970 the picture began to shift.

First, women stopped gaining ground on men. Between 1977 and 1980 the male/female ratio for age-adjusted mortality stabilized at about 1.8 (Verbrugge, 1985a). Then the trend actually began to reverse, as men's longevity continued to advance while women's stagnated. By 1985 the sex-mortality ratio rate had dropped to 1.75 (Verbrugge 1989). Changing smoking patterns—the focus of this case study—are widely believed to be the prime underlying reason for the recent trend (Waldron 1976, 1982, 1986).

Thus the driving interest behind research on gender and health has been to shed light on these two seemingly contradictory observations—that women appear healthier than men in terms of mortality but sicker in terms of morbidity—and to assess to what extent, and why, recent social trends may be causing these patterns to change. One motivating force behind these questions is the longstanding belief that a better understanding of the differential mortality and morbidity experiences of the two sexes might unearth new gender-specific risk factors that could be prevented. That question becomes especially salient in periods of rapid change in gender roles and relationships, as in the current entrance of women into the labor force in unprecedented numbers and roles.

In fact, writings on gender and health have often implicitly assumed that "the liberation of women"—improvement of their social and economic standing vis-à-vis men—will somehow deprive them of whatever it was that shielded them against earlier death. The historical image of women as the weaker sex, in need of extra protection against the brutalities of worldly life, and the related view of disease as a consequence for women who deviate from cultural norms, have been axiomatic in Western culture. Much of the fascination with gender differences in health, then, either emanates from or struggles to debunk deep-seated prejudice about women's limited native capacities and circumscribed "natural" roles.

Epidemiological Studies of Sex Differentials in Health: Biology or Society?

In 1938, Dorothy Wiehl, a demographer, made the case that the encouraging progress in overall mortality in the United States (1920–1935) was masking important inequalities, notably growing excess mortality among males. Drawing on aggregate mortality data from 24 state death registries, broken down by age and by calendar periods but not by cause of death, she demonstrated that from 1920 to 1935 excess mortality for males jumped from 6 percent to 24 percent. Wiehl offered no speculation about the reasons for the trend, but did recommend a medical specialty to care for men, comparable to the practice of gynecology for women (Wiehl, 1938). These findings were updated and confirmed in a 1943 paper (Yerushalmy, 1943), and again in a 1950 study showing that the gap had widened continuously from 1900 to 1945 (Bowerman, 1950).

Madigan extended the analysis in a 1957 study showing that from 1900 to 1950 the mortality advantage of white females over white males had doubled from 2.85 to 5.80. He questioned whether these growing sex-mortality differentials were biologically ordained or "chiefly reflections of the greater sociocultural pressures and strains which our culture lays upon male shoulders." In his framing of the problem, Madigan laid the substrate for a research agenda directed at improving the health of men. If the differences were a function of social pressures, he asserted, short of a "profound cultural revolution" not much could be done. But if the male mortality disadvantage had biological origins (as his analysis of the comparative mortality rates of priests and nuns seemed to indicate), "medical research can isolate the factors responsible for greater female viability, and use this knowledge to advantage in the treatment of middle-aged and old men" (Madigan, 1957, p. 203). The (untested) assumption in Madigan's work that biologically targeted interventions are more feasible than targeting social arrangements has been a longstanding justification for biologically reductionist research.

Enterline's 1961 epidemiological analysis began to break down the problem by major disease entities, and challenged the emerging consensus around a biological explanation of women's mortality advantage. He showed that divergence in mortality rates by sex had begun around 1922 and continued fairly steadily thereafter. By calculating the relative contribution of selected causes of death in given age cohorts, he was able to trace the widening sex-mortality difference to improvement in conditions that especially affected women (tuberculosis, maternal mortality, uterine cancer, and hypertension-related diseases) and increases in male death rates from motor vehicle accidents, lung cancer, and coronary heart disease. From these findings, Enterline drew the crucial inference that "environmental factors" were more important than biological ones (Enterline, 1961).

Thereafter the corpus of epidemiological work seeking to explain gender differences in health expanded rapidly. The simple dichotomy between biology and society yielded to more complex classification schemes, which Verbrugge has systematized in a remarkable series of papers (Verbrugge 1976a, 1976b, 1978, 1979, 1980a, 1980b,

1982a, 1982b, 1983a, 1983b, 1985a, 1985b, 1986, 1988, 1989; Verbrugge and Madans 1985; Verbrugge and Wingard, 1987). She organized the many hypotheses advanced to explain sex differences in health into five broad categories, ranked in descending order of apparent overall contribution to sex differences in health: (1) risks acquired through roles, stresses, lifestyles, and long-term preventive health practices; (2) illness experiences and behaviors that stimulate awareness of symptoms and health-oriented action; (3) exposure to prior health care, through its influence on a lifetime of acquired risk, health behavior, and health; (4) biological factors, especially those related to reproduction and health conditions specifically related to the sex organs; and (5) reporting artifacts, which have a small effect.

Summarizing the evidence, Verbrugge advanced four hypotheses. First, men have higher incidence and prevalence rates of serious morbidity as a function of both biological and acquired risks. For reasons that are less clear, women have higher rates of most nonfatal chronic conditions and acute time-limited illness, and more health problems in any time frame—daily, yearly, and lifetime. This distinction, she pointed out, explains the apparent paradox of longer life for women but better health for men: men have higher rates of fatal illness.

Second, women are more attentive to their bodies, more aware of symptoms, more inclined to assess them as serious, and quicker to yield to them for longer convalescence periods. The effects of help-seeking and sick-role propensities pertain mainly to minor health problems; major illness mutes the effect of gender.

Third, men and women differ little in their recall ability and motivation to report major health problems, although women are fuller reporters of minor ailments and of emotional content. Proxy reporting by women respondents to household surveys probably does produce a little underestimation of men's health problems. Fourth, women do seek more medical care, which may diminish the severity of conditions they develop and therefore help extend their lives. In future studies of these and other hypotheses, Verbrugge concluded, we need sturdier "theoretical banisters" (1985a).

Theoretical Underpinnings of Research on Gender and Health

The theoretical perspective that has dominated discourse to date is social-role theory. Social roles, variously defined, have been explored as mechanisms through which men and women acquire differential risks that produce distinctive health outcomes. Social roles have also been examined as sources of gender-specific perceptions of illness, resistance resources, and coping styles, and of gender-tinctured responses from medical-care providers. Role theory takes largely for granted the underlying social stratification processes that sort people into categorical and static roles. It tends, therefore, to reify and reinforce roles, rather than exposing them as negotiated and malleable. Asymmetries of power are seldom the overt focus of studies anchored in role theory.

An early and influential application of social-role theory to explain gender disparities in health appeared in the sociological literature in 1973 (Gove, 1973), and stimulated a trend in empirical work that harkened back to Durkheim. In an analysis of 1970 national health survey data on white adults, Walter Gove (1973) adduced evidence that marriage was protective against death for both men and women, but far more so for men. He saw this variation as most pronounced in conditions for which mortality might plausibly be mediated by psychological states of mind, either directly (as in suicide, homicide, and accidents), or indirectly through a risk behavior (such as alcohol abuse) or a help-seeking behavior (such as submitting to prolonged treatment for tuberculosis or diabetes). He examined and rejected selection and economic arguments, and concluded that his findings were best understood in terms of the nature of marital roles (Gove, 1973).

Four distinct lines of work on gender and health subsequently developed, each revolving more or less loosely around some notion of a social role:

1. One very active strand of research explored the impact of women's "role density" (LaRosa, 1988) or *multiple-role occupancy* (wife, mother, worker) as a potential generator of both stress and strength.
2. A subset of research on role occupancy focused on the *role of worker*, and investigated whether women's and men's labor-force participation and differential work experience was a particular source of risk and/or reward.
3. A very substantial social-psychological literature pursued the internalization of *feminine and masculine roles*, how such roles affect stress and coping, the resources and repertoires men and women summon in times of duress or illness, and the implications for health and mental health.
4. A line of thought strongly rooted in feminist theory found its strongest expression in political organizing for women's health. It emphasized sexual politics in *caretaking roles*, with an accent on power relationships, both within the health and medical professions and more broadly in medical/social control of deviance.

What follows is an encapsulation of those four large bodies of work, drawing on review articles whenever available. Our object is to set the stage—to gather analytic props that may prove useful—for sketching a more complete picture of how gender dynamics cut across health and health care, and how gender structures produce particular understandings about health.

The Multiple-Role Literature

Reviewing the literature on gender disparities in health through the mid-1970s, Nathanson (1975) was surprised that sociologists had paid little attention to what then seemed an intriguing contradiction in women's mortality advantage and morbidity disadvantage. She identified three broad explanatory models to account for sex differences in illness experience, all involving role theory: (1) reporting illness is more acceptable for women, in that the feminine role applies a less "adult" standard of health;

(2) assuming the sick role is more feasible for women, in that they have more flexible roles, more fluid schedules, fewer time demands; and (3) living is more stressful for women, in that they suffer from special strains inherent in their biological and social roles. The literature seemed to be moving toward the third model—that is toward a theory of the feminine role, specifically the role of wife, as uniquely frustrating and confining.

When men and women were compared, Nathanson found the evidence for all three models skimpy and contradictory. But when the three models were held to a different test—how well they explained gradations of illness experience *among* women—only the second model (compatibility between the feminine role and the sick role) seemed to find a modicum of empirical support. Among all women, relatively lower levels of morbidity were reported by those who were married (unless unhappily), employed, and/or mothers of preschool children, a finding that suggested that demanding role obligations deterred or distracted them from assuming the sick role. In a more recent study examining time use, however, Bird and Fremont (1991) present evidence contradicting the notion that women's schedules are more elastic than men's: such work presses investigators of multiple roles to measure the actual demands of particular roles.

On the question of multiple roles, a variety of studies have implicitly or explicitly tested a "scarcity hypothesis" (more roles produce more demands on scarce personal resources) versus an "expansion hypothesis" (more roles produce expanded horizons and greater actualization) (Froberg et al., 1986). This line of research has tended to confirm that in both sexes better health prospects accompany employment, marriage, and parenthood (in that order, with respect to both the strength of the association and the consistency of the evidence). In many studies the causal dynamics are circular, and in most they are clouded by the respondent's expectations. Still, the evidence does suggest that married workers are healthier than people who function in only one of the two roles (spouse/worker). Single working mothers report more illness than single working nonmothers, but parenthood seems not to affect the health status of married working women (Verbrugge, 1985a). There is some evidence too that the quality of the role matters; for instance, divorced women seem to be healthier than those who remain unhappily married (Wingard, 1984). Recent research attempts to measure the effect of qualitative differences in the experience of various roles.

Occupying multiple roles is thought to increase women's opportunities to learn; to develop self-efficacy and self-esteem; to build social networks and gain access to informational, instrumental, and emotional support; and to buffer life's stresses and strains. Rodin and Ickovics (1990) suggest one possible link between multiple roles and enhanced health: a more diversified self-concept should provide "cognitive cushioning" and alternative sources of self-esteem and gratification when things go poorly in one life domain (Rodin and Ickovics, 1990). Sorensen and Verbrugge (1987) observe that the various configurations in the "role-expansion model" may be additive or interactive, but note that the evidence is "surprisingly slim."

Social support may figure more prominently (or just differently) in the stress process for women than for men, and may be a two-edged sword for at least some women in some circumstances (Gove and Hughes, 1979; Gore 1989). The causal pathways have yet to be fully mapped, and selection factors have seldom been adequately controlled. Still, multiple roles do seem to have additive positive effects, and concern that the combination of employment, marriage, and motherhood might threaten women's health seems to have been convincingly laid to rest for now (Froberg, 1986; La Croix and Haynes, 1987). Rodin cautions, however, that all these findings are culture- and cohort-bound, and that it may be too soon to see the negative health effects of multiple roles until the "baby-boom generation" reaches old age (Rodin and Ickovics, 1990).

In the meantime, investigators are questioning whether categorical measures of social role (father, worker, husband) capture a meaningful reality without further specification of the conditions, contexts, burdens, and demands of such roles; and the attitudes, expectations, and satisfactions of individual role incumbents (Hall, 1992; Froberg, 1986; Waldron et al., 1982). Bird and Fremont (1991) fault previous studies for using "crude and indirect measures" of role pressures. They use a 1981 data set on time-use to model the effects of role demands, measured in hours per week, on self-rated health. Employing this operational definition of social role reverses the apparent effects of gender on health, suggesting that the male morbidity advantage may be largely a function of gender differences in the actual time demands of social roles. This finding is consistent with Verbrugge's 1989 study, using categorical definitions of social roles (1989). Both economic and health benefits accrue to men by virtue of more advanced education, higher wages, and more time spent in paid work and less in housework and child care. Were gender roles to be equalized along these dimensions, Bird and Fremont speculate, women would not only outlive men, they would enjoy better health along the way.

The Work Role, Gender and Health

Sorensen and Verbrugge (1987) identify three competing perspectives as having been advanced to explain how working may affect women's health. The role-expansion model places work in a broader context, whereas the other two models address the job itself as potentially harmful (the "job-stress model"), or protective (the "health-benefits model").

The possibility that exposure to harmful work might explain differential health outcomes for men and women has been taken seriously since such differences were first noticed. It was initially assumed that the male's shorter life span must be a function of his heavier burdens as economic provider. This belief prompted the prediction that women would lose their mortality advantage as they entered the workforce and assumed demanding jobs.

As evidence undermining this prediction began to accumulate (LaCroix and Haynes, 1987), a fall-back assumption was voiced that women's jobs must be inherently safer (Barnett et al., 1987, p. 1). This is partly true. Men do experience greater exposure to occupational hazards, including carcinogens, and their job accident rates are considerably higher. Waldron estimates that these factors jointly account for about 5.1 percent of excess male mortality in the United States (Waldron, 1991).

In fact, as Barnett et al. (1987) and Hall (1991) have argued, a longstanding male bias in stress research has depicted the workplace as inherently stressful and home as a sanctuary. But some newer studies suggest that women may be more susceptible to stress emanating from the family than from work, while the opposite may be true for men. For women the workplace may be a haven in which "the balance of psychological demands and control is more favorable than at home" (Barnett et al., 1987), a possibility that remains to be demonstrated convincingly.

Another possibility awaiting empirical confirmation is that women's work may be concentrated in the low-control/high-demand quadrant of the job-strain model that Karasek and colleagues (see Karasek and Theorell, 1990) have used to predict cardiovascular risk. There is limited evidence that from a job strain perspective, women's work may on average be more hazardous than men's (Hall, 1991). This may prove to be the critical dimension if Syme (1991) is correct that psychosocial job stressors have a greater health impact than physical ones in modern postindustrial society.

Hall (1991) emphasizes, however, how little we know about characteristics of women's jobs or the impact of work on women's health. The U.S. labor force is nearly half (45.4 percent) female, but it remains strikingly segregated by sex. The potential hazards of female-dominated occupations have scarcely been noticed and are probably underappreciated (Klitzman et al., 1990). "Women's jobs" are typically less differentiated than "men's jobs," which means that more occupations are dominated by men than by women. The relative homogeneity of women's employment offers some obvious targets for research but makes it harder to study how work affects women's health across a wide spectrum of exposures (Moser et al., 1988).

Investigations of occupational hazards have typically emphasized high-profile toxic materials, such as asbestos and coal dust, in male-dominated industries. The male has thus become the *de facto* model for assessing work-related health risks, without recognition that responses could differ in women. Although the small numbers of women employed in heavy industry make it difficult to determine the risks associated with their employment in "men's jobs," it cannot safely be assumed that models of exposure derived from studies of men necessarily apply to women (Moser et al., 1988).

Women's patterns of employment also differ from men's by virtue of the multiple roles they play at home and on the job. These demands have forced many women to work part-time, to move in and out of the labor force, and to take jobs unrelated to their training or skills. Ascertainment of occupational exposures is more difficult among workers in less stable and less predictable jobs, a pattern more common among women than men (Bond et al., 1987). Furthermore, available information on risks associated with women's occupational exposures is limited by the types of questions typically asked. For example, death certificates in Great Britain list the husband's employment but not the wife's, unless she was employed full-time when she died (Moser et al., 1988).

Thus, occupational sex segregation complicates research on the health effects of women's work. More important, there has been persistent sex bias in the basic premises that govern choices of outcome variables and study designs. With very few notable exceptions, Hall (1991) points out, occupational health studies linking job strain to physical health outcomes, especially cardiovascular mortality and morbidity, have been employed on male samples, establishing men's experiences as the implicit "gold standard." Studies of women and work, by contrast, have tended to look backward from mental distress, as Aneshensel and Pearlin (1987) observe, seeking psychological insight into the question of why women report more distress than men.

Hall (1991) argues that the literature is fundamentally skewed, because studies of women workers overlook structure and dwell on contextual and emotional issues while studies of men tend to do just the reverse. The result of this pervasive bias in the way questions are framed is that "available evidence" on the physical health impacts of work is almost completely limited to men (Hall, 1991). The literature is still haunted by the theoretical ghosts of Dorothy Wiehl (1938) and her successors, who set the agenda as a quest for explanations of women's longevity advantage despite their apparently heavier emotional burdens.

Internalized Roles and Responses to Stress and Illness

Gender differences in psychological distress have been extensively studied over the years (Cleary, 1987; Barnett et al., 1987). It is now well established that women experience more depression, demoralization, unhappiness, and general dissatisfaction with life, although the social construction and medicalization of women's psychic distress has also been exposed (Chesser, 1972). Women's greater dissatisfaction has often been said to reflect the more limited and frustrating range of their social roles—the boredom, undervaluation, social isolation, and lack of challenge of the homemaker role, and the role conflict and insufficient support accorded working mothers who come home each night to work the "second shift" (Hochschild, 1989). In addition, it is felt, women's orientation toward nurturing may prompt them to do "emotional work" (Hochschild, 1989) for others, without reciprocation or compensation (Gore, 1989).

The frequent assertion that women's coping styles are less damaging to their long-term health than men's is unsubstantiated, in part because the physiological mechanisms linking stress and illness are still imperfectly understood. It is true that women's informal social networks tend to be larger, and their ties more intimate and active, than men's. Mounting evidence from longitudinal research showing that social ties extend health and longevity (Berkman, 1984; Gore, 1989) suggests that women's mortality advantage may be accounted for in part by their closer social ties. Caring is, however, not without costs; its psychic and physical demands can seem incessant (Wetherington et al., 1987).

Rodin posits that social support and a sense of control are the key psychosocial mechanisms that mediate stressors and stress responses differently for women and men. She cites mounting evidence that lack of control has a direct psychobiological effect on cardiovascular disease (probably through elevated stress hormones, particularly catecholamines and cortisol) and on tumor growth and proliferation (perhaps through vascular flow, steroids, and prolactin) (Rodin and Ickovics, 1990). These interesting hypotheses about the conduits linking psychological inputs to physiological outputs have generally not been accompanied by equally imaginative research into the conduits at the macrosocial end of the continuum.

Caretaking Roles, Sexual Politics, Power, and Health

In a genre far removed from epidemiological investigations of relative risk, important conceptual groundwork was being laid for an analysis of gender and health that does begin at the social and cultural end of the continuum. Strikingly different in form and substance from the literature reviewed so far, this work makes a useful bridge from an epidemiological to a social-structural perspective on women's health. Like the three bodies of work on gender and health we have already examined, it too takes off from an analysis of sex-typed social roles. The difference is that this line of inquiry challenges the underlying assumptions about what constitute natural roles.

In a pair of widely circulated pamphlets published in the early 1970s, just as contemporary feminism was awakening, Ehrenreich and English (1973) articulated some radical ideas about women and health that have powerfully influenced the women's-health movement. The Industrial Revolution in nineteenth-century America, they argued, generated a dual ideology of sexism to justify two very different divisions of labor.

Upper-class women, who were needed to function as a "client caste" for the growing (male) medical profession, were seen as frail and delicate, perpetually ill and inherently sick. Working-class women, whose labor the economy required, were viewed as the obverse—inherently healthy and robust, except when, through their own sloth and ignorance, they contracted and became carriers of infectious disease. These two social constructions, Ehrenreich and English pointed out, embodied "two ancient strands of sexist ideology: contempt for women as weak and defective, and fear of women as dangerous and polluting" (1973, p. 14). Both held women in a position of subservience to men, limiting their social and economic mobility and power.

Other than indirectly, attention to such questions of socioeconomic power has been implicit or absent in most epidemiological research on social roles and acquired health risks and/or vulnerability to stress. But power is the central focus of the active efforts to organize around women's health issues that have accompanied the rebirth of feminism, notably the women's health movement and ongoing struggles for control of conception, childbirth, research protocols, and priorities. Activist movements have stretched the seams of conventional thinking and scholarship on gender issues in health.

In the late 1960s, through consciousness-raising groups, white middle-class women began to develop a fundamental critique of medicine, focusing initially on indignities, insensitivities, and irrationalities of gynecological, reproductive health, and maternity services designed and dominated by men. *Our Bodies, Ourselves*, first published by the Boston Women's Health Book Collective in 1971, has sold over 3 million copies in more than 12 languages. A women's self-help movement that began in California in 1971 spread across the country and beyond; while outrage over the inadequacies of contraceptive research gave rise to national organizations emphasizing consumer protection.

Some of these groups joined in broader and more radical efforts to organize community health centers, free clinics, worker health groups, and to provide access to affordable primary care and reproductive health services. As the rising conservative tide rendered the politics of abortion progressively more incendiary and antiestablishment, however, it became clear that more inclusive coalitions would be needed to secure basic "reproductive rights." The difficulties of forming such coalitions made it abundantly clear that women's interests were less uniform than they may have seemed in the early days of consciousness raising among homogeneous affinity groups.

Organizing for freedom of choice required finding common ground shared by establishment women and working-class, minority, and poor women, whose priorities were bread-and-butter issues like welfare rights, day care, entry-level jobs in the health-care system, and an end to sterilization abuse (Rodriguez-Trias, 1984). These agendas broadened the concerns that had initially animated the women's health movement— concerns for greater responsiveness to women's perspectives, less medical control of women and less male domination of medicine, a reconciliation of the private and public worlds, and a recognition of how the body shapes identity (Zola, 1991).

Throughout the 1980s politicized women struggled to find a common voice across lines of race, ethnicity, class, and privilege, and to develop a shared vision of a more responsive, healthier, and safer society. Animating this movement was what Adrienne Rich, the feminist poet and essayist, has characterized as "the consciousness of self as Other which Simone de Beauvoir has described . . . [the knowledge that makes women] potentially the deepest of all questioners of the social order created by men" (Gelpi, 1975). From such questioning has evolved feminist thinking on gender and power that stands in opposition to orthodox epidemiological models of gender and health.

Gender, Society and Power

R. W. Connell (1987), an Australian sociologist, has proposed a "large synthesis" of the literature on gender and power, beginning with "the nature of social reality itself" and exploring unspoken premises about what is biological or natural and what is social. Asserting that much previous work on gender falls into the trap of viewing the biological as somehow more real than the social, Connell has channeled his efforts into the elaboration of a *social* theory. His synthesis is thus especially valuable for understanding gender and health, since it is all too easy to fall back on physiological explanations for conditions whose ultimate manifestations are somatic.

Several strands of intellectual history meet in Connell's analysis. One is Freud's attention to the social contexts of emotional growth and to "femininity and masculinity as psychological forms constructed by social processes." Another is the theory of social structure supplied by the turn-of-the-century Utopian socialists. The socialist women's movements that developed in Europe and the United States in the early 1900s brought the oppression of women into sharp relief, and called attention to the need for an intellectual explanation of what is now called "the sexual division of labor." As the radical tide ebbed in the 1920s, debates about gender receded into the backwaters of academia and shrunk down to a sterile and confining (in Connell's view) concept of "sex role." The fact that we take for granted the existence of sex roles—but not of race roles or class roles—bears witness, Connell asserts, to a persistent inability to grasp that gender, like race and class, is socially constructed, not biologically given.

Another strand picked up by Connell was the ground-breaking work, at mid-century by Simone de Beauvoir. *The Second Sex* was among the first analyses to point out clearly the importance of power imbalances in the subordination of women. Then, with the resurgence of feminism in the 1960s, interest in gender revived in the social sciences, this time with de Beauvoir's appreciation of power and inequality at its very core. New ideas (particularly about the nature of femininity, power relations between men and women, and the socialization of children) were now linked not only to social theory but also to politics and programs for the radical transformation of patriarchal gender relationships.

By the mid-1980s, according to Connell, the field was in a state of paradox. On the one hand, it was "difficult to think of any other field of social science in which such penetrating and original work [had] been going on." On the other, because converging and integrative synthesis were still starkly lacking, incompatible interpretations of data and issues continued to appear and to remain unresolvable. Connell's project, then, was to reconsider available theories in search of an integrative theory that would arrange the building blocks already assembled.

Previous research, according to Connell, points to two fundamental structures that explain and constrain the relationships between women and men: structures of labor and structures of power. The *division of labor* includes the organization of housework and child care, the distinction between paid and unpaid work, the segregation of labor markets and the creation of "men's jobs," discrimination in training and promotion practices, and inequalities in wages. *Power structures* supply the machinery of authority, control, and coercion. They include government and business hierarchies, institutional and interpersonal violence, sexual regulation and surveillance, and the dynamics of authority within domestic relationships. The two structures are different—each follows a distinct historical trajectory and has its particular effects on shaping masculinity and femininity—but they are tightly intertwined.

Another major structure, Connell argues, defines the social patterning of relationships that are sexual or based on emotional attachment. The dynamics of desire and desirability are organized around a structure Connell calls (borrowing from Freud) the *structure of cathexis* (1987). This structure produces laws, taboos, and prohibitions that define normalcy, restrain sexuality, and proscribe certain kinds of sexual acts and attachments (such as incest, rape, homosexuality, and under-age sex).

The structure of cathexis shores up a cultural norm in which important emotional relationships are defined dichotomously in terms of the opposition of highly standardized forms of masculinity and femininity. It idealizes sexual practice within stable couple relationships, and defines hetero- and homosexuality as binary categories and specifies the relations between them. It gives rise to gender antagonisms (man-hating, woman-hating, self-hating) and undergirds the trust and distrust, jealousy and solidarity in a wide variety of emotional relationships, including those organized around raising children. The structure of cathexis is clearly bound up with the division of labor and the structure of power. Most sexual and emotional attachments, however complex and multilayered, are anchored in a division of labor and an imbalance of power—physical, social and/or economic—that maintains the male partner's ultimate dominance.

Connell posits that these three structures should be evident at different levels of social organization, and proposes two types of structural analysis at two different levels. At the high level of logical abstraction that characterizes historical, cross-cultural, and international comparisons, he sees structural "models" as useful rubrics (also see Frenk et al., 1991). He also suggests conducting "inventories" of structural forces at two levels of logical complexity.

First, a whole society has a "gender order"—a "pattern of power relations between men and women and definitions of femininity and masculinity"—that can be inventoried. The gender order changes slowly and writes the terms and conditions for ordinary practice. At a lower level of generality, specific "gender regimes" can also be subjected to inventory through local customs and informal rules in a variety of mediating structures and institutions (families, schools, worksites, communities, voluntary and formal organizations). Gender regimes comprise the daily practices through which the gender order is negotiated, institutionalized, and sometimes gradually changed.

The distinction between underlying structure (in gender order) and surface practice (particular gender regimes) is an elegant solution to a problem that has bedeviled social theory for at least the last 30 years: how to reconcile the determinism inherent in the concept of social structure with the consciousness, voluntarism, pluralism, and motivation necessary to account for personal agency and social change. Paying attention to both levels reveals interconnections between structure and practice: how "people in their daily lives constitute the social relations they live in," however complex, ambiguous, and contradictory their actions may seem or be (Connell, 1987).

As an illustration, the sexual division of labor operates at the level of the gender order as a constraint or norm (specifically, a segregation rule) allocating people among job categories and erecting corollary constraints that maintain occupational sex segregation: discrimination in vocational and training, job placement, and career tracking, unequal pay for comparable work, and bias in the valuation of boys' and girls' skills. The sex-segregated status quo continues to be reinforced by male solidarity, even across class lines, and by the consistent allocation to women, even as they are absorbed into the permanent labor force, of uncompensated household and child-care responsibilities. At the level of the gender regime, the sexual division of labor not only limits but also focuses daily practice, in particular occupations or places of work, producing minor skirmishes as men and women impose or resist sex bias in, for example, the distribution or design of jobs.

Even now, to extend the example, a young woman who thinks of becoming a neurosurgeon typically receives well-meaning advice (a practice) from official and self-appointed career counselors who dwell on the sacrifices and difficulties she will face. Unspoken but unmistakably present is an enduring ideology, built into the gender order, about women's psychological unsuitability for certain kinds of (men's) work. Physical unsuitability is taken for granted too, which is why it took a court-supervised consent decree to impress on AT&T ergonomists that women moving into highly paid outdoor craft work were at risk of falling from telephone poles, not because of insufficient strength but because the climbing tool the company had used for over 70 years was too long to fit the leg of the average female employee (Walsh and Egdahl, 1980). The existence of federal antidiscrimination legislation constitutes evidence that the gender order is somewhat tractable over time.

As Connell stresses, and these examples attest, different occupations and different workplaces may employ very different mechanisms (gender regimes) for sustaining segregation and imbalance of power (the gender order). And the gender order itself is part of a larger pattern of production, consumption, and distribution. In fact, Connell argues, gender divisions are a deep-seated feature of production itself, a central organizing principle of modern industrial society. This is not to deny that the global pattern (subordination of women in society as a whole) is sometimes contradicted in particular families, workplaces, or other settings. Such departures may or may not arouse policing efforts to reimpose the global pattern as a local norm, according to Connell: they may even signify structural tension that could eventually lead to large-scale social change. But the deeper structures continue to bound daily life.

Connell's three underlying structures—division of labor, power structures, and the structure of cathexis—are easily discerned in the health domain. The sexual division of labor is evident in the uneven distribution of men and women in the health-care professions, in the myriad ways that women's health is defined in terms of their assigned social function as childbearers and nurturers, and in the occupational sex segregation that produces different health risks for women and men.

The impact on health of masculine authority is manifest in the medicalization and social control of women's deviance and distress; in the feminization of poverty, sexual abuse, and domestic violence; and in the proliferation of technology and the degradation of the ecosystem, insofar as these trends reflect an "aggressive masculinity" (Connell, 1987) that fosters brute competition and needless destructiveness.

Finally, the structure of cathexis lies at the heart of the growing epidemics of sexually transmitted diseases, including AIDS. It undergirds sexual abuse, interpersonal violence, and pornography, contributes to eating disorders and substance abuse, and is the basis of many advertising campaigns promoting consumer products that have health consequences.

As valuable as these concepts are for describing the social dynamics of health, illness, and well-being, they are seldom evident in serious research on gender issues in health. That research has focused chiefly on explaining women's mortality advantage over men, men's morbidity advantage, and trends in these relationships. The comparative epidemiological framework observes the very real possibility that both men and women might be healthier in a social order better structured for economic and social equity, shared power and responsibility, and tolerance of diversity in sexuality and other realms of personal expression. Instead of framing questions built on the categorical premise that the social progress of one group is achieved at the expense of another, we need a framework that raises larger questions about the kind of society that can maximize health and quality of life for all its members.

Alternative Theoretical Lenses on Gender and Health

So far we have undertaken a cursory review of two literatures—one on gender and health, the other on gender and power. Integrating the two reveals limitations and silences in the conventional discourse on gender and health. Investigators have looked at gender dynamics in health through a number of lenses, which can be loosely arrayed along a continuum from macro to micro levels of organization and analysis, as Figure 5–1 shows (also see Allison, 1971; Tesh, 1988; Stallones, 1980).

The different disciplinary lenses used to examine whether and how gender affects health not only produce different answers to similar questions but, more importantly, bring different basic questions to the fore (Allison, 1971). None gives a correct or complete picture in itself; each brings a certain set of details into sharp focus while relegating others to a blurry background. Starting from different assumptions about the origins of disease, each produces its own justification for a particular program of intervention in the name of health. A full rendering of the complex mix of gender dynamics in health would be more like an album of photographs taken from a variety of angles, depths of field, resolutions, and perspectives than a single wide-angle picture, or, to quote Verbrugge, more like a quilt than a tapestry (personal communication October, 1993).

The Biomedical Lens

At the micro level, the biomedical lens focuses on biophysiological theories of disease causation and the effects on health of biomedical interventions. We tend to assume, in this scientific age, that illness is nothing more than biology gone awry. Among the questions about gender and health that occupy the foreground at this level of analysis

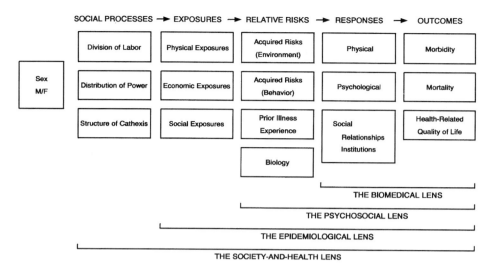

Figure 5-1. Alternative disciplinary lenses for analyses of relationships between gender and health.

are whether women have greater intrinsic protection against mortality through X-chromosome-linked genes and female sex hormones, whether men benefit from inherent differences in reproductive anatomy and physiology, and how these physiological differences manifest in relative morbidity and mortality rates.

Because it traces causation within the physiological organism, the biomedical lens produces health improvement programs that emphasize individual properties and deficiencies—genetic predispositions, biochemical departures from normalcy, signs, symptoms, and physical syndromes amenable to medical intervention. The biomedical lens also raises questions about whether and how gender differences in health might be a function of systems and styles of medical practice: whether, for example, women's more active use of medical care helps explain their greater longevity by speeding recovery, slowing chronic disease, facilitating earlier detection and better treatment, or rendering them more astute judges of signs of disease and available services. A related topic of increasing concern is whether, and if so how, treatment strategies and protocols are distorted by gender bias (e.g., see Nathanson, 1975; Verbrugge, 1978; Verbrugge and Steiner, 1981; Roter et al., 1991; Ayanian and Epstein, 1991; Steingaart, 1991).

The Psychosocial Lens

Continuing to focus on the individual, but at the intrapsychic and interpersonal levels, the psychosocial model raises questions about individual and social behavior, personality structures, coping repertoires and resources, sense of control and self-efficacy, and gender differences in the experience and reporting of signs and symptoms. The kinds of questions that arise include the following: Do specific health behaviors serve different psychosocial functions for women and for men? Which personality constructs and psychological processes—rebelliousness, sensation-seeking, external locus of control, self-efficacy—put men or women in harm's way? How are these attributes and predispositions distributed by the gender order and within local gender regimes? Are men more confident of their ability to make specific changes in behavior, and/or less likely to attribute lapses to personal failure in a self-defeating cycle?

Do women and men respond differently to discomfort? Do they have different thresholds for taking action in the face of symptoms or threats to health?

Do women and men in different social strata and life stages call on different coping and resistance resources when faced with stress and strain? Do they maintain and use social networks, social supports, and lay referral systems differently, with different implications for health? And how do race and/or ethnicity, age, and class cut across the gender divide? Is gender alone a meaningful organizing frame, or do within-gender gradations and interactions with other factors (such as education or class) make all the difference?

The prescriptions for action that emanate from these analyses still focus on the individual, but at the levels of cognition, information processing, and decision-making. They include educational programs, psychotherapy, skill-building workshops (for example, in stress management), mutual aid, and support groups. Implicitly or overtly, these programs are built on social-psychological models and theories that range from classic psychoanalytic thinking to the more socially conditioned perspectives exemplified by social-cognitive theory (Bandura, 1986). With or without attention to a social context, however, these action plans are aimed ultimately at individual transformation and change.

The Epidemiological Lens

At the next higher level of generality, an epidemiological risk factor model begins with disease patterns in populations or groups and seeks to parse out differential risk factors, including biological predispositions and markers, as well as behavioral and environmental exposures. Methodological issues in the statistical assessment of risk arise in this domain as well.

Because it seeks pathways from relative risk to specific disease endpoints, the epidemiological lens continues to focus on personal behavior as a mediating mechanism that translates broad environmental exposure into what Verbrugge calls "acquired risk." Whether harmful (like smoking and alcohol abuse) or protective (like exercise, balanced diets, and preventive health regimens), personal behavior has become the prime focus of epidemiological questions about gender and health.

Do men engage more often in known risk behaviors such as smoking, drinking, and frequent or careless driving? (Yes.) Do women outperform men in preventive health behaviors, including vitamin use, home dental care, regular physical checkups, and consumption of foods believed to lower risk of heart disease and cancer? (Again, yes, although men are better at maintaining a regimen of vigorous exercise.) How much do these preventive health behaviors contribute to gender differences in longevity and illness incidence, functioning and well-being?

To what extent are there inherent differences in the subjective experiences of health and illness? To what extent are other apparent differences spurious? Do women really have more illness, or are they just better equipped with a language to speak of it and/or retain it in memory?

As the core discipline of public health, epidemiology should in theory lead to social, not individual, action plans. Yet modern epidemiological studies have tended, though they draw their inferences from broad patterns within populations, to aim at explanations that endorse the importance of individual decisions in minimizing personal risk. Epidemiological studies bearing on gender and health may identify broad classes of environmental exposure to potential risk—exposures related to occupation or family roles, for example—but the prevailing impulse is to assign groups of individuals to specific risk categories and trace the biological pathways to ultimate health outcomes, rather than to characterize the mechanisms through which social groups are sorted differentially into risk categories.

For example, an enormous investment has been made in studies specifying minutely all the ways in which tobacco smoke can compromise health. Much less effort has been dedicated to understanding all the sources and manifestations of the tobacco industry's economic and political power, and all the impacts of its $3.9 billion outlay for advertising and promotion of cigarettes.

The Society-and-Health Lens

By contrast, a society-and-health lens brings to the foreground large-scale cultural, social, economic, and political processes and seeks to understand the pathways through which they produce differential risks. What is most distinctive about this perspective is its emphasis on how health concerns, responses to risk factors, signs, and symptoms, as well as the social construction of knowledge about health, are ordained and constrained by crucial mechanisms of social control and distribution of resources and power. Current epidemiological research on gender and health takes for granted a social-stratification system that allocates resources and power on the basis of gender-determined social roles, and leaves the underlying social processes unidentified, unquestioned, and unexplored.

Explanations of risk that are founded on notions of socialization and social roles, and traced through causal pathways that highlight lifestyle and personal choice, assume more latitude for personal agency than the social order—as characterized in works like Connell's—may actually permit. Adopting a society-and-health perspective means raising questions about how social structure may affect personal choice—how the division of labor, the distribution of authority and power, and the stereotypes endemic to these power and authority relations may themselves constitute a social environment fully as palpable and pathogenic as the physical world.

Seeing health in broad social-structural terms is difficult in several respects. First, social structures are abstract and elusive, while psychological evidence is immediately available. Popular psychological explanations for behavior appear self-evident; to construct situational explanations requires imagination. Second, we have ingrained habits of mind, and cultural tendencies get in the way of seeing large social forces. Westerners tend to explain a situation in terms of the personal dispositions of the participants (someone was stupid, or venal, or ambitious or a hero), whereas adults in certain non-Western cultures (Indians, for example) are more likely to offer situational explanations (someone had a competing role obligation, or there was a technological failure, or miscommunication occurred). Westerners also have an analytic bias in favor of reductionism at the expense of integrative, intuitive, and convergent styles of knowing.

The third and most serious impediment to seeing health in social terms is the sense of powerlessness that often results. If we recognize, for example, that high smoking rates among children who are failing in school are a function of basic political and economic arrangements in our society, and of implicit value choices about who will have opportunities, where do we go from there? Such an acknowledgement seems either a call to revolution or an admission of defeat; locating explanations in individual or institutional failures leads to much more manageable action plans, even if we grant that they are less effective than they could be if they were rooted in a deeper and more richly nuanced understanding of fundamental causes and meaning systems. The question for policy is whether deeper social analysis can lead to more promising action plans.

A Society-and-Health Perspective on Gender and Cigarettes

Cigarette smoking serves as an appealing case for exploring deeper social questions about gender and health. First, smoking matters. It is the leading cause of preventable mortality, accounting for over 400,000 deaths in 1990 (Centers for Disease Control, 1992). Second, gender-related patterns of tobacco use are strongly influencing trends in sex-specific morbidity and mortality (Waldron, 1986; Verbrugge, 1989). Unraveling the influences of patriarchy on smoking—sometimes overprotecting women, sometimes heightening their risk—should help strengthen our grip on more general relationships between gender and health. Third, gender patterns in smoking rates have been changing markedly, offering a kind of natural experiment that could produce intriguing insights into how change in gender relations occurs. Fourth, women's smoking has become an urgent public health concern now that lung cancer has overtaken breast cancer as the leading cause of cancer death among women. Fifth, the lessons of smoking can be generalizable to other important health risks, such as alcohol and drug abuse, obesity and nutrition, physical inactivity and violence. Finally, existing efforts to address women's smoking seem to have reached an impasse, raising the question of whether a society-and-health perspective can shed new light on questions of etiology and/or avenues to effective action.

Cigarette smoking had become common among American men by the end of World War I. For several decades thereafter, gender was the decisive axis dividing smokers and nonsmokers. Women, especially younger women, began to take up smoking in the 1920s, but the steepest increase in smoking rates among women occurred during World War II. Women as a group still have not caught up to men; aggregate rates of smoking in the United States have always been higher among men than women. But with each successive birth cohort from World War II on, women's smoking-related characteristics (average age at onset, numbers and types of cigarettes smoked, cessation attempts) became more and more like men's.

Scientific reports about the harmful effects of smoking began to appear in the late 1950s. In the wake of the highly publicized Surgeon General's Report on Smoking and Health in 1964 (U.S. Department of Health, Education and Welfare, 1964), overall smoking prevalence began to decline, reflecting increased cessation by current smokers and a decrease in new smokers. Prevalence rates among both men and women peaked in 1964–1965, when over half of men (51 percent) and about a third of women (34 percent) actively smoked (Gritz, 1987). As Figure 5–2 shows, the subsequent de-

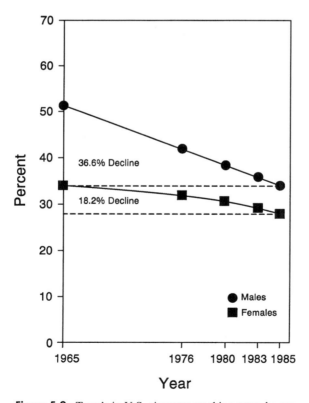

Figure 5-2. Trends in U.S. cigarette smoking rates, by sex.

cline in prevalence rates occurred in both sexes, but at a slower pace among women than men (Fiore et al., 1989). As of 1985, 32 percent of men and 28 percent of women smoked. The 1991 smoking prevalence rates, 28 percent for men and 23 percent for women, suggest a slight relative increase in the rate of decline among women over the last 6 years (Centers for Disease Control, 1992).

These patterns and trends can be partially understood in terms of the sexual division of labor, the gender-based structure of power, and normative role prescriptions defining sexually attractive behavior among women and men. We will discuss power first, in accordance with our view of power as the primary structure on which the others rest.

Structures of Power, Gender, and Smoking

Power discrepancies in relations between the sexes influence smoking in several ways. First, "permission" for women to smoke has been withheld and granted over the years by male authority. Smoking has consistently served as a symbol in sexual politics and in struggles over social control. Second, smoking rates reflect patterns of inequality, historically in gender relationships, and more recently in social-class divisions. Third, on a more macro plane, these shifting patterns and rates have reflected political accommodations to the evolving marketing needs of the tobacco industry, with its enormous socioeconomic power in the (male-dominated) capitalist system.

Smoking, Patriarchy and Social Control

Definitions of patriarchy extend back at least to Engels (1884), who connected the patriarchal family organization to hunger, slavery, war, exploitation of the weak and the modern state. Adrienne Rich defines patriarchy as "any kind of group organization in which males hold dominant power and determine what part females shall and shall not play, and in which capabilities assigned to women are relegated generally to the mystical and aesthetic and excluded from the practical and political realms" (Rich, 1979). Authority and legitimate power are viewed in masculine terms. Trends in smoking by gender have long reflected these forces.

A critical dimension of power—in close personal interactions and within small and large groups—is the license and the ability to control others' behavior. Women's lack of power has often translated into constraints and controls on their behavior, at times crude and violent, at other times subtle and indirect. The more brutal and coercive forms of control (like domestic violence and rape) serve a latent enforcement function for the more genteel forms.

When tobacco first came into wide-spread use in turn-of-the-century America, it immediately became embedded in identity politics and lines of demarcation between women's moral and aesthetic sphere and the practical world of men. Condemnation of smoking by women at the beginning of the century can be seen as part of a system of male-dominated social control, enforced through strict rules of decorum and gender-appropriate behavior. This is where the structures of power and cathexis most clearly overlap. Powerful and powerless women were the exceptions who proved the rule that power was deeply at issue. The President's daughter and other elite women (puffing in their carriages on the way to the opera, according to one press report) could smoke with impunity in the early 1900s; otherwise, smoking was reserved for women in the lowest classes. Among "respectable" women of the middle class—where power boundaries were being drawn and negotiated in local gender regimes—public smoking was subject to social sanction and even prohibited by law in cities like Chicago and New York (Ernster, 1987).

As women's roles expanded, restrictions on their behavior were gradually relaxed and smoking became socially acceptable though not unequivocally so. A recent study of attitudes among high-school seniors found that they attribute more negative characteristics to girls who smoke than to boys who do (Elkind, 1985). Other research has shown that parents more often disapprove of smoking by their daughters than by their sons (Waldron et al., 1991). Historically, males have experienced greater social pressure to smoke than have females, but these norms are undergoing change. A sample of 6-grade boys rated girls who smoked more attractive and more desirable as friends than nonsmokers (Barton et al., 1982), suggesting that in some (but only some) local gender regimes, smoking may be a rational strategy for girls to seek social approval (Gilchrist et al., 1989). The subgroups in which this is true are defined, increasingly, in terms of social class.

Smoking and Inequality

Recent trends in cigarette smoking reveal complex interactions among gender, education, other indicators of social class, and the imbalances of power that attend these social locations. As the hazards of cigarettes have become almost universally known (if not always consistently accepted), smoking—once a behavior that cut across all socioeconomic strata and was much more widespread among men than women—has become concentrated in less-advantaged social groups. These groups are now defined less by gender than by income and education (except in the lowest strata of income and education, where men are still much more likely than women to smoke). Between 1974 and 1985, as Figure 5–3 indicates, smoking prevalence declined five times faster among higher-educated groups: the decline in smoking prevalence over the decade was 2 percentage points among high-school dropouts (36 percent to 34 percent), and 10 percentage points among college graduates (29 percent to 18 percent) (Pierce et al., 1989). By 1991, 32 percent of the least-educated group smoked, compared to 14 percent of college graduates (Centers for Disease Control, 1992).

Gender differences in smoking interact with education: the male-female gender gap in smoking prevalence is wider for high-school graduates (37 percent versus 27 percent) than for holders of college or advanced degrees (15 percent versus 12 percent). This phenomenon reflects somewhat higher adoption rates among male high-school graduates: among young people aged 20 to 24 in 1990, 37 percent of men and 33 percent of women with a high-school degree started smoking, compared to 16 percent of

Society and Health

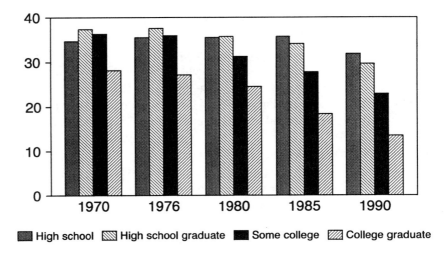

Figure 5-3. Smoking prevalence (in percentages) among adults 20 and older, 1970–1990. *Sources:* Centers for Disease Control, 1992. Cigarette Smoking Among Adults—United States, 1990. Morbidity and Mortality Weekly Report, 41 (20):354–362. U.S. Department of Health and Human Services, 1989. Reducing the Health Consequences of Smoking: 25 Years of Progress. A Report of the Surgeon General, pp. 259–376.

men and 14 percent of women who had advanced to or through college (Centers for Disease Control, 1992). High-school dropouts had by far the highest initiation rates— 55 percent for men and 47 percent for women. Rates of smoking by income, like the education rates, exhibit a clear social-class gradient, with rates decreasing at each increment of additional education.

Meanwhile, women have increasingly become the nation's poor. Poverty is overwhelmingly a condition of women and their children in the contemporary United States: two of three adult Americans living in poverty are female. The "feminization of poverty" (Pearce, 1978) reflects certain recent changes, notably the dismantling of social-welfare programs in the 1980s and rapid growth in the numbers of female-headed households, whose poverty rate—27 percent overall, 52 percent for blacks and 53 percent for Hispanics—was five times that of intact families in 1984. But it also reflects an enduring underlying gender order: a dual labor market and a heavy burden of unpaid domestic labor, both of which profoundly disadvantage women in national and world economies (Sidel, 1986). These forces could continue to accelerate women's smoking rates in relation to men's, although there are complexities. Gender issues in health are inextricably bound up with disparities in income and social class. This is one of the ways in which the structure of power overlaps with and reinforces the gender-based division of labor and the structure of cathexis. As smoking is driven into lower social strata, it encounters more restrictive cultural norms about women's behavior. Thus, there are two opposing forces, one militating for relatively more smoking by women than men, the other for less. The feminization of poverty places more women than men in the higher-risk income groups, but, in at least some of those groups, traditional gender roles still put brakes on women's smoking.

A number of hypotheses have been advanced to explain the distillation of smoking in lower socioeconomic groups. One common explanation, a human-capital argument that speaks indirectly to issues of power, draws on the concept of discounting to explain why "those with more favorable life prospects" would be "more sensitive to information about behaviors that affect mortality late in life" (Schelling, 1992, p. 431). This theory is consistent with the observation that the gender gap in smoking is closing fastest among more-educated segments of the population because it is in these groups that women's "life prospects" relative to men's are improving the most.

A second hypothesis, again related to power, is that education and cosmopolitanism confer a greater opportunity to "receive and appreciate and understand health messages from credible sources" (Schelling, 1992, p. 433). This argument builds on the concept, in diffusion theory, that early adopters of an innovative practice have easier access to new ideas because of their social position and mobility (Rogers, 1983). Ferrence (1988) draws on diffusion theory to compare smoking trends among women and men, arguing that because of their superior social power, higher incomes, and greater time spent away from home, men were in a position to adopt smoking earlier than women early in the century. As evidence of health hazards began to mount in subsequent decades, men were again earlier adopters of the "innovative" response, smoking cessation.

Waldron (1991) notes, however, that diffusion theory fails to adequately explain at least three historical facts: (1) higher rates of quitting among men during the 1960s and early 1970s, despite good evidence that women were fully as cognizant of the risks, (2) women's earlier and more complete adoption of the innovation of filter cigarettes, and (3) women's almost total imperviousness, over a very long period, to the "innovations" of smokeless tobacco, cigars, and pipes. Diffusion theory, which would have predicted a different result in all three instances, (Waldron, 1991) falls short here because it fails to take adequate account of external social and economic forces.

The Economic and Political Power of the Tobacco Industry

Tobacco products are not as easily mapped as "innovations" that follow a natural diffusion curve through society because the natural forces are dramatically distorted and amplified by the economic power and political economy of the tobacco industry. These forces have been crucial in shaping the changing gender distribution of cigarette use. As male smoking rates have gradually declined, tobacco marketing has become more aggressive and segmented, with a special emphasis on recruiting women and ethnic minorities (Davis, 1987). The tobacco industry has monitored, promoted, and capitalized on evolving social norms defining women's smoking as a badge of autonomy and social power.

Although studies have produced conflicting evidence on the direct impact of advertising and marketing, cigarette companies have worked hard and effectively to associate themselves with the women's movement and with symbols of women's equality and liberation. Industry advertising constantly links smoking to symbols of independence and success, portraying cigarette smoking as a "torch of freedom" and an emblem of women's having "come a long way." Tobacco interests contribute funds to women's groups, particularly leadership groups in politics, business and professional affairs, and minority concerns (Berman, 1987), probably distorting their agendas. The editorial policies of women's magazines have been influenced by their financial dependence on tobacco advertising (Warner, 1986).

Industry sponsorship of women's sports links cigarettes to young, healthy women, and to images of vitality, resilience, and self-determination. As one of many examples, Philip Morris donates about $12 million each year to the Virginia Slims women's tennis tournament, indispensable support that would be difficult or impossible to raise from other sources. The object is to associate cigarettes in the public mind with vital, strong-minded female athletes. The tobacco interests have effectively aligned themselves with women's struggles against the patriarchy.

The Division of Labor, Gender, and Smoking

The division of labor influences smoking in at least four ways. First and foremost, it shapes the overarching gender order and the distribution of wealth and power. As a result, it interacts with and reinforces the structure of power discussed earlier. Second, within local gender regimes, the historical patterns of men's and women's smoking emerged in the context of a gender-defined division of labor, and were affected by changing patterns in labor-force activity (Ernster, 1987). Third, according to some hypotheses about gender factors in smoking, divisions of labor in the workplace and family domains cause women to experience more stress because of their gender-defined social roles. Finally, the division of labor defines women's unique role in reproduction, thereby placing their smoking in a special class from the standpoint of social control and policy.

Smoking and the Gender Order

The gender order sharply demarcates men's and women's work, and, through a "gendered logic of accumulation" (Connell, 1987, p. 105), excludes women from opportunities to amass wealth and/or to move up career ladders to a level in which they would control significant capital and wield important power. The U.S. labor force is nearly half (45 percent) female, and yet it remains highly sex-segregated. Women are 99 percent of secretaries but 19 percent of lawyers, 95 percent of nurses but 20 percent of physicians, 97 percent of child-care workers and 2 percent of fire-fighters.

More than half (53.7 percent) of adult American women worked for wages outside the home in 1991 (U.S. Department of Labor, 1994), compared to only 34 percent in

1959. This represents a jump between 1959 and 1983, from 34 percent to 54 percent. Between 1959 and 1983, women's overall work burdens increased relative to men's. Including hours spent in paid work, housework, and child care across the labor force aged 25–64, the female-to-male ratio of total hours worked flipped from 0.91 to 1.04. During these same years, as women's time spent in paid work increased (by 357 hours, from 572 to 929), their time spent in housework and child care declined (by 236 hours, 171 for housework and 65 for child care) but not sufficiently to offset the effects of their increased time at work (Fuchs, 1986). Many contemporary women still go home to work the "second shift" (Hochschild, 1989).

Smoking and Labor-Force Participation

Perhaps this is why, today, whether women are in or out of the paid labor force does not seem to predict their smoking status (Waldron, 1986). Historically, smoking emerged in the context of a status-distinction system in which women's ability to bear and nurse children justified a gender role designed to keep them at home and out of harm's way (Waldron, 1986). In the first decade of the century, men went to work and, later, to war, where smoking was normative, while respectable women did not smoke; they tended home and hearth, where probity, aesthetic virtues, and moral rectitude held sway.

As consumer markets expanded, the division of labor adapted. Increasingly, women's participation was needed in the consumption of luxury goods, including alcohol and cigarettes. Men were the producers for the expanding capitalist system; women were its consumers. This meant that strictures against women's drinking and smoking needed to be relaxed, and, gradually, they were. As early as 1919, the Lorillard Company ran a series of advertisements showing women smoking (Ernster, 1987). A double standard did linger for a very long time, but tobacco industry advertising chipped away at it, at first by indirect suggestions that kept the division of labor intact. Chesterfield, for example, ran an advertising series in the 1920s in which a nonsmoking young woman seductively asked her male companion to "blow some [smoke] my way" (Ernster, 1987). Estimates of the proportion of cigarettes consumed by women increased, between 1923 and 1929, from 5 percent to 12 percent (Ernster, 1987). But widespread cigarette use by women lagged behind men by 25 to 30 years.

The biggest jump in the prevalence in women smokers came when a large proportion of the 1910–1919 birth cohort of women was recruited into nontraditional occupations as jobs were vacated by soldiers who had gone off to World War II. Even then, women smokers, on average, consumed fewer cigarettes than men, inhaled less deeply, and had shorter smoking histories, so their mortality rates were correspondingly lower.

This lighter exposure among women may have fed into a gender bias in research on smoking and health. (The absence of women investigators—the division of labor in science—probably had an effect.) The famous "MRFIT" (multiple-risk factor intervention trial to reduce the risk of cardiovascular disease among a large cohort of men) is perhaps the most blatant example of a major study that specifically excluded women, but there were others. Of the eight large prospective epidemiological studies specifically designed to ascertain the health effects of cigarettes, only five included women (U.S. Department of Health and Human Services, 1980). Throughout the 1960s and 1970s, studies of smoking-related illness and of smoking-cessation strategies, as well as public-information campaigns, focused almost exclusively on men. Not until 1980 did the U.S. Surgeon General's report on smoking and women's health attempt to lay to rest once and for all "the fallacy of women's immunity" to the ravages of smoking (U.S. Department of Health and Human Services, 1980).

A number of investigators hypothesize that the scarcity of clear health warnings directed specifically at women may account for men's much higher cessation rates during the 1960s and 1970s (Waldron, 1991; Ferrence, 1988). Although women knew that smoking was harmful to health, they argue, the risk had not been personalized for them to the degree that it had for men.

Smoking Cessation, Stress and Work

If women's protected status within the traditional division of labor postponed their initial exposure to cigarettes, and if sex bias in scientific research impeded an aggressive response, their slower cessation rates have also been ascribed to the heavy burdens they are presumed to carry in the modern era. This stress hypothesis is rooted in observations about inequities in the division of labor. Men's higher cessation rates were first documented in the 1950s (Heanszel et al., 1956), though subsequent research showed that the differences were less clear-cut when length and strength of exposure were taken into account. Even after controlling for exposure, though, as well as for attempts to quit, women do seem to have lower rates of successful quitting (Blake et al., 1989).

Gritz (1987) hypothesizes that women's smoking is strongly maintained by the stress of multiple roles and by the function cigarettes serve for them as a "time marker or validation for time off" from work. But Waldron (1991) raises a caution about the lack of empirical support for stress-based explanations of gender differences in smoking. Studies do show that smoking is often used to regulate negative affect and reduce stress. Women do generally report more stress. And some studies do suggest stronger links among women than men between smoking adoption and stress reduction. However, the evidence is mixed on whether women have more trouble with smoking cessation because of a greater tendency to use cigarettes for tension reduction (Waldron, 1991). Nor is it at all clear whether or how these factors relate to women's work, even though the hypothesis draws on the "scarcity" notions of the multiple-role perspective. More research on this question is needed.

Smoking and the Division of Labor in Production and Reproduction

Another dimension of growing policy concern over women's smoking—the effects of cigarette smoke on reproduction and the fetus, and during lactation, and the consequences of exposing vulnerable young children to environmental tobacco smoke—

harks back to very old themes about the sexual division of labor. One of the five rotating warning labels on cigarette packaging and advertising reads: SURGEON GENERAL'S WARNING: Smoking By Pregnant Women May Result in Fetal Injury, Premature Birth, And Low Birth Weight." Neither this nor warnings on alcohol packages mentions documented effects on sperm, male sex hormones, and male reproductive functioning. "It is the potential to independently incubate and nurture the youngest members of the newest generations that separates the girls from the boys," according to one (woman) obstetrician-gynecologist in a recent call for special attention to women's smoking (Dorfman, 1987, p. 12).

Comments like this reinforce a court-endorsed position that the reproduction of the human species is women's work. Women who use cocaine during their pregnancies are being criminally prosecuted for harming their fetuses, even though treatment programs for pregnant addicts are entirely inadequate. A Chicago woman who used cocaine during pregnancy was charged with involuntary manslaughter when her baby died 2 days after birth. In rare instances, pregnant women who use alcohol have been placed in "preventive detention," jailed for minor offenses, charged with child abuse, or neglect and threatened with manslaughter charges should they abort spontaneously (French, 1992).

Maternal smoking is a well-established and powerful risk factor for low birth weight and infant mortality (Institute of Medicine, 1985). Inexpensive smoking cessation programs for pregnant women have been developed but are to date inadequately disseminated. This is a clear and promising target for public health intervention, but smoking programs targeting pregnant women need to be embedded into a broader social context. Otherwise, they will fall into the trap of taking for granted a sex-segregated division of labor. They will overlook the importance of the father's health and well-being in the reproduction and nurturing of the young (Mannino et al., 1994), and of the mother's health long before she becomes pregnant. They will also obscure the importance of women's health and well-being independent of their reproductive functions.

Cigarette Smoking and the Structure of Cathexis

Popular culture, the entertainment industry, and the mass media routinely sexualize women as standardized objects of male desire to a degree, and with an intensity, far beyond any comparable stereotypification and objectification of male sexuality. This basic difference in the portrayal of women and men in American popular culture is rooted in unequal exchange and an imbalance of social power.

Smoking patterns—and the themes promoted in cigarette advertising campaigns— dramatically illustrate the structure of cathexis. First, cigarettes have always been sold by linking them with highly diversified themes of sex appeal. Second, the industry's marketing has emphasized a specific and vital connection between smoking, body weight, and images of sexual attractiveness. These images emanate from a system of patriarchal control of women's bodies, their self-conceptions, and (importantly) their actual life options. The crucial link between smoking and weight forges a link between the structures of power and cathexis. Third, cigarettes have been carefully positioned in relation to conventional gender norms as a symbol of both conformity and rebellion, two contradictory impulses the tobacco industry has successfully exploited especially among the young.

Cigarettes as Sex Appeal

Images of sexual attractiveness have always been widely and effectively used as vehicles to promote smoking. The "Marlboro man," for instance, is as enduring and pervasive a cultural symbol of rugged masculinity as Madison Avenue has ever produced. Cigarette advertising campaigns invariably seek to portray smoking as glamorous, sexually attractive, sophisticated, romantic, fun, healthy, sporty, sociable, relaxing, calming, emancipated, rebellious and/or slimming. Film stars, fashion models, prominent socialites, and attractive women surrounded by admiring men have appeared in cigarette advertising since the late 1920s (Ernster, 1987; U.S. Department of Health and Human Services, 1980). Sexual innuendo has also consistently been a feature of cigarette advertising. Research has suggested that young girls use cigarettes as emblems of sophistication and sexual attractiveness, while young boys use them to demonstrate masculinity and male assertiveness (Gilchrist et al., 1989).

Smoking for Weight Control

As early as 1928, Lucky Strike was promoting smoking for women for weight control with the famous campaign slogan "Reach for a Lucky instead of a sweet." The new "women-only" cigarette brands use advertising and packaging to emphasize feminine beauty and positive female images; virtually all promote the potential "slimming" effects of smoking. Many of the models in cigarette ads directed at women are astoundingly thin; they look like the "social X-rays" described in *Bonfire of the Vanities* (Wolfe, 1987).

These advertisements are rooted in the structure of cathexis. Women consistently diet more and show greater concern about their weight than men do, although in most social groups obesity is no more prevalent among women and sometimes considerably lower. Women's preoccupation with weight reflects gender norms about attractiveness that are reinforced by the structure of power. Physical appearance is more laden with consequence for women than men, and the double standard has psychological and material consequences.

Society exacts a higher price for overweight from women than from men (Attie and Brooks-Gunn, 1987). Research on stereotypes of physical attractiveness has shown that women's physical appearance, far more than men's, affects the degree to which others perceive them as intelligent, well-educated, effective, personable, and desirable as a friend or colleague. In girls but not in boys, one study showed, overweight is significantly associated with not attending college (Canning and Mayer, 1966). Rothblum (1990) argues that a feminine norm of extreme slimness tends to reemerge during historical periods of organized feminist activity, and is part of a systematic backlash against women's progress toward social parity.

Studies indicating that women are more likely than men to use smoking for weight control, and that women's slower cessation rates may be related to concerns about weight gain demonstrate the implications for smoking of such norms (Waldron, 1991). Female smokers attach special importance to the fact that smokers tend to weigh less than nonsmokers and to gain weight when attempting to quit (Gilchrist et al., 1989). Much more research is needed on the relationships among women's smoking, concerns about weight control, and sex discrimination.

Smoking as Conformity and as Rebellion

Two other mechanisms may link gender-role identity to smoking, among both women and men. "Congruence" mechanisms reflecting a desire to conform to sexual norms and "deviance" mechanisms reflecting a desire to escape the restraints of convention have been partially traced with reference to alcohol. Because heavy drinking is strongly associated in most cultures with masculinity, alcohol use has been studied from the perspective of sex-role orientation and androgyny (Wilsnack and Wilsnack, 1978; Huselid and Cooper, 1992). Since both congruence and deviance themes are evident in cigarette advertising, it is likely that smoking behavior serves both functions for different smokers and for the same person at different times.

If a congruence model were operative, girls and women would be expected to smoke only if they considered smoking consistent with conventional sex-stereotypic notions of feminine behavior. In a deviance model, females would use smoking to express their rebellion against convention and their defiance of normative role prescriptions. Both themes have long been evident in cigarette advertising, which portrays women as sex objects but also as "flouters of old-fashioned ways" (Ernster, 1987). The tobacco marketers have hedged their bets; they address appeals to both trend-setters and resisters of normative change. This double-barreled approach may be an especially effective strategy for recruiting young smokers, since during adolescence desires to conform are powerful but also volatile and ambivalent.

Cigarettes, Gender and Power: Summing Up

Women's smoking—like smoking in general—has been addressed through a variety of public health strategies, from information-based educational campaigns, to counteradvertising and persuasive efforts seeking to alter the social norms, and to formal rules, laws, ordinances, and policies restricting smoking or the latitude of the tobacco industry (Walsh and Gordon, 1986). When well-designed, these initiatives have had an effect, and substantial progress has been made against smoking in the past quarter century. Still, there remains a large minority of refractory heavy smokers, and sizable new cohorts of smokers are being recruited every year. Young girls with limited horizons are especially vulnerable to taking up smoking, and women smokers seem less decisive and less successful than men in their quit attempts (Blake et al., 1989). Few serious policy efforts and far too little research have directly addressed the issue of gender and smoking. Attempts to position smoking as a feminist issue have mostly fizzled.

The impediments to gender-based antismoking efforts are easier to understand when they are seen to reflect fundamental social processes that subsume and transcend physiological addiction, psychological dependence, and personal motivation, as intricate and important as these biological and psychosocial mechanisms certainly are. Interventions directed at individual smokers are being played out against a panoply of shifting social norms and claims defining the relative power of women and men; their options for action and influence in the material, commercial, and political realms; and sex-appropriate behavior in their intimate relations. And these gender regimes operate within a larger gender order in which it is understood that women's behavior must, in the final analysis, remain acceptable to men.

At the same time, there is much more to smoking than gender effects alone. In recent years, as we have seen, education has become the cardinal predictor of smoking status (Pierce et al., 1989). Also, smoking patterns by race and ethnicity have been changing. In 1990, for the first time since monitoring began in 1965, the prevalence of smoking was comparable in blacks and whites (26 percent and 26 percent) (Centers for Disease Control, 1992). According to 1991 data, however, the gap appears to be opening again, with 25 percent of whites and 29 percent of blacks reporting smoking (Centers for Disease Control, 1992). Between 1974 and 1985 the smoking rate among blacks dropped from 44 percent to 35 percent compared to a more modest drop from 36 percent to 29 percent among whites. However, gender continues to be a factor here too: among women, the rate of decline has not been faster for blacks than for whites (Fiore et al., 1989). These bivariate relationships between smoking and race are further confounded by income and education.

Hispanic-Americans as a group appear to smoke relatively less (20 percent in 1991) than the other large race/ethnic groups for whom data are collected in National Health Interview Surveys. (Asian/Pacific Islanders report the least smoking at 16 percent). However, much lower rates among Hispanic women mask much higher rates among Hispanic men. Recent special surveys using bilingual data-collection protocols and more refined sampling procedures are uncovering potentially worrisome trends among Hispanic-American males: age-adjusted smoking rates of 42.5 percent, 39.8 percent, and 41.6 percent respectively among Mexican-, Puerto Rican- and Cuban-American men aged 20–74. By contrast, Hispanic women in the same subgroups had much lower rates: 23.8 percent, 30.3 percent, and 24.4 percent respectively (Haynes et al., 1990). Cultures with traditional attitudes toward gender roles (including Hispanic-Americans) tend to restrict women's smoking suggesting that the forces of modernization have a built-in dynamic toward greater smoking among women. Aggressive marketing of Western tobacco products throughout the Third World is exacerbating the tendency for modernization and Westernization, a mixed blessing for the health of women, since this trend is reducing maternal mortality but increasing other risks.

Certain limitations of the Connell framework become increasingly nettlesome as we try to account for the powerful interactions in the smoking data among gender, social class, education, and culture. Connell's work has been criticized as "a white social theory of gender" (West, 1989). The structure of cathexis occupies a strategic place in his typology, picking up on Juliet Mitchell's call in *Woman's Estate* (1971) for "making an analysis of sexuality central to understanding gender" (Aulette, 1991). Cathexis underscores the importance of sexuality and sexual relations in the development and maintenance of sexism. The concept of cathexis, however, serves less well than the other two structures to illuminate general social processes involved in health and health care, where the effects of sexism are accompanied and confounded by racism, classism, and ageism, all of which strongly influence population health.

To broaden the framework and make it more useful for understanding health, then, we will take some liberties and expand the structure of cathexis to encompass the phenomenon of stereotype: values and social rules that are established and perpetuated by a ruling group or class, and sustained and maintained by structures of production and power. Stereotypes protect and perpetuate existing power structures; they function as mechanisms for social control and the management of deviance. They produce unquestioned rules and behavioral norms surrounding relations not only between and among the sexes, but also within and across cleavages of age, race, ethnicity, and class. In all cases, they render the broad social order extremely resistant to change.

This occurs because the structure of stereotype shapes our perceptions of ourselves and others, and also limits and distorts our actual experiences of reality. Sexual segregation of the labor force, for example, begins with stereotypes about women's natural capacities and abilities, and then limits their access to just those kinds of experiences in the workplace that would challenge the stereotypes. Stereotyping has a built-in circularity that perpetuates unequal access to economic, political, and social power, and it functions in similar ways with reference to gender, race, ethnicity, class, and age.

The structure of stereotype shapes the phenomenological experience of gender, race, class, age, and other social categories: what it means to be a woman who passes a whistling, leering construction crew on its lunch break, a homosexual or lesbian on the alert for "gay bashers," a black male who notices a white woman crossing the street or locking her car door at the sight of him, a low-income white woman who buys groceries with food stamps and senses others unspoken disapproval of her food selections, or an isolated and devalued "senior citizen."

In short, the distribution of power throughout a society—replicated at lower levels of organization in more proximal institutions and smaller social groups—supports a hierarchical division of labor and a set of rules of decorum. All these structures interact to sustain a broad social order, establish the bounds of appropriate behavior for various social subgroups, create a differential sorting mechanism with an inherent selection bias, and produce and perpetuate stereotypes that call up visceral and emotional reactions in day-to-day interactions. And these three sorting processes profoundly affect health. Figure 5–4 attempts to summarize some of these relationships

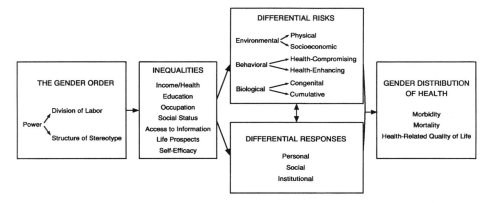

Figure 5-4. A schematic model of important relationships between gender and health.

and connect them back to epidemiological understandings of gender differences in health.

Gender, Society and Health: Summary and Conclusions

In reviewing the literature on gender and health, we have drawn on Connell's analysis of gender and power to extract four disciplinary lenses, or traditions, through which the intricate and fluid relationships between gender and health can be viewed. Next, we have argued that a "society-and-health" lens is both more encompassing than the bio-medical, psychosocial, and epidemiological lenses that have dominated research on gender and health, and better positioned to expose unstated assumptions and biases about the ways in which the dynamics of gender influence practices in health. Finally, we have refracted gender issues in cigarette smoking through a particular society-and-health lens, in an effort to explore its utility. How useful is it?

Implications for Understanding

First, as a heuristic or critical stance, the society-and-health lens does offer a useful corrective. Untested assumptions about gender and health are so deeply rooted in our culture, so implicit in our causal maps, and so routinely taken for granted that they often go entirely unnoticed and are in some ways inaccessible to empirical testing. For this reason, one of the major contradictions or puzzles in the literature on gender and health is the difficulty of constructing a convincing empirical case that patriarchy and sexism are damaging to women's health.

We know that the patriarchal gender order has disempowering and dehumanizing effects on women in particular. With the influx of American women into the paid labor force, their situation, at least, should be improving. But between 1959 and 1983 the relative economic standing of U.S. women *declined*. Some growth in wages was offset by less leisure, greater financial responsibility for children, and more dependence on their own incomes; as a result, overall and relative to men, they enjoyed 4–15 percent less access to goods, leisure, and services in 1983 than in 1959 (Fuchs, 1986).

The argument that these sex-based inequalities are harmful to health is supported by women's heavier burden of acute and chronic disabling conditions, higher rates of mental illness, and greater use of medical care. At the same time, the argument is deeply undermined by women's longer lifespans and lower age-adjusted rates of most life-threatening diseases, and by the inference from their greater utilization of medical services that they have easier access to care then men do. This hardly sounds like the profile of a downtrodden group. Without the comparison point of a nonpatriarchal society, one can speculate that women have a biological mortality advantage that is being eroded by sexism—that the sex-mortality ratio would be even wider in a more egalitarian society. But this proposition is difficult or impossible to test convincingly. The usefulness of broad comparative studies of men and women is inherently undermined by the pervasiveness of patriarchy across space and time.

The smoking case shows, first and foremost, that analyses of gender and health have to be historically and culturally specific and have to take account of interactions between gender and class, however class is defined. At the same time, it sheds light on the more global question of why male domination appears not to have put women at a relative disadvantage for early mortality. It demonstrates how women's smoking behavior—the risk factor to which epidemiologists attribute much of the gender differential in longevity—has been shaped in very complex ways by patriarchy. Paradoxically, women's social disadvantage in the era when smoking first became popular turned into a major health advantage: the social discrimination that restricted women's access to cigarettes before it was understood that tobacco was lethal mitigated the effect of smoking on women's mortality. By the time women's social power had begun to expand, it was becoming clear that smoking was a serious health risk, and women have yet to catch up to men in their overall smoking rates.

As the harmful effects of smoking have become known, the patterns of smoking behavior have gradually shifted. These shifts shape and are shaped by local regimes. The economic forces affecting the manufacture, marketing, regulation, and taxation of tobacco products are the fundamental forces. Changing occupational structures of the labor force and evolving rules about working and smoking have an influence, as do cost pressures on the public and private medical and welfare systems. There is a cultural lag in some ethnic subgroups, where gender gaps remain very wide. School-based educational programs and prohibitions are affecting smoking norms, as is the greater willingness to restrict smoking as it has become marginalized in subgroups with little socioeconomic and political power. The society-and-health perspective looks to these broad social forces for explanations of the ways in which cigarette smoking interacts with relationships between gender and health. Such an analysis is illuminating but where does it lead?

Implications for Research and Action

The biological and psychosocial lenses remain focused at the level of the individual. Even the more wide-angle epidemiological lens assigns behavioral and psychological factors to a strategic position as mediators between social location and relative risk. Conventional epidemiological models tend to test for psychological and behavioral factors as suspected risks and to control for the effects of social constructs like gender, race/ethnicity, and class. The central assumption that pervades the literature on gender and health is that the most fundamental and useful explanations for health differences between women and men are properties of individuals. This assumption has led to programs that emphasize voluntary individual action to promote improvements in health.

Public health interventions, including those directed at smoking, have faltered or failed when they have ignored the social environment. Health promotion initiatives that ignore contextual factors are plagued by high recidivism, refusal rates, and dropout rates because they demand concerted and sustained personal effort without providing adequate environmental and social support. But strategies that rail at large structural inequities without proposing practical programs of social change seem equally futile. In raising questions about how the social structures limit the range of personal choice, and about how people in their daily practice can and do maneuver within these structures and even sometimes force them to change, Connell's thinking may suggest a middle course between the two extremes of structural determinism and thwarted individualism.

With regard to smoking, epidemiological research has made enormous strides in sorting data on the health of large-scale populations and specifying the ways in which exposure to tobacco smoke poses risks to health. Left largely unexplored, though, is why smoking patterns are distributed as they are within population subgroups. Our cursory examination of changing smoking patterns demonstrates how consistently social variables (like gender, education, and social class) have influenced the distribution of this "risk factor" within populations. To date research on smoking and health has either given short shrift to these social factors or has merely controlled for their effects.

What we need now are studies that seek to conceptualize and measure the important social variables, and to trace how they produce differential rates of smoking initiation, maintenance, and cessation. A better understanding of the mechanisms will lead to more effective action plans. Macro-level investigation is needed of forces that divert resources and priorities away from aggressive and effective public policies of prevention for the many, into high-technology late-stage medical treatment for the few. We need studies of the forces that reinforce the tendency to assign the causes of illness to individuals, stigmatizing victims and deterring them from fighting the problem on a social or political plane. Most of all, we need elegant intervention and policy research that systematically tests alternative strategies for mobilizing social power in local gender regimes. We need strategic efforts to understand and to change the social structures—especially the power arrangements—that place disadvantaged groups (whether lower-class women at the turn of the century or high-school dropouts now) at higher risk for cigarette smoking and a vast array of socially generated and socially reinforced threats to their health, their dignity, their communities, and their quality of life.

References

Allison, G. 1971. *Essence of Decision: Explaining the Cuban Missile Crisis.* Boston: Little Brown.

Aneshensel, C. S., and L. I. Pearlin. 1987. Structural contexts of sex differences in stress. In R. C. Barnett, L. Biener, and G. K. Baruch (eds.), *Gender and Stress*, pp. 75–94. New York: Free Press.

Aulette, J. 1991. Gender and power: Society, the person and sexual politics. *Soc. Forces* 69:953–954.

Ayanian, J., and A. Epstein. 1991. Differences in procedures between men and women hospitalized for coronary artery disease. *N. Engl. J. Med.* 325:221–225.

Attie, I., and J. Brooks-Gun. 1987. Weight concerns as chronic stressors in women. In R. C. Barnett, L. Biener, and G. K. Baruch (eds.), *Gender and Stress*, pp. 219–256. New York: Free Press.

Bandura, A. 1986. *Social Foundations of Thought and Action: A Social Cognitive Theory.* Englewood Cliffs, NJ: Prentice-Hall.

Barnett, R. C., L. Biener, and G. K. Baruch (eds.). 1987. *Gender and Stress.* New York: Free Press.

Barton, J., L. Chassin, C. C. Presson, and S. J. Sherman. 1982. Social image factors as motivators of smoking initiation in early and middle adolescence. *Child Dev* 53:1499–1511.

Berkman, L. 1984. Assessing the physical health effects of social networks and social support. *Ann. Rev. Public Health* 5:413–32.

Berman, A. 1987. Women's smoking behavior: A summary. Smoking Behavior and Policy Discussion Paper Series. Harvard University, J.F. Kennedy School of Government, Institute for the Study of Smoking Behavior and Policy. Cambridge, MA.

Bird, C., and A. M. Fremont. 1991. Gender, time use and health. *J. Health Soc. Behav.* 32:114–129.

Blake, S. M., K. I. Klepp, T. F. Pechacek. 1989. Differences in smoking cessation strategies between men and women. *Addict. Behav.* 14:409–418.

Bond, G. G., E. A. McLaren, J. B. Cartmill, K. T. Wymer, T. E. Lipps, and R. R. Cook. 1987. Mortality among female employees of a chemical company. *Am. J. Ind. Med.* 12:563–578.

Bowerman, W. G. 1950. Annuity mortality. *Actuarial Society of America Transactions* 2:76–102.

Canning, H., and J. Mayer. 1966. Obesity: Its possible effect on college acceptance. *N. Engl. J. Med.* 275:1172–1174.

Centers for Disease Control. 1992. Cigarette smoking among adults—United States, 1990. *M.M.W.R.* 41:354–362.

Chesser, P. 1972. *Women and Madness.* New York: Doubleday.

Cleary, P. D. 1987. Gender Differences in stress-related disorders. In R. C. Barnett, L. Biener, and G.K. Baruch (eds.), *Gender and Stress*, pp. 39–74. New York: Free Press.

Connell, R. W. 1987. *Gender and Power.* Stanford, CA: Stanford University Press.

Davis, R. 1987. Current trends in cigarette advertising and marketing. *New Engl. J. Med.* 316:725–732.

De Beauvoir, S. 1949. *The Second Sex* (reprinted 1972). Harmondsworth: Penguin.

Dorfman, S. 1987. Tobacco, Women, and Health. In *Proceedings of Not Far Enough: Women vs. Smoking.* A Workshop For Women's Group and Women's Health Leaders, pp. 11–14. Boston, MA: Harvard University Institute for the Study of Smoking Behavior and Policy.

Ehrenreich, B., and D. English. 1973. *Complaints and Disorders: The Sexual Politics of Sickness*, Glass Mountain Pamphlet No. 2. New York: The Feminist Press.

Elkind, A. K. 1985. The social definition of women's smoking behavior. *Soc. Sci. Med.* 20:1269–1278.

Engels, F. 1884. *The Origin of the Family, Private Property, and the State* (trans. by Evelyn Reed, 1972). New York: Pathfinder.

Enterline, P.E. 1961. Causes of death responsible for recent increases in sex mortality differentials in the United States. *Milbank Q.* 39:312–322.

Ernster, V. L. 1987. Mixed messages for women: A social history of cigarette smoking and advertising. In *Proceedings of Not Far Enough: Women vs. Smoking.* A Workshop for Women's Group and Women's Health Leaders, pp. 4–10. Boston, MA: Harvard University Institute for the Study of Smoking Behavior and Policy.

Ferrence, R. G. 1988. Sex differences in cigarette smoking in Canada, 1900–1978: A reconstructed cohort study. *Can. J. Public Health* 79:160–165.

Fiore, M. C., T. E. Novotny, J. P. Pierce, E. J. Hatziandreu, K. M. Patel, and R. M. Davis. 1989. Trends in cigarette smoking in the United States—the changing influence of gender and race. *JAMA* 261:49–55.

French, M. 1992. *The War Against Women.* New York: Summit Books.

Frenk, J., J. L. Bobadilla, C. Stern, T. Frejka, and R. Lozano. 1991. Elements for a theory of the health transition. *Health Transition Rev.* 1:21–38.

Froberg, D. 1986. Multiple roles and women's mental and physical health: What have we learned? *Women and Health 11*:79–96.

Fuchs, V. R. 1986. Sex differences in economic wellbeing. *Science* 232:459–464.

Gelpi, A. C. 1975. *Adrienne Rich's Poetry: Texts of Poems, the Poet on Her Work; Reviews and Criticisms*, New York: Norton.

Gilchrist, L. D., S. P. Schinke, and P. Nurious. 1989. Reducing onset of habitual smoking among women. *Prev. Med.* 18:235–248.

Gore, S. 1989. Social supports and social networks in health care. In H. Freeman and S. Levine (eds.), *The Handbook of Medical Sociology*, 4th Edn.; pp. 306–331. Englewood Cliffs, NJ: Prentice-Hall.

Gove, W. R. 1973. Sex, marital status and mortality. *Am. J. Soc.* 79:45–67.

Gove, W. and M. Hughes. 1979. Possible causes of the apparent sex differences in physical health: An empirical investigation. *Am. Soc. Rev.* 44:126–146.

Gritz, E. R. 1987. Which women smoke and why? In *Proceedings of Not Far Enough: Women vs. Smoking.* A Workshop for Women's Group and Women's Health Leaders, pp. 15–19. Boston, MA: Harvard University Institute for the Study of Smoking Behavior and Policy.

Haenszel, W., M. B. Shimkin, and H.P. Miller. 1956. *Tobacco Smoking Patterns in the United States.* U.S. Department of Health, Education, and Welfare, Public Health Service, Monograph No. 45, Washington DC: U.S. Government.

Hall, E. 1991. Gender, work control and stress. A theoretical discussion and an empirical test. In J.V. Johnson and G. Johansson (eds.), *The Psychosocial Work Environment: Work Organization, Democratization and Health*, pp. 89–108. Amityville, NY: Baywood.

Hall, E. 1992. Double exposure: The combined impact of the home and work environments on psychosomatic strain in Swedish men and women. *Int. J. Health Serv.* 22:239–260.

Haynes, S. G., J. Odenkirchen, and J. Heimendinger, 1990. Worksite health promotion for cancer control. *Seminars in Oncology* 17:463–484.

Hochschild, A. 1989. *The Second Shift.* New York: Viking.

Huselid, R. F., and M. L. Cooper. 1992. Gender roles as mediators of sex differences in adolescent alcohol use and abuse. *J. Health and Soc. Behavior* 33:348–362.

Institute of Medicine. 1985. *Preventing Low Birthweight.* Committee to Study the Prevention of Low Birthweight. Division of Health Promotion and Disease Prevention. Washington, DC: National Academy Press.

Karasek, R., T. Theorell. 1990. *Healthy Work: Stress, Productivity and the Reconstruction of Working Life.* New York: Basic Books.

Klitzman, S., B. Silverstein, L. Punnett, A. Mock. 1990. A women's occupational health agenda for the 1990's. *New Solutions* 1:7–17.

LaCroix, A. Z., and S. G. Haynes. 1987. Social roles, gender, and psychological distress. In R. C. Barnett, L. Biener, and G. K. Baruch (eds.), *Gender and Stress*, pp. 96–121. New York: Free Press.

LaRosa, J. H. 1986. Cholesterol and smoking education programs—applications to the workplace. *AAOHN* 34:326–32.

Madigan, F. C. 1957. Are sex mortality differentials biologically caused? *Milbank Q.* 35:202–225.

Mannino, D. M., R.M. Klevens, and W. D. Flanders. 1994. Cigarette smoking: An independent risk factor for impotence? *Am. J. Epidem.* 140:1003–1008.

Mitchell, J. 1971. *Woman's Estate,* New York: Pantheon.

Moser, K. A., H.S. Pugh, and P.O. Goldblatt. 1988. Inequalities in women's health: Looking at mortality differentials using an alternative approach. *Br. Med. J.* 296:1221–1224.

Nathanson, C. A. 1975. Illness and the feminine role: A theoretical review. *Soc. Sci. Med.* 9:577–62.

Pearce, D. 1978. The feminization of poverty: Women, work, and welfare. *Urban Soc. Change Rev.* 11:28–36.

Pierce, J. P., M. C. Fiore, T.E. Novotny, E. J. Hatziandreu, and R. M. Davis. 1989. Trends in cigarette smoking in the United States—Educational differences are increasing. *JAMA* 261:56–60.

Rich, A. 1979. *On Lies, Secrets, and Silence: Selected Prose 1966–1978.* New York: Norton.

Rodin, J. and J. R. Ickovics. 1990. Women's health: Review and research agenda as we approach the 21st century. *Am. Psychol.* 45:1018–1034.

Rodriguez-Trias, H. 1984. The women's health movement: Women take power. In W. Victor and R. Sidel (eds.), *Reforming Medicine*, pp. 107–128. New York: Pantheon.

Rogers, E. 1983. *Diffusion of Innovations.* New York: Free Press.

Roter, D., M. Lipkin, and A. Korssgaardd. 1991. Sex differences in patients and physicians' communication during primary care visits. *Med. Care* 29:1083–1093.

Rothblum, E. D. 1990. Women and weight: Fad or fiction. *J. Psychol.* 124:5–24.

Rowley, B. D., D. C. Baldwin, Jr., and M. McGuire. 1991. Selected characteristics of graduate medical education in the United States. *JAMA* 266:933–943.

Schelling, T. C. 1992. Addictive drugs: The cigarette experience. *Science.* 255:430–433.

Sidel, R. 1986. *Women and Children Last.* New York: Penguin.

Sorensen, G. and L. M. Verbrugge. 1987. Women, work and health. *Annu. Rev. Public Health* 8:235–251.

Stallones, R. A. 1980. To advance epidemiology. *Ann. Rev. Public Health* 1:69–82.

Steingaart, R. 1991. Sex differences in the management of coronary artery disease. *N. Engl. J. Med.* 325:226–230.

Stellman, J. M. 1984. Personal protective equipment for women. In D. A. Atwood and C. McCann (eds.), *Proceedings of the International Conference on Ergonomics*, Vol. 1.

Syme, S. L. 1991. Social epidemiology and the work environment. In J. V. Johnson and G. Johansson (eds.), *The Psychosocial Work Environment: Work Organization, Democratization and Health*, pp. 21–31. Amityville, N.Y.: Baywood.

Umberson, D., C. B. Wortman, and R. C. Kessler. 1992. Widowhood and depression: Explaining gender differences in vulnerability. *J. Health Soc. Beh.* 33:10–24.

U.S. Bureau of Census. 1992. Statistical Abstract of the United States (112th edition), Washington, DC: U.S. Government.

U.S. Department of Health, Education and Welfare. 1964. *Surgeon General's Report on Smoking and Health*. Report of the Advisory Committee to the Surgeon General. Washington DC: U.S. Public Health Service.

U.S. Department of Health and Human Services. 1980. *The Health Consequences of Smoking for Women*. A Report of the Surgeon General. USDHHS, Public Health Service, Office on Smoking and Health, p. 47.

U.S. Department of Health and Human Services. 1989. *Reducing the Health Consequences of Smoking: 25 Years of Progress*. A Report of the Surgeon General. USDHHS, Public Health Service. Washington, DC: U.S. Government.

U.S. Department of Labor. 1994. *Employment and Earnings*. Bureau of Labor Statistics, U.S. Department of Labor, Washington, DC: U.S. Government.

Tesh, S. N. 1988. *Hidden Arguments*. New Haven: Yale University Press.

Verbrugge, L. M. 1976a. Sex differentials in morbidity and mortality in the United States. *Soc. Biol.* 23:275–296.

Verbrugge, L. M. 1976b. Females and illness: Recent trends in sex differences in the United States. *J. Health Soc. Behav.* 17:387–403.

Verbrugge, L. M. 1978. Sex and gender in health and medicine. *Soc. Sci. Med.* 12:329–333.

Verbrugge, L. M. 1979. Female illness rates and illness behavior: Testing hypotheses about sex differences in health. *Women Health* 4:61–79.

Verbrugge, L. M. 1980a. Comment on Gove and Hughes, 1979. *Am. Soc. Rev.* 45:507–513.

Verbrugge, L. M. 1980b. Recent trends in sex mortality differentials in the United States. *Women Health* 5:17–37.

Verbrugge, L. M. 1982a. Sex differentials in health. *Public Health Rep.* 97:417–437.

Verbrugge, L. M. 1982b. Sex differences in legal drug use. *Journal of Social Issues* 38:59–76.

Verbrugge, L. M. 1983a. Multiple roles and physical health of women and men. *J. Health Soc. Behav.* 24:16–30.

Verbrugge, L. M. 1983b. Women and men: Mortality and health of older people. In M. W. Riley, B. B. Hess, and K. Bond (eds.), *Aging in Society: Selected Reviews of Recent Research*, pp. 139–174. Hillsdale, NJ: Lawrence Erlbaum.

Verbrugge, L. M. 1985a. Gender and health: An update on hypotheses and evidence. *J. Health Soc. Behav.* 26:156–182.

Verbrugge, L. M. 1985b. Triggers of symptoms and health care. *Soc. Sci. Med.* 20:855–876.

Verbrugge, L. M. 1986. Role burdens and physical health of women and men. *Women Health* 11:47–77.

Verbrugge, L. M. 1988. Unveiling higher morbidity for men: The story. In M. W. Riley (ed.), *Social Structures in Human Lives*, Vol. 1, *Social Change and the Life Course*, pp. 138–160. Newbury Park, CA: Sage.

Verbrugge, L. M. 1989. The twain meet: Empirical explanations of sex differences in health and mortality. *J. Health Soc. Behav.* 30:282–304.

Verbrugge, L. M., and J. H. Madans. 1985. Social roles and health trends of American women. *Milbank Q.* 63:691–735.

Verbrugge, L. M., and R. P. Steiner. 1981. Physician treatment of men and women patients—sex bias or appropriate care? *Med. Care* 12:103–145.

Verbrugge, L. M., and D. L. Wingard. 1987. Sex differentials in health and mortality. *Women Health* 12:103–145.

Waldron, I. 1976. Why do women live longer than men? *Soc. Sci. Med.* 10:349–362.

Waldron, I. 1982. An analysis of causes of sex differences in mortality and morbidity. In W. R. Gove and G. R. Carpenter (eds.), *The Fundamental Connection between Nature and Nurture*, pp. 69–115. Lexington, MA: Lexington Books.

Waldron, I. 1983a. Sex differences in human mortality: The role of genetic factors. *Soc. Sci. Med.* 17:321–333.

Waldron, I. 1983b. Sex differences in illness incidence, prognosis, and mortality: Issues and evidence. *Soc. Sci. Med.* 17:1107–1123.

Waldron, I. 1986. The contribution of smoking to sex differences in mortality. *Public Health Rep.* 101:163–173.

Waldron, I. 1991. Patterns and causes of gender differences in smoking. *Soc. Sci. Med.* 9:989–1005.

Waldron, I., J. Herold, D. Dunn, and R. Staum. 1982. Reciprocal effects of health and labor force participation among women: Evidence from two longitudinal studies. *J.O.M.* 24:126–132.

Walsh, D. C., and R. H. Egdahl. 1980. *Women, Work, and Health: Challenge to Corporate Policy.* Heidelberg, Germany: Springer-Verlag.

Walsh, D. C., and N. D. Gordon. 1986. Legal approaches to smoking deterrence. *Ann. Rev. Public Health* 7:127–149.

Warner, K. E. 1986. *Selling Smoke: Cigarette Advertising and Public Health.* Washington, DC: American Public Health Association.

West, C. 1989. Gender and power: Society, the person and sexual politics (book review). *Am. J. Soc.* 94:1487–1489.

Wethington, E., J. D. McLeod, and R. C. Kessler. 1987. The importance of life events for explaining sex differences in psychological distress. In R. C. Barnett, L. Biener, G. K. Baruch (eds.), *Gender and Stress*, pp. 144–158. New York: Free Press.

Wiehl, D. G. 1938. Sex differences in mortality in the United States. *Milbank Q.* 16:145–155.

Wilsnack, R. W., and S. C. Wilsnack. 1978. Sex roles and drinking among adolescent girls. *J. Stud. Alcohol* 39:1855–1874.

Wingard, D. L. 1984. The sex differential in morbidity, mortality and lifestyle. *Ann. Rev. Public Health* 5:433–458.

Wolfe, T. 1987. *Bonfire of the Vanities*, New York: Bantam.

Yankelovich, S. and W. Ino. 1977. A study of cigarette smoking among teenage girls and young women: Summary of the findings. Department of Health, Education and Welfare, U.S. Public Health Service, Department of Health, Education and Welfare, Publication No. (NIH) 77-1203. Washington DC: U.S. Government Printing Office.

Yerushalmy, J. 1943. The age-sex composition of the population resulting from natality and mortality conditions. *Milbank Q.* 21:37–63.

Zola, I. K. 1991. Bringing our bodies and ourselves back in: Reflections on a past, present, and future medical sociology. *J. Health Soc. Behav.* 32:1–16.

6

Explanations for Social Inequalities in Health

MICHAEL MARMOT, MARTIN BOBAK, and GEORGE DAVEY SMITH

Britain's secretary of state for health recently published her strategy for improving health in England, *The Health of the Nation* (Secretary of State for Health, 1992). Among the sillier responses to this publication was one along the line of, "Health is improving anyway—why do we need to take action to improve it further?"

It is true that there have been dramatic across-the-board improvements in life expectancy in industrialized countries. However, two phenomena stand in stark contrast to this general trend: marked divergence in life expectancy among industrialized countries, and persistent, even widening, social inequalities in health within countries. These realities made only fleeting appearances in the British government's health strategy. Gender, ethnic, and regional variations in mortality also persist.

Inequalities in health within and between countries are of profound significance to public health, and hence to society in general. It is important to understand them, both because they may enhance understanding of disease etiology and because improving the health of nations requires that such inequalities be addressed. Our work seeks explanations for social inequalities within countries, but we speculate that inequalities between countries may have a similar set of explanations.

When reviewing this subject five years ago (Marmot et al., 1987), we noted the tendency in the literature to treat social class, or socioeconomic status, as a mere confounding factor. If smoking rates and disease rates both differ among social classes, for instance, the association between smoking rates and disease must be adjusted for the "effects" of social class. As we shall discuss, it may sometimes be appropriate to adjust for social class in order to examine independent effects. Our aim, however, is not to treat social class as a nuisance variable that messes up statistical analysis, but to understand the links between social position and health. In short, it is to trace how the powerful influence of society on health operates, not to explain it away statistically.

The observations that sparked our own interest in this—published as the Whitehall Study of British civil servants (Marmot et al., 1978a)—are illustrative. Conventional wisdom held that heart disease was a disease of stressed business executives; indeed, this was Osler's description (Osler, 1910). Because we were interested in the causes of coronary heart disease, we examined mortality rates using grade of employment as a measure of social position. The results are shown in Figure 6–1, updated from previous reports (Marmot et al., 1984a).

The striking step-wise relation between grade of employment and mortality shown in this figure has influenced our approach to social inequalities. The Whitehall Study consists of a group of people of relatively uniform ethnic background, all employed in stable office-based jobs and not subject to industrial hazards, unemployment, or extremes of poverty or affluence; all live and work in Greater London and adjoining areas. Yet in this relatively homogeneous population, we observed a gradient in mortality—each group experiencing a higher mortality than the one above it in the hierarchy. The difference in mortality between the highest and lowest grades was threefold. The question is not merely why people at the bottom have worse health, but why social differentials in health are spread across the entire society. Our starting position has been that there is no biological reason why those in the lowest grades of the civil service should not enjoy the same health status as those in the highest grade.

A second provocative finding from the Whitehall Study is that social differentials in mortality apply to most of the major causes of death (Marmot et al., 1984a). This observation broadens the explanatory task beyond the one with which we began—the social gradient in coronary heart disease—to the social gradient in a wide variety of other

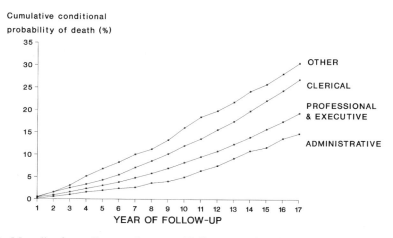

Figure 6-1. Mortality from all causes by year of follow-up and grade of employment, in Whitehall (U.K.) male civil servants, initially aged 40–64. *Source:* Marmot et al., 1991.

diseases. In recent years there has been considerable interest in measuring and, to a lesser degree, understanding social inequalities in health (Baker and Illsley, 1990; Wilkinson, 1986a; Goldblatt, 1990; Fox, 1989; Bunker et al., 1989; Blane et al., 1992a; Blaxter, 1991; Black et al., 1988). We will draw heavily on these reviews and use our own studies to show that inequalities in health persist in a range of countries and in different times. We then discuss the issues of poverty or inequality, and go on to discuss possible explanations. First, however, some introductory observations may be useful.

Are social inequalities an appropriate topic for scientific study? Some have their doubts. One version of this viewpoint is that "the poor are always with us"; in all societies, some are better off than others; if this results in differences in health, there is little that can be done about it. As we shall show, although inequalities in health are widespread, they are not of fixed magnitude. If they can vary, we need to seek reasons for this variation with the ultimate aim of reducing it.

A second objection is that the situation is too complex: the mass of intercorrelated variables will never allow us to sort out explanations for inequalities in health (Secretary of State for Health, 1992). The Black Report (Black, 1988) took the lead in sorting through categories of explanation. Our view is that the situation is complex, but that understanding of possible reasons for inequalities in health has increased.

Inequalities or social inequalities? George Orwell notwithstanding, all people are not born equal. Individual differences in genetic endowment may well contribute to differences in life expectancy. Even if all individuals were subject to the same set of environmental influences, they would not all flourish, age, and die at the same rate. As Rose (1992) has made clear, however, the determinants of individual risks of disease— why one individual gets sick and another remains healthy—may be different from the determinants of population rates of disease. By extension, the causes of social inequalities in health are likely to be different from the causes of individual differences, in which genetic factors will play a bigger role.

Le Grand and Illsley (LeGrand, 1989; Illsley and LeGrand, 1987), for example, have focused on individual differences in life expectancy. Having shown (using Gini coefficients) that variability of age at death has narrowed, they argue that inequality in society has decreased. This focus on individuals, however, is a different topic than the one we address: differences in health among social groups. If the determinants of variations between individuals are different from the determinants of variations among social groups, it is quite possible for there to be no reduction in *relative* differences in health between social groups despite a general improvement in health. If fewer people die prematurely, for instance, variation in age at death will decrease. This reduction, however, may still be distributed unequally across social groups.

There are other sources of inequality in society, among them gender, and race/ethnicity. Gender differences are of great interest and importance but have been treated by others (Chapter 5). In England and Wales at least, ethnic differences in mortality cannot easily be explained on the basis of conventional social class descriptions (Marmot et al., 1984b). There must be other explanations of ethnic differences but these will not be reviewed here.

Equality or equity? Implications for action. The Black Report spoke of "inequalities in health." Subsequent work in this tradition also uses the word *inequality*. The World Health Organization has adopted as its number one target of Health For All 2000, equity in health (World Health Organization, 1986). The term *equity* is commonly used by economists in discussing fair allocation of resources. Why bother with this semantic distinction? Culyer and Wagstaff (1991) argue that it is worth making a distinction between fairness in distributing resources (equity) and equal distribution of health states (relative equality). They specify four approaches to equity in distributing health care:

1. Equality of expenditure per capita
2. Distribution according to need
3. Distribution according to health status
4. Equality of access

The crucial distinction here is between health status and capacity to benefit from health care. In Culyer and Wagstaff's view, people may be sick and untreated but not "in need" of medical care if their conditions, and medical technology, are such that they have no capacity to benefit. They show that applying the principle of equity of distribution of resources according to need may actually increase inequalities in the "outcome" health status. Consider the prognosis of cancer. People of lower socioeconomic status have worse prognoses from cancer than people of higher status (Leon and Wilkinson, 1989). If, as the evidence suggests, this cannot be explained by worse medical care (Kogevinas et al., 1991), delivering the same "amount" of medical care to all patients with the same diagnosis will lead to increased social inequality in the outcome, in this case survival. This is presumably due to some greater capacity to respond to treatment on the part of more advantaged people. (This analysis assumes, of course, that medical care offers some benefit, however defined, in such cases. If it does not, there is no "need" for it.) Anti smoking campaigns, when they have been effective, appear to have resulted in increased social inequalities in smoking rates.

In our opinion, social inequalities in health cannot be explained by inequity in the distribution of health care. Even so, the general point may still be of profound importance. Suppose that what is true of cancer treatment is true of education, and that we define the "outcome" of education as fitness for a career or acquisition of life-management skills. It is possible, indeed likely, that an equity principle, distribution of expenditure on education according to need, may increase social differences in career prospects or life-management skills. Due to differential capacity to benefit, social background will be a potent predictor of outcome (Wadsworth, 1991). In sum, equity in the distribution of certain services will not solve the problem of inequalities in health, unless their root causes are understood and addressed. Without such understanding, action based on an equity principle may well lead to increased inequalities.

Inequalities in health or inequalities in disease? Like almost everyone, we speak of inequalities in health when we mean inequalities in death or disease. Antonovsky (1989) has argued that a clear distinction between the two, and a deliberate focus on health, might lead to a different set of explanations for social inequalities. If health is not merely one end of the spectrum of disease but a different spectrum, the determinants of health may well be different from the determinants of disease. A complete lack of connection between health and disease, and hence no overlap in their determinants is unlikely. Nevertheless, our justification for focusing on disease is in part pragmatic, rather than theoretical. First, large bodies of data exist on disease rates but very little on rates of health. Second, although health may not be merely the absence of disease, absence of disease is a high priority for people and governments throughout the industrialized world.

If we are then to focus on disease, which disease? The most remarkable finding about social inequality is that it interacts with most of the major causes of morbidity and mortality. It also applies throughout the life span. We shall concentrate on adult health, invoking earlier influences only insofar as they affect adult health. The production of social inequalities in health during childhood has been well documented (Power et al., 1991).

Persistent Social Differences in Mortality

Since they were first collected, routine health statistics have been used to demonstrate socioeconomic differentials in mortality in England and Wales. Chadwick reported the average age at death in several occupationally defined groups in 1942 as follows: "gentlemen and persons engaged in professions, and their families . . . 45 years; tradesmen and their families . . . 26 years; mechanics, servants and labourers, and their families . . . 16 years" (Chadwick, 1965). Mortality data on broad occupationally based social-class groups (Pamuk, 1985) have been available since 1921, a unique historical record that demonstrates the persistence of socioeconomic differentials in mortality risk, despite overall improvement in life expectancy.

Table 6–1 shows mortality in England and Wales for men of working age, according to the Registrar General's classification of social classes (Blane, 1992b). This classification standard in British statistics, categorizes occupations according to status and level of responsibility. Standardized mortality ratios (SMRs)[1] allow for comparisons of relative differences in death rates in a given period; they show trends over time in relative differences, not in absolute rates. What these data do not show is that the widening of mortality differentials between the 1930s and the 1980s took place against a background of falling death rates.

When social-class differences in mortality in Sweden are compared with those of

---

1. The SMR is a ratio; each groups mortality rate is compared with a standard England and Wales 100, after adjusting for age differences.

Table 6-1 Mortality[a] of Men Aged 15–64 by Social Class, England and Wales, 1930–1982

Social Class		1930–1932	1949–1953	1959–1963[b]	1970–1972	1979–1980/ 1982–1983[c]
I	Professional	90	86	75	77	66
II	Intermediate	94	92	81	81	76
IIIN	Skilled nonmanual	97	101	100	99	94
IIIM	Skilled manual	97	101	100	106	106
IV	Partly skilled	102	104	103	114	116
V	Unskilled	111	118	127	137	165

a. Standardized mortality ratios, all men = 100.

b. Adjusted figures: occupations reclassified according to 1950 classification.

c. Men aged 20–64. (Note: deaths for 1981 were not collected.)

Source: Blane et al., 1992b.

England and Wales (Vagero and Lundberg, 1989), Sweden exhibits a similar gradient of progressively higher mortality as one descends the social scale, though the gradient appears to be shallower than in England and Wales. Such comparisons are made difficult, however, by possible noncomparability of the classification systems: the social status and material conditions of life of a given occupation may vary between countries.

Potential Problems in Interpretation of Data

Apart from the difficulty of international comparisons, interpreting these data from England and Wales presents several potential problems including lack of comparability between numerator and denominator, changing class composition, and doubt about the appropriateness of Registrar General's social classes and of the classification for women. There is also the question of whether differences in mortality are an effect of belonging to a certain class, or whether degree of healthiness determines both occupational class and mortality risk—selection for class on the basis of health?

The numerator/denominator argument arises because death records are not linked to census data that supply estimates of population at risk (Office of Population Censuses and Surveys, 1978). The recording of occupation, and hence assignment to social class, at death may differ from that at the census, leading to biased estimates of mortality ratios. While this argument may apply to data in the Registrar General's supplements on occupational mortality, it cannot apply to longitudinal studies such as the Whitehall Study (Marmot et al., 1984a) or the Office of Population Censuses and Surveys (OPCS) Longitudinal Study, which follows a 1 percent sample of the census. Comparison of the OPCS Longitudinal Study and the Registrar General's Decennial Supplement "cross-sectional" approach to social inequalities shows that the relative differences between each pair of classes is similar, as is that between the top class and lower class (Office of Population Censuses and Surveys, 1978; Goldblatt, 1990).

A version of the numerator/denominator issue was raised as casting doubt on time trends. It was argued at the time of production of the 1979–1983 Decennial Supplement that the size of the numerator/denominator bias may have changed between 1971 and 1981 (Office of Population Censuses and Surveys, 1986). If, for example, some people whose occupation would have been classified as unskilled manual (Class V) in 1971 were classified as semiskilled (Class IV) in 1981, the apparent size of the denominator in Class V would shrink. If no similar change was imposed on coding of occupation at death, the numerator in Class V would not be reduced in the same way. This discrepancy could account for the apparently increasing relative mortality disadvantage in Class V, from an SMR of 137 to 165.

One way of addressing this issue was simply to combine the three nonmanual and three manual classes into two groups (Marmot and McDowall, 1986). Misclassification of manual and nonmanual is highly unlikely. Analyses confirm that for total mortality and for lung cancer, coronary heart disease and stroke, the social differential in mortality has widened for both men and women (Marmot and McDowall, 1986). Estimates have been calculated using the 1979–1983 rates as standard, allowing comparison of absolute as well as relative changes in mortality over time. Mortality has declined over the 10-year period, while the gap between nonmanual and manual classes has widened. For example, mortality for men from all causes has dropped from 130 to 120 for manual workers, and from 100 to 80 for nonmanual workers, while the relative difference has grown from 30 to 40.

Similar changes have been found in Finland (Valkonen et al., 1990). Using linked data—i.e., death records linked to census information—Valkonen has shown a clear inverse association between an occupation-based measure of social class and mortality. These differences increased over the period 1971–1985 (Fig. 6–2).

Illsley argues that the relatively high death rates of Class V apply to a decreasing proportion of the population, and the low death rates of Class 1 to an increasing proportion (Illsley, 1986; Strong, 1990). It is therefore difficult to assert that inequalities have increased or even changed in magnitude over time. This observation is less applicable to a comparison of manual and nonmanual classes: in 1971, 60 percent of men were in manual occupations; in 1981, 55 percent were. The widening gap in mortality therefore applies to groups of nearly similar size.

Pamuk (1985) dealt with changing class composition and changes in classification over a longer period by reclassifying occupations and constructing an index of inequality that takes into account both relative mortality and the relative sizes of classes. She concluded that class inequality in mortality in England and Wales narrowed in the 1920s and increased again during the 1950s and 1960s, such that by the early 1970s it was greater than it had been early in the century in both absolute and relative terms.

The question of the extent to which this social gradient in mortality could be produced by selective social mobility will be dealt with more fully in a later section, as well the appropriateness of the classification for women.

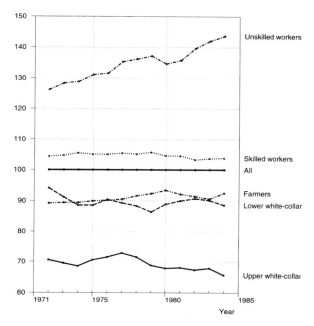

Figure 6-2. Relative probability of death by occupational class in Finland, 3-year moving averages, men aged 35–64 (all men = 100). *Source:* Valkonen et al., 1990.

Measures of Social Differences in Mortality

Occupation-Based Measures of Class

The customary British approach to social-class analysis, using the Registrar General's classification of occupations, has also been subject to other criticism (Bunker et al., 1989; Illsley, 1986; Strong, 1990). The measure is said to lack theoretical content—that is, it is not clear what it signifies. It may not apply to people outside the labor force: people below working age have to be classified by their parents' occupation, and those who are retired, or otherwise unemployed, by their previous employment. And women may not be well classified, especially housewives.

These issues have been comprehensively addressed by the OPCS Longitudinal Study (Goldblatt, 1990). Goldblatt notes that the classification was developed by Stevenson for the 1921 Decennial Supplement on Occupational Mortality (Stevenson, 1928) to indicate way of life. He quotes Stevenson (Goldblatt, 1990):

Classification of individuals by income was not possible under present conditions in this country, though it had been employed on a very limited scale in America. Estimation of poverty by housing conditions was very unsatisfactory, as bad housing was only one of the handicaps of poverty, so that it was impossible to determine how far the excess of mortality associated with bad housing was due to poverty and how far to the direct effects of overcrowding, etc. Even if full details of income were available, these in themselves would not provide an ideal basis for classification, as it was probably the cultural associations of wealth which promoted longevity rather than wealth itself. The method advocated for meeting the conditions to be considered was that of inferring social position from occupation. By this means regard could be paid to (average) culture as well as income. (Stevenson, 1928)

This passage contains the seeds of arguments that continue to flourish: the extent to which we should be seeking to measure material well-being or lifestyle—"culture," in Stevenson's terms; and the degree to which we want a measure of poverty or of social position more generally.

Social Class and Household Measures of Social Circumstances

Classification based on occupation has served well to predict differences in mortality across the social spectrum, as shown in Table 6–1. The OPCS Longitudinal Study, which has been following a 1 percent sample of the 1971 census has explored the use of this and other methods of social classification based on the material conditions of households: housing tenure and access to cars. Both measures are strongly related to household income. The relation of these measures to mortality in men aged 15–64 is shown in Table 6–2 (Goldblatt, 1990): social class, housing tenure, and access to cars all predict mortality.

One criticism of current analyses of social class is that in this type of analysis the extremes of mortality apply to small groups of the population. Indeed, Table 6–2 shows that the SMR of 67 in Class 1 applies to only 5 percent of the expected deaths; the SMR of 125 in Class V applies to only 7 percent. The analysis by access to cars deals with this criticism: the SMR of 122 for those with no access to cars applies to 33 percent of deaths.

The Longitudinal Study also addressed the question of applying social classifications to people of different ages. Figure 6–3 shows that each of the three measures—social class, housing tenure, and access to cars—makes an independent contribution to the prediction of mortality at working age, and that each continues to predict beyond working age (Goldblatt, 1990). Lack of access to a car is less predictive at age 75 and above, in keeping with the low percentage of people with access to a car beyond age 75.

Applying Measures of Social Classification to Women

Using the Registrar General's social classes to examine mortality among women is more problematic. Married women who are not employed outside the home are classi-

Table 6-2 Mortality of Men Aged 15–64 by Alternative Social Classifications, 1976–1981

Social Classification	SMR	(%)[a]	SMR	(%)[a]	SMR	(%)[a]
Occupation-based						
Social class[b]						
I	67	(5)				
II	77	(20)	75	(24)	84	(35)
IIIN	105	(10)				
IIIM	96	(37)				
IV	109	(17)				
V	125	(7)	114	(24)	103	(61)
Other	189	(4)				
Household-based						
Private households						
Tenure						
Owner-occupied	85	(51)				
Privately rented	108	(16)	114	(47)		
Local authority	117	(31)				
Car access						
Two or more	77	(15)				
One	90	50	87	(65)		
None	122	(33)				
Non-private households	162	(2)				
All men aged 15–64	100	(100)				

a. Figures in parentheses represent percentages of expected deaths attributed to each group.

b. Classification as in Table 6–1.

Source: Goldblatt, 1990

fied provocatively, as "unoccupied," and are therefore difficult to assign to a social class. Furthermore, if occupational class is supposed to provide a guide to culture as well as income, as Stevenson posited, a married woman's occupation will provide only part of the picture. The family's circumstances will more often be misclassified if only the woman's occupation is known than if only the man's is known. Figure 6–4 shows that, for married women, social class based on husband's occupation predicts mortality better than social class based on the woman's own occupation (Moser et al., 1990). According to the figures showing proportions of expected deaths, approximately 41 percent of deaths are expected to befall women who are "unoccupied" (mostly housewives). Husband's social class predicts mortality more strongly among these women, than among other women. For single women, their own social class is a powerful predictor. For example, the SMR among such women in nonmanual occupations is 81, and among manual occupations it is 156 (not shown in the figure).

Housing tenure and access to cars predict mortality both at working age, and among older women, showing an overall pattern similar to men's. One feature of these measures for use with women is that they do not require a distinction between married and unmarried women (Goldblatt, 1990). As in the case of men, they also distinguish mortality differences among groups that make up large proportions of the total population.

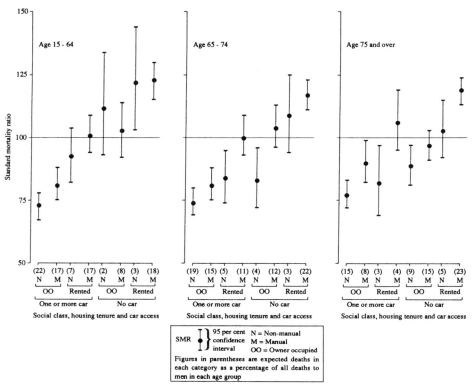

Figure 6-3. Mortality of men by social class, housing tenure, access to cars and and age at death, 1976–1981. Longitudinal study, England and Wales. *Source:* Goldblatt, 1990.

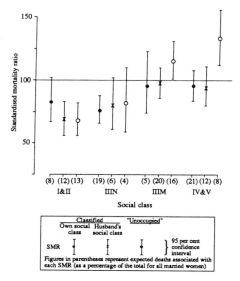

Figure 6-4. Mortality in 1976–1981 among married women aged 15–59 by (a) own social class and (b) husband's social class, for those with a classified occupation, and by (c) husband's social class for those "unoccupied" in 1971. *Source:* Moser et al., 1990.

Education

Another approach to measurement of the social gradient in mortality is to use education as a predictor. Valkonen (1989), has used education to compare socioeconomic
differences in mortality in various European countries in the 1970s (Fig. 6–5). For
men, the slope of the relation is remarkably similar in Scandinavian countries, in England and Wales, and in Hungary: the more years of education, the lower the mortality
rate. The relationship is similar among women, but the slope of the lines varies. With
regard to education as well as social class based on occupation, a woman's material income and wealth tend to be determined not only by her own characteristics but also by
her husband's. The degree to which this is so may vary from country to country and
this variation accounts to some extent for the variation in slopes.

Valkonen (1989) points out that the apparently fixed nature of the relationship between education and mortality for men should not be taken as a general rule. The slope
became steeper in England and Wales, for instance, between 1971–1975 and
1976–1981. This observation is consistent with the findings occupational social class
(Marmot et al., 1987).

Similar findings come from the United States. Kitagawa and Hauser found a strong
and consistent inverse association between education and mortality in the 1960s (Kitagawa and Hauser, 1973). More recently, Feldman and colleagues (1989) showed that
the decline in mortality in the United States varied substantially by education: the more
years of education, the steeper the decline in death rates for three age groups (55–64,
65–74, 75–84).

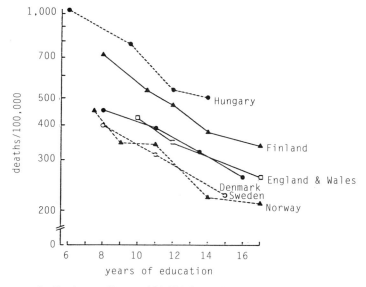

Figure 6-5. Age-standardized mortality per 100,000 from all causes of death by years of education and country, males aged 35–54, log scale. *Source:* Valkonen, 1989.

Area-Based Measures of Material Circumstances

A very different approach to measuring inequalities in health is to classify areas rather than individuals. To some extent area-based measures have been used as a proxy for individual-based measures, where the latter are not available. The use of such measures has also been justified on theoretical grounds. Townsend, one of the authors of the Black Report, developed census-based measures of social deprivation specifically to examine the effect on mortality of material circumstances (Townsend et al., 1988). His index of deprivation consisted of the proportion of households with access to cars, percent unemployed, percent of owner-occupiers, and crowding. In the Northern Region of England, this measure was strongly related to mortality: the greater the deprivation, the greater the mortality (Townsend et al., 1988). In Scotland, a similar measure of deprivation was strongly related to area differences in mortality (Carstairs and Morris, 1991).

We have applied the Townsend measure of deprivation to census tracts (population approximately 7,000) throughout England (Eames et al., 1993). The relationship of deprivation scores to mortality from all causes is shown in Figure 6–6. The figure illustrates the continuous relationship between deprivation and mortality: the more deprived have higher mortality. There are alternative interpretations of this gradient in the relationship of deprivation to mortality. One interpretation is that deprivation is a misleading term and that, as in the case of data on occupation-based social class, we

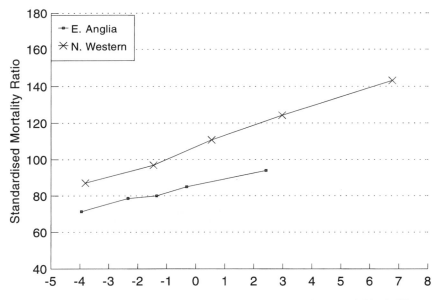

Figure 6-6. Mortality from all causes for males in two regions of England, North Western and East Anglia. *Source:* Eames et al., 1993.

are dealing not with the effects of poverty but with relative social position—that is, there is a social gradient in mortality. According to this interpretation, most residents of wards classified in the second or third quintiles in Figure 6–6 are not deprived, yet their mortality rate is higher than that of people in the least-deprived quintile. This interpretation suggests that relative deprivation is being measured rather than absolute material disadvantage.

An alternative interpretation posits a dichotomy between deprived and nondeprived: above the threshold of deprivation, mortality is elevated relative to below the threshold. This interpretation would suggest that each successive quintile contains a greater proportion of deprived households with higher mortality rates, hence the appearance of a gradient in mortality. It is not easy to distinguish between these two interpretations on the basis of ecological studies. Nevertheless, the studies based on classification of individuals, reviewed above, suggest strongly that the relationship between social position and mortality is graded and not a threshold effect.

A second observation drawn from Figure 6–6 involves regional differences in mortality within England. The North Western Region has higher mortality than East Anglia, and a greater range of deprivation, yet the regional difference in mortality persists at comparable levels of deprivation. Furthermore, the slope of the relationship between deprivation and mortality appears to differ between regions. This observation suggests that the "meaning" of the deprivation index differs depending on the context, or that some other factor(s) modifies the effect of deprivation on mortality within a given region, and contributes to regional differences in mortality independent of deprivation.

These area-based studies may be important for reasons other than the insight they provide into the socioeconomic status of individual residents. The Human Population Laboratory in Alameda County, California, has shown that people living in a poor area experienced a higher mortality rate than people living in nonpoor areas, independent of a wide range of personal characteristics including income and health behaviors (Haan et al., 1987).

Choosing Between Measures

Stevenson based his social-class measure on occupation because he wanted it to signify status in the community: a mixture of material conditions and culture. To the alternative methods of classifying social position discussed above, we should add income, commonly used in the United States (Bunker et al., 1989). How are we to choose between measures? There are two types of criteria: prediction and explanation.

Let us take prediction first. The OPCS Longitudinal Study shows that household measures—housing tenure and access to cars—predict mortality independent of social class and are more appropriate for married women. Education also predicts mortality. As Valkonen and colleagues (1990) discuss with reference to Finland, where a majority of the middle-aged population falls into a single educational category, education distinguishes better among higher-status groups than lower-status groups. A similar consideration limits the use of education in census-based studies in Britain (Goldblatt, 1990).

The question of the best socioeconomic predictor is a pragmatic one, and will be answered differently depending on circumstances. In the special circumstances of the Whitehall Study, for example, employment grade serves as a precise social classification that is a powerful predictor of mortality. This particular measure is highly correlated with salary and material conditions, such as housing tenure and access to cars (Davey Smith et al., 1990), and with "culture" as well as years of education.

These correlations raise the more difficult question of explanation. One should be wary of the temptation to use a standard multivariate analysis as a way of determining which of a number of socioeconomic indicators is most important in the causal network (Marmot, 1989). For example, suppose mortality were analyzed using a statistical model in which the predictors (independent variables) included education, social class (based on occupation), housing, cars, income, and area deprivation score. Years of education might demonstrate the strongest ability to predict value simply because it was measured more precisely than the others. One should be wary of concluding that education offers the best prospects for intervention to reduce social inequalities. Education may be a precise marker of social position and hence good as a predictor, but may not itself be a determinant of health status. We will look further at the question of explanations in a later section.

International Variations in Mortality

We in developed countries have grown accustomed to the expectation that health will improve continually. Mortality statistics from WHO for men and women aged 30–69 (Uemura and Pisa, 1988) and figures for life expectancy at birth (World Bank, 1991) show that this expectation is justified in most countries, although there is significant heterogeneity. The main exceptions are the postcommunist countries of Central and Eastern Europe. Between 1965 and 1989, life expectancy for men increased by 1 year in Czechoslovakia and Poland, and not at all in Hungary; the decline in infant mortality was counterbalanced by the rise in mortality from chronic diseases mainly cardiovascular disease, in middle age. In the same period, by contrast, life expectancy in men improved by 4 years in neighboring Austria, 5 years in the United Kingdom, and an astonishing 8 years in Japan. Japan now has the longest life expectancy in the world: 76 years for men and 82 for women. It appears from these data that inequalities in mortality are increasing internationally just as they are within countries.

In developed countries, trends in mortality from all causes will, by and large, be duplicated in trends in mortality from the major chronic diseases. In the Whitehall Study, for example, grade of employment showed an inverse association with most major causes of death (Marmot et al., 1984a). National variations in this pattern, however, may prove enlightening. Leclerc (1984, 1989) compared mortality by occupational class in France and in England and Wales. The magnitude of the relative difference between unskilled and higher-status workers varies with different causes. Cirrhosis of the liver is the disease that most sharply distinguishes the French mortality data from the English: mortality from cirrhosis is about 15 times higher in France than in England and Wales, and it is the disease with the steepest social gradient in France. Similarly, mortality from respiratory disease is high in England and Wales compared to France and most other European countries, and it is the disease with the steepest social gradient in England and Wales. These international differences in disease-specific mortality rates are probably related to environment and lifestyle. It is therefore interesting to speculate that the same factors that account for international variation in disease rates account for the social variation within countries.

Coronary Heart Disease as an Illustration of the Influence of Social Change on Disease

Although coronary heart disease (CHD) currently fits this pattern at higher rates in lower socioeconomic groups, there is evidence that the pattern has changed. As CHD rose to epidemic proportions in England and Wales, it first affected the higher classes disproportionately (Marmot et al., 1978a). The subsequent decline in CHD appears to have begun first in the same classes (Marmot and McDowall, 1986). A similar pattern had been observed for peptic ulcer (Susser and Stein, 1962).

Other countries report a similar pattern (Mackenbach and Kunst, 1992; Vagero and Lundberg, 1992). The overall pattern can be ideally illustrated as in Figure 6–7. As the rate of CHD rises, it appears to affect those of higher socioeconomic status first; at an intermediate stage, there is little social-class difference; subsequently there is an inverse association with social position. Data from Hong Kong (Wong and Donnan, 1992), Puerto Rico (Sorlie and Garcia-Palmieri, 1990), and India (Sarvotham and Berry, 1968) show higher rates of CHD in higher-income groups. These countries are, presumably, at the left-hand side of the curve. Poland, which has shown a marked increase in CHD mortality, also shows a slightly higher mortality rate in groups with more education (Krzyzanowski and Wysocki, 1986). England and Wales occupied the flat part of the curve between the early 1950s and the 1960s. The social-class transition actually began before the overall mortality rate began to fall, but the decline in mortality appeared first in higher-status groups in both England (Marmot and McDowall, 1986) and the United States (Feldman et al., 1989).

As is true of mortality from all causes, inequalities within countries are paralleled by inequalities between countries. Thom (1989) has demonstrated marked divergence in trends in CHD mortality among European countries for both men and women. Figure 6–8 lists CHD death rates for men. The countries of the West show decreases, while the countries of Central and Eastern Europe—at the time under Communist governments—all show increases (Uemura and Pisa, 1988).

A comparison of mortality from CHD at one point in time replicates the pattern

CHD MORTALITY

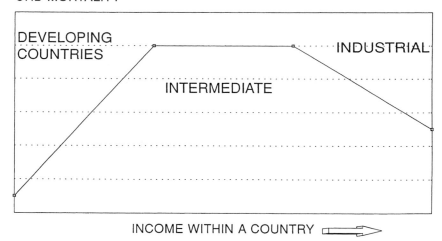

Figure 6-7. An idealized model of the relationship between income and mortality from coronary heart disease.

shown in Figure 6–7. In Figure 6–9, we have divided countries into those with per-capita GNP above and below $6,000. As an index of prosperity, we have used the proportion of total household income not spent on food. In countries with low average incomes, there is a positive relation between prosperity and CHD rates. Among higher-income countries, there is little relationship (Feachem et al., 1992; World Bank, 1992).

These results support the hypothesis that inequalities between countries and within countries share a common set of factors. Before discussing what these factors might be, let us consider a framework for examining these international trends in CHD. How can we synthesize these findings? If we ask why central and eastern European countries present an epidemiological picture like that of England and Wales several decades ago, it is not fanciful to suggest that this pattern may reflect their relative state of economic development. Those countries may have reached the point in industrialization and economic development that coincided in the West with the initial upswing of the CHD epidemic (Marmot, 1992).

What does development mean in this context? Internationally, there is a correlation between CHD mortality and both smoking rates and consumption of dietary fat. Smoking rates are certainly high in Hungary and Czechoslovakia, as is intake of dietary fat. Data from the WHO MONICA study show that Hungary and Czechoslovakia have about 80 percent higher CHD mortality rates than the western part of Germany (MONICA, 1987). Our own calculations using MONICA data suggest that differences in smoking and plasma cholesterol account for 35 percent of the excess in

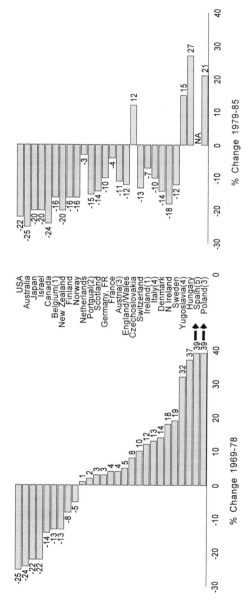

Figure 6-8. Percent change in death rates from CHD in two time periods for men and women aged 45–64 by country (1) 1979–84; (2) 1971–78: 1980–86; (3) 1980–86; (4) 1979–83; (5) 1979–85 not available. *Source*: Thom, 1989.

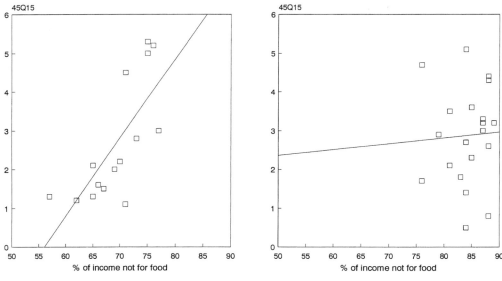

Figure 6-9. Probability of death between ages 15 and 60 according to level of personal prosperity in low-income and high-income countries. Low-income countries are defined as those with per capita Gross Domestic Product less than $6,000. *Source:* World Bank, 1992; Feachem, 1992.

CHD rates in Czechoslovakia and 24 percent in Hungary (Bobak and Marmot, unpublished report).

In inquiring what may account for the remaining excess, it is instructive to look at Japan, where over the 20-year period (1965–1985) life expectancy increased by an astonishing 7.5 years—the equivalent of abolishing heart disease and cancer from Britain (Marmot and Davey Smith, 1989). The two major causes of death, stroke and stomach cancer, have declined markedly, and mortality from heart disease—always low in Japan—has continued to decline. Japan's low rate of heart disease is likely to be related to its low-fat diet. Diet does not offer an easy explanation for these trends, however, in that mortality from heart disease continued to decline despite a doubling of fat intake. Important as smoking is as a cause of premature mortality, it does not help explain the Japanese mortality record, since two-thirds of Japanese men smoke. Over this 20-year period, however, Japan has experienced an unequalled rise in prosperity. Not only has its gross national product (GNP) increased markedly, according to World Bank figures; this income is also more equitably distributed than in any other Organisation for Economic Co-operation and Development (OECD) country (see below). These observations suggest three broad classes of influence on the rise and fall of CHD rates: nutrition, smoking, and factors related to socioeconomic level. This hypothesis is consistent with findings from within-country studies. Our task is to determine what the factors related to socioeconomic level might be.

Social Differences in Morbidity

Because of relative lack of data, there has been less study of social-class differences in morbidity than in mortality. Existing data have been well reviewed by Blaxter (1991), who discusses the problems associated with self-reported ill health but shows that in Britain there is a consistent inverse association between social class and reported morbidity in national surveys.

We have addressed morbidity in our two large studies of British civil servants. The first Whitehall study examined 18,000 men aged 40–69, in 1967–1969, and has continued to follow the cohort for mortality. The Whitehall II Study examined 10,314 men and women aged 35–55, in 1985–1988, nearly 20 years later. As in the case of mortality, the indicator of social class we have used is grade of employment. This is a precise social classification; it corresponds closely to salary and is related to position in the employment hierarchy.

Table 6–3 shows the prevalence rate of various indicators of morbidity in different employment grades in the Whitehall II Study (Marmot et al., 1991). The two top levels of the civil service, here called 1 and 2, correspond to administrators in the original Whitehall Study. In general, the lower the employment, the higher the prevalence of ischemic heart disease. Women report higher prevalence of angina than men, despite a lower prevalence of ischemic electrocardiograms (ECGs). The excess of abnormal ECGs in men is greater for probable ischemia (Q-waves) than it is for possible ischemia (S-T and T-wave changes).

Among men, there is an inverse association between employment grade and (1) number of symptoms reported in the last 14 days, (2) health problems in the last year, (3) likelihood of rating health as "average" or "poor," as opposed to "good" or "very good," (4) a prior diagnosis of hypertension or diabetes, and (5) prevalence of cough with phlegm. This is in addition to the inverse association with prevalence of ischemia.

Women, in general, report a higher level of morbidity than men. The relation with employment grade was less consistent. In addition to a higher prevalence of premenstrual bloating, lower-grade women were more likely to report premenstrual irritability and breast tenderness.

For comparison with the Whitehall results from 1967–1969, Figure 6–10 restricts the 1985–1988 data to men aged 40–54, grouped into three broad classes by employment grade. The figure shows prevalence rates for ECG abnormalities, angina pectoris, chronic bronchitis, and smoking in these two cohorts of civil servants in the studies separated by 20 years.

A lower prevalence of ischemia would be expected in the first Whitehall Study, in which limb leads only were used for ECGs compared with the full 12-lead ECGs used in Whitehall II (Marmot et al., 1991). There is no evidence, however, of a diminution

Table 6-3 Morbidity Prevalence by Civil-Service Grade of Employment[a]

	Sex	1	2	3	4	5	6	Total Sample	Test for Trend
				Employment Grade+					
Number of men and	M	1026	1627	1228	1496	881	642	6900	
women in grades	F	122	264	198	480	660	1690	3414	
Age (mean)	M	46.9	44.2	43.5	42.5	43.4	44.6	6900	***
	F	44.1	43.0	42.1	42.9	45.5	46.7	3414	***
Probable ischemia	M	1.3	0.9	1.1	1.2	1.4	2.1	6896	(*)
on ECG[b] (%)	F	0.0	0.0	0.7	0.1	0.7	1.1	3412	*
Probable/possible	M	6.4	4.9	5.0	6.5	6.7	10.5	6896	***
ischemia on ECG[b] (%)	F	3.6	3.3	3.0	6.5	7.8	7.3	3412	**
Angina by	M	1.7	2.4	2.5	3.1	1.9	2.9	6835	ns
questionnaire (%)	F	1.8	1.6	2.9	3.3	5.8	4.0	3351	*
Probable/possible	M	7.6	7.0	7.3	9.3	8.4	12.3	6835	***
ischemia on ECG[b] or angina (%)	F	4.5	5.0	5.5	9.8	13.3	11.1	3357	***
History of diabetes	M	0.3	0.6	0.8	0.8	1.7	1.7	6852	***
(%)	F	0.9	0.6	0.0	0.0	0.8	1.4	3386	*
Mean number of	M	2.1	2.4	2.5	2.5	2.6	2.6	5151	***
symptoms	F	3.2	3.3	3.1	3.1	3.2	3.0	2442	ns
Self-rated health	M	15.3	19.5	21.5	22.8	27.5	33.7	6874	***
average or worse (%)	F	26.2	25.5	28.7	28.9	34.4	42.1	3404	***
Regular cough with	M	6.7	7.3	6.9	9.2	11.0	10.9	6850	***
phlegm in winter (%)	F	4.2	6.1	10.3	6.4	6.5	8.6	3364	(*)
Longstanding	M	29.9	30.4	30.1	31.6	31.8	36.4	5157	**
illness (%)	F	30.2	35.8	26.7	33.7	31.6	30.5	2485	ns
Any health	M	69.0	68.0	67.3	67.7	66.5	70.7	5148	ns
problems last year (%)	F	69.8	70.6	73.5	72.3	75.3	75.6	2463	*
Drug therapy for	M	2.1	2.1	2.1	2.7	4.8	5.2	6673	***
hypertension (%)	F	3.7	4.4	4.1	2.9	3.5	4.3	3338	ns
Premenstrual bloating (%)	F	2.2	8.6	9.6	10.9	16.8	19.6	1939	***

a. Age-adjusted figures.

b. Probable ischemia is defined as the presence of Q-waves on electrocardiogram (Minnesota codes 1:1, 1:2). Possible ischemia is the presence of S-T abnormalities on electrocardiogram (Minnesota codes 4:1, 4:2, 4:3, 5:1, 5:2, 5:3) or left bundle branch block (Minnesota code 7:1).

+*Grade categories*
Grade 1 - Unified Grades 1–6
Grade 2 - Unified Grade 7
Grade 3 - Senior Executive Officer ⎫
Grade 4 - Higher Executive Officer ⎬ and professional equivalents
Grade 5 - Executive Officer ⎭
Grade 6 - Clerical Officer / Office Support

P-values
ns P >0.10
(*) 0.05 < P ≤ 0.10
* 0.01 < P ≤ 0.05
** 0.001 < P ≤ 0.01
*** P ≤ 0.001

Source: Marmot et al., 1991.

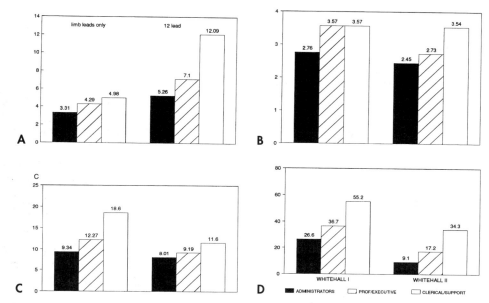

Figure 6-10. Prevalence of cardiorespiratory disease and smoking among men aged 40–54 in the Whitehall I (1967–1969) and Whitehall II (1985–1988) studies (age-adjusted percentages) A, Probable and possible ECG ischaemia; B, angina pectoris; C, chronic bronchitis; D, current cigarette smokers. *Source:* Marmot et al., 1991.

in the grade difference in prevalence of ischemia over the 20 years separating White-hall and Whitehall II (Marmot et al., 1991). The relative difference between clerical officers and administrators appears to have increased. For angina pectoris the questionnaire was identical in the two studies, and the difference between grades has changed little. For chronic bronchitis—cough with phlegm production—the prevalence rate among men aged 40–54 is considerably lower in Whitehall II than in the first Whitehall Study, but the relative difference between the grades is similar. Both the grade differences in chronic bronchitis and the diminution in prevalence rates between the 1960s and the 1980s are likely to be related to smoking. Figure 6–10 also shows that smoking prevalence among civil servants has decreased, but the striking inverse association with grade of employment persists.

Poverty or Inequality

Much of the preceding discussion of social inequalities in health has concentrated on the health disadvantage of those at the bottom (M'Gonigle and Kirby, 1937). This is analogous to interpreting pervasive social problems as particularly harmful to a disadvantaged minority. There is little doubt that poverty or deprivation is likely to be harmful, to health among other things. But our Whitehall data on mortality (Fig. 6–1) and morbidity (Table 6–3) suggest that something other than absolute poverty is at work here. Even clerical officers—who are far from well-off, with earnings at or below the national average–are not poor by the standards of England at an earlier period in its history, or those of developing countries. The crucial point is that each grade has worse health and higher mortality rates than the grade above it. Executive-grade civil servants are not poor by any absolute standard, yet they have higher mortality rates than administrators.

This social gradient in mortality suggests the operation of factors that cut across the entire society. Whether we are speaking of relative deprivation or relative lack of access to the fruits of a wealthy society, it is clear that explanations for socioeconomic differentials in Britain in the 1990s must be broader than the notion of poverty advanced earlier in the century (M'Gonigle and Kirby, 1937). International data suggest conclusions that are congruent with the findings of within-country comparisons. Wilkinson (1992) argues that there is a relationship between per-capita GNP and life expectancy at birth only in poor countries: in 1984, below a threshold of about $5,000 in per capita GNP, few countries had a life expectancy of 70 years or more. Above that level, however, there is little relationship between GNP and life expectancy (Wilkinson, 1986a,b). The relationship is much closer with measures of income dispersion. In Figure 6–11 the measure of equality of income distribution is the share of total post-tax household income received by the least-well-off 70 percent of families; the higher this percentage, the more equal is income distribution. There is a striking correlation

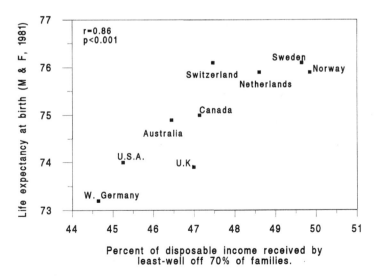

Figure 6-11. Relationship between life expectancy at birth (male and female combined) and percentage of total post-tax and benefit household income received by the least-well-off 70% of families, 1981. *Source:* Wilkinson, 1992.

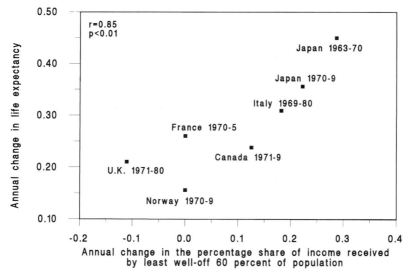

Figure 6-12. Annual change in life expectancy and in percentage of income received by least-well-off 60% of population. *Source:* Wilkinson, 1992.

with life expectancy. Wilkinson (1992) tried several measures of income distribution, including the share of total income received by the least-well-off 10 percent, 20 percent, 30 percent, and so on. He found that the correlation with life expectancy increased progressively until the bottom 60–70 percent was reached—that is, the higher the share of total income enjoyed by the bottom 60 or 70 percent, the longer the average life expectancy. This suggests that the correlation between income inequality and life expectancy is not the result only of the income level of those at the bottom (e.g., the lowest 10%).

As a further test of the income-inequality hypothesis, Wilkinson plotted changes in life expectancy against changes in income distribution in six countries for which such data were available (Figure 6–12). Japan experienced both the greatest increase in equality of income distribution and the greatest increase in life expectancy. As we have noted, Japan now enjoys the most equitable distribution of income and the longest life expectancy of any OECD country. In the United Kingdom, by contrast, the bottom 60 percent of households received a declining share of total income, and the population as a whole experienced a relatively small increase in life expectancy.

Potential Explanations of Social Inequalities in Health

How are we to explain the relationship between income inequality and life expectancy? One hypothesis is that greater income inequality implies a greater proportion of the population in poverty. If there were a nonlinear relationship between income and life expectancy—stronger at lower incomes than at high—the apparent relationship between income inequality and life expectancy could possibly be explained by variations in the proportion of those in poverty. Wilkinson (1992) points out that this is not the most likely explanation. When the criterion of income inequality is the share of income received by the bottom 10 percent, the relation with life expectancy is far weaker than when the criterion is the share received by the bottom 60–70 percent. Even if increased income inequality did result in more households in poverty, the proportion of absolute poor is still too small in OECD countries to account for the magnitude of the relation between income inequality and life expectancy. In order to do so, income inequality must have an effect on the bulk of the population. In other words, its influence on life expectancy among rich countries is likely to be a matter of relative rather than absolute deprivation.

Medical Care

One explanation for social inequalities in health might be inequity in the distribution of medical care. Indeed, a committee was appointed in the United Kingdom in 1978 to investigate the persistence of social inequalities in health 30 years after the establishment of the National Health Service. In keeping with McKeown's (1979) conclusions on the limited contribution of medical care to improvements in life expectancy, the Black Committee did not attribute inequalities in health to inequity in the distribution of medical care.

This issue has also been examined by looking at mortality due to causes considered be amenable to medical care. Figure 6–13, which extracts data from a report by Mackenbach et al. (1989), shows that the relative decline in mortality from causes amenable to medical care may have been slightly greater in Social Class I than in Class V, an observation consistent with inequity in medical care. Amenable causes are, however, a small proportion of the total. In absolute terms the widening gap in mortality between the classes is clearly the result of a decline in nonamenable mortality in the higher classes and lack of decline in the lower classes.

Within Britain, an analysis of data from the OPCS Longitudinal Study shows that social class differences in cancer mortality are largely the result of differences in the incidence of cancer. Differentials in survival contribute minimally to overall cancer mortality (Kogevinas et al., 1991).

Analogous to the limited role of medical care in generating social inequalities in health is its limited role in generating international differences. When comparing Japan to England and Wales, for example, we noted that both nations spend a relatively small proportion of GNP on medical care. Furthermore, the decline in mortality in Japan was observed to pertain to both amenable and nonamenable causes of death (Marmot and Davey Smith, 1989). Thus it is hard to argue that differential access to medical care is responsible for inequalities in health in European countries.

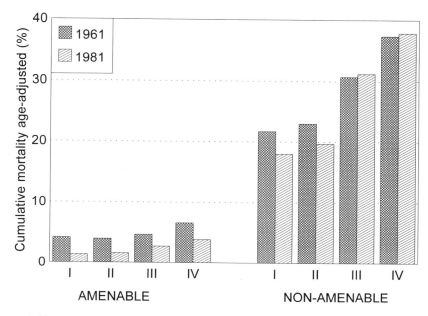

Figure 6-13. Mortality amenable and nonamenable to medical care, in England and Wales, for men aged 15–64, by social class. *Source:* Mackenbach et al., 1989.

Health Selection

It has been hypothesized that health may determine social position, rather than vice versa. This thesis was considered and rejected by the Black Committee as a major cause of social inequalities in health (Black et al., 1988). There are several periods during the life course when such selection could operate, as well as several potential mechanisms with varying degrees of plausibility and supporting evidence (Blane et al., 1992a).

The most straightforward suggestion is that the sick drift down the social hierarchy, producing social groups at the bottom characterized by a disproportionate number of unhealthy individuals. Three pieces of evidence bear on whether such intragenerational selection is an important contributor to mortality differentials. First, in the OPCS Longitudinal Study—a follow-up of 1 percent of the population from the 1971 census—social-class mortality differentials after 1981 for subjects who belonged to the same social-class groups in 1971 and 1981; and therefore could not have experienced health-related social mobility—were identical to those for the whole population (Goldblatt, 1989). Second, in the same study, mortality differentials between social classes persisted beyond age 75, long after retirement (Fox et al., 1985). Social class in retirement is based on last occupation; by definition, health after retirement cannot cause downward social drift since the classification is fixed. Third, in participants free of

manifest disease at entry into the Whitehall Study, mortality differentials by employment grade are essentially identical to those of the study population as a whole. Since
social position is not reclassified after entry into the study, mobility caused by health
status, at least as measured, cannot account for the mortality gradient (Marmot et al.,
1978a).

It has recently been speculated that selection at an earlier age—between early childhood and labor-market entry—is an important determinant of health inequalities (Illsley, 1986; West, 1991). Such selection could occur if health status in childhood determines both health and social class in early adulthood; or if a common antecedent
determines both adult health status and future adult social class. There is evidence that
ill health in childhood is associated with downward social mobility, but the effect is
minor (Wadsworth, 1986). Studies that relate health in childhood to health in early
adulthood similarly fail to account for class differences in health in adulthood (Power
et al., 1990; Lundberg, 1991).

Factors Operating Early in Life

A different version of the selection hypothesis posits that, though social selection
based on health status is not a crucial contributor to health differentials, common background factors determine both social position and health in adulthood. This theory of
"indirect selection" (Wilkinson, 1986c) recognizes that people carry into adulthood the
results of earlier influences: genetic factors, biological results of early experiences, and
educational, cultural, psychological, and social factors. It has been argued that the
major influences on health in adulthood operate early in life (Barker, 1989), and it is
also possible that both social position and health in adulthood are determined by the
same early-life influences. On the other hand, this focus on the childhood origins of
adult disease has been faulted precisely because early influences shape the lives people
lead and the social environments in which they live and work as adults: if it is these
conditions of adult life that are related to ill health, the role of childhood conditions
may be indirect (Ben-Shlomo and Davey Smith, 1991). Clearly it is not easy to separate the direct effects on health of early and later life experiences.

One useful indicator is height. In his studies in Aberdeen, Scotland, Illsley (1955)
showed that women who were upwardly mobile—whose husbands' social class was
higher than their fathers'—were taller than women who married within their class.
More recent work, analyzing data from the 1958 birth cohort in the UK, confirms that
social mobility between birth and age 23 is selective with respect to height, although
mobility did not account for social gradients in height (Power et al., 1990, 1991).
Whitehall data relating height to mortality may provide some insight into the separate
effects of current and past environment. Height is influenced by environment as well as
by genes. As Table 6–4 shows, height is related to social status as measured by employment grade. Modest height also predicts adult mortality independent of grade of
employment (Marmot et al., 1984a), and it is reasonable to speculate that this correla-

Table 6-4 Physiological Measurements, Health Behaviors, and Family History by Grade of Employment[a]

| | Sex | Employment Grade+ | | | | | | Total Sample | Test for Trend |
		1	2	3	4	5	6		
Physiological Measurements									
Mean cholesterol	M	6.05	5.97	5.93	6.02	6.00	6.00	6865	ns
	F	5.79	5.85	5.80	5.80	5.90	5.86	3375	ns
Mean systolic blood	M	124.3	124.6	123.9	124.8	125.4	125.4	6886	**
pressure	F	117.6	120.5	120.6	119.2	119.7	119.5	3413	ns
Mean diastolic blood	M	77.6	77.5	77.6	77.9	78.8	79.1	6886	***
pressure	F	74.0	75.2	75.3	74.3	74.8	74.9	3412	ns
Mean body mass	M	24.6	24.4	24.6	24.5	24.8	25.1	6888	***
index	F	23.7	23.7	24.3	24.1	24.5	25.3	3412	***
Obesity (%)	M	4.1	3.7	4.6	5.1	6.0	10.7	6888	***
	F	7.4	4.6	7.9	7.8	10.3	13.2	3412	***
Mean height	M	177.8	177.1	176.9	176.3	174.3	172.9	6890	***
	F	165.5	165.1	165.3	163.1	162.8	160.7	3413	***
Health Behaviors									
Current smoking (%)	M	8.3	10.2	13.0	18.4	21.9	33.6	6892	***
	F	18.3	11.6	15.2	20.3	22.7	27.5	3408	***
Mean units of	M	14.6	12.6	12.9	12.9	11.6	10.1	6845	***
alcohol in last 7	F	12.1	9.8	9.3	7.0	5.2	3.6	3375	***
days									
No moderate or	M	5.1	5.4	4.9	7.5	16.2	30.5	6662	***
vigorous exercise	F	12.0	14.7	10.8	13.2	19.7	31.1	3221	***
(%)									
Customary use of	M	44.2	39.3	35.1	31.8	27.8	21.2	6869	***
skim or semi-skim	F	39.5	48.3	49.8	46.2	40.5	34.4	3389	***
milk (%)									
Customary choice of	M	47.7	45.2	43.6	37.2	37.5	32.2	6867	***
wholemeal bread	F	57.2	52.9	58.2	55.4	43.8	35.5	3380	***
(%)									
Consumption of	M	34.0	39.6	40.6	47.9	52.5	61.7	6881	***
fresh fruit or	F	17.7	20.4	28.4	29.7	36.4	43.6	3400	***
vegetables less									
than daily (%)									
Family History									
Parent with history	M	26.1	28.1	26.1	26.1	24.0	22.5	6649	**
of heart attack	F	39.2	36.4	24.7	29.8	22.6	24.5	3234	***
(%)									
Sibling with history	M	2.0	2.3	2.7	3.2	4.4	3.8	5496	**
of heart attack	F	0.8	1.7	1.0	4.3	4.8	6.4	2804	***
(%)									

a. Age-adjusted figures.

+*Grade categories*
Grade 1 - Unified Grades 1–6
Grade 2 - Unified Grade 7
Grade 3 - Senior Executive Officer ⎤
Grade 4 - Higher Executive Officer ⎬ and professional equivalents
Grade 5 - Executive Officer ⎦
Grade 6 - Clerical Officer / Office Support

P-values
ns P $>$ 0.10
(*) 0.05 $<$ P $\leq$ 0.10
* 0.01 $<$ P $\leq$ 0.05
** 0.001 $<$ P $\leq$ 0.01
*** P $\leq$ 0.001

Source: Marmot et al., 1991.

tion may in part reflect a persistent influence from early life. Grade of employment, which is to some extent an index of current social influences, in turn predicts mortality independent of height. Thus two sets of influences may affect mortality risk: those from early life and current influences. As we have seen, this is an oversimplification: one's current social situation is influenced by one's prior experiences. Nevertheless it is valuable to attempt to distinguish these two sets of influences, since their relative contribution is crucial to identifying interventions that could both improve overall adult health and reduce socioeconomic differentials. Current research may reduce the degree of polarization between those who think future health status is virtually programmed in early life (Barker, 1990) and those who emphasize influences acting in later life (Elford et al., 1991).

General Susceptibility or Specific Causes

A striking feature of social-class differences in health is their generalizability across diverse pathological conditions. In the Whitehall Study, the higher risk of death in the lower employment grades applied to deaths from lung cancer, other cancers, CHD, cerebrovascular disease, other cardiovascular disease, chronic bronchitis, other respiratory disease, gastrointestinal disease, genitourinary disease, accidents, and violence (Marmot et al., 1984a). Findings such as these, have prompted speculation that there may exist factors that increase general susceptibility to ill health (Berkman and Syme, 1979; Cassel, 1976).

An alternative to such a general–susceptibility hypothesis is the possibility that a set of specific factors explain social-class differences in mortality. This view is supported by the fact that some cancers, notably those of the colon, brain, prostate, hematopoietic system, and breast, and melanoma, do not show the same social-class variation as those listed above (Davey Smith et al., 1991).

Confronted with two conflicting alternatives such as these, it is reasonable to hypothesize that both are correct. A general-susceptibility hypothesis implies that, whatever causes are operating, certain groups will be at higher risk of death; it does not deny the operation of specific causes. Diseases linked to smoking, such as chronic bronchitis and lung cancer, show a particularly strong social-class gradient—stronger than do cancers and other diseases not linked to smoking. But the latter too show a social-class gradient. To put it another way, the general-susceptibility hypothesis posits the operation of factors that cut across our current system of classifying diseases, and that increase risk of death over and above the effects of known factors such as smoking. This thesis would account for the fact that an administrator who smokes 20 cigarettes a day has a lower risk of lung-cancer mortality than a lower-grade civil servant who smokes the same amount (Marmot et al., 1984a), even after pack-years and tar content are taken into account. It would also account for the gradient in mortality from CHD even among nonsmokers. Figure 6–14 illustrates this point (Davey Smith and Shipley, 1991).

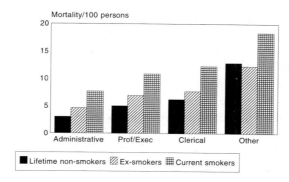

Figure 6-14. Ten-year mortality risk by smoking behavior and employment grade (age-adjusted figures) of Whitehall male civil servants. *Source:* Davey Smith and Shipley, 1991.

This apparently increased susceptibility may well be a socially induced phenomenon. The life-courses of people in different social groups are different from beginning to end, and insults to health may accumulate over the entire span from birth to death. That these influences on health cluster in such a way as to produce differing degrees of disadvantage with respect to most diseases in different social groups is undeniable. But our current level of knowledge about this general susceptibility does not allow us to venture far beyond this empirical observation.

Health-Related Behaviors and Biological Risk Factors

The possible role of health behaviors and other established biological risk factors in generating social inequalities in health is illustrated by Table 6–4, which presents, by grade of employment, various differences found in the Whitewall II Study (Marmot et al., 1991). Plasma cholesterol levels do not differ by grade, and the small inverse association between grade and blood pressure observed in men in the original Whitehall Study is still present but now even smaller. There is a significant inverse trend in mean body-mass index (BMI: weight/height^2) by grade but the differences are small, especially in men. Distribution of body mass is different, however: obesity (BMI>30) is more prevalent in the lower grades, strikingly so in the clerical grade. As in the original Whitehall Study, the higher the grade, the taller the man or woman.

The most striking risk-factor difference among grades was smoking (also see Fig. 6–10). Women also smoke more than men in all but the lowest grade (clerical and office support). The proportion of men and women who do not perform moderate or vigorous exercise in their leisure time is higher in the lower grades. Consumption of skim and semi-skim milk, wholemeal bread, and fresh fruit and vegetables—a rough indicator of dietary patterns—is higher in the higher grades. Average alcohol consumption is reported to be higher in the higher grades among both men and, more strikingly, women.

Reports of parents having had a heart attack were more frequent in the higher grades; a positive family history among siblings was more common in the lower grades. This finding is in keeping with data suggesting a possible recent social-class crossover in CHD risk (Marmot et al., 1978b).

There is thus a range of possible explanations for grade differences in mortality, only some of which were measured in the first Whitehall Study. As discussed earlier, differences in smoking patterns were insufficient to account for differences by grade in mortality from smoking-related diseases (Marmot et al., 1984a, b). Differences in blood pressure between grades were minimal, and plasma cholesterol levels were higher in higher grades. The main coronary risk factors could therefore account for little of the gradient in mortality by grade of employment. Some of the other factors listed in Table 6–4 may provide part of the explanation.

To the extent that behavior does account for social gradients in health, a new set of questions arises: Why is there a social gradient in behavior? It is worth dwelling on the implications of the smoking rates in Figure 6–10. The baseline investigations for the first Whitehall Study, conducted in 1967–1969, found a clear social gradient in smoking. Twenty years later, the prevalence of smoking has declined across the entire society, and a new cohort of civil servants, different people from those examined 20 years earlier, reproduces the social gradient.

To focus on behavior as an explanation for social inequalities in health is to take a step backward along the causal chain. Why are there social inequalities in behavior? The comments at the beginning of this paper about treating social class as a confounding variable are relevant here. It is reasonable to "control for" smoking if one is examining the extent to which smoking accounts for social-class differences in disease. Similarly, an analysis of the health risks of smoking will be flawed if it fails to take into account that smoking is associated with social position, which is in turn associated with adverse health for other reasons besides smoking (Davey Smith and Shipley, 1991). To understand the pathways by which social inequalities in health are generated, however, one needs to examine the links in the chain, e.g., between social position and smoking, not to control for their effects.

Material Conditions

The Black Report (Black, 1988) emphasized the importance of material conditions in explaining social inequalities in health. Specifically, Black referred to materialist or structural explanations, emphasizing hazards to which some people have no choice but to be exposed given the present distribution of income and opportunity. This thesis can be interpreted more broadly to apply not simply to material conditions but also to psychosocial influences inherent in one's position in society.

In the working population that makes up the Whitehall cohort, employment grade is a guide to material conditions in that it is a proxy for salary, which in turn helps determine circumstances outside work. It is not surprising that in Whitehall II, the lower the employment grade, the greater the frequency of reported financial problems.

In the OPCS Longitudinal Study, as we have seen, other measures besides social class based on occupation predicted mortality, among them housing tenure (ownership) and household access to cars. These factors are clearly indicative of material conditions. In the Whitehall Study, car ownership predicted mortality independent of grade of employment (Davey Smith et al., 1990). In addition, men who reported engaging in gardening had lower mortality than other men. The link between gardening and lower mortality is open to a variety of interpretations, among them that possessing a house with a garden is a measure of wealth. These data are consistent with the link between deprivation and mortality found in the geographic-based studies reviewed earlier.

The difficulty posed by material explanations is understanding how they operate. When poor living conditions meant polluted water, crowded and unsanitary housing with high rates of cross-infection, inadequate diet, and appalling conditions of employment, it was not difficult to see why there would be worse health among the socially deprived. As conditions improved, mortality rates fell in all social groups. But why do the social gradients persist? Are we to understand that residual effects of bad housing, as well as air pollution and other material conditions, still affect the lower social classes, though less than they used to? If there are such residual effects, it is no surprise that they do not affect all social strata equally. Can this be the whole explanation?

The Whitehall data are relevant here, as are Wilkinson's data on income inequalities. In both Whitehall studies, morbidity and mortality varied linearly with grade of employment. It is possible that the gap between the second-highest and highest grades could be the result of worse housing, poorer diet in childhood, or greater pollution, but it seems unlikely that comfortable "middle-class" people in Britain are suffering from the effects of material deprivation. Similarly, comparing rich countries, Wilkinson showed that it was not differences in wealth that predicted differences in life expectancy, but differences in inequality of income distribution.

One is drawn to the view that, in addition to the multiple influences we have already discussed, relative position in society must have an impact—not absolute deprivation, in other words but relative deprivation. This thesis would account for a social gradient in ill health because each group, while not necessarily suffering from greater effects of bad housing and the like, will have "less" than the group above it. This hypothesis would also account for social inequalities in health in societies with very different levels of health. The social gradient in ill health will vary in magnitude depending on the magnitude of relative differences in deprivation.

In a society that has met the subsistence needs of its members, what do we mean by "less," or by "relative deprivation?" In addition to the factors explored above, let us look at psychosocial factors for part of the answer.

Psychosocial Factors

The potential importance of psychosocial factors in explaining social gradients in health may be illustrated by data from the Whitehall II Study. Table 6–5 shows differences in psychosocial characteristics by grade of employment. The lower grades report

Table 6-5 Psychosocial Characteristics by Grade of Employment[a]

	Sex	Employment Grade+						Total Sample	Test for Trend
		1	2	3	4	5	6		
Work Characteristics (upper third of distribution)									
High control over	M	59.3	49.7	43.1	31.6	24.7	11.8	6877	***
own work (%)	F	51.2	45.4	47.1	31.2	20.1	10.2	3341	***
Varied work (%)	M	70.5	52.1	41.9	27.1	18.2	3.9	6875	***
	F	71.2	55.2	40.5	31.7	14.0	4.7	3356	***
Fast pace (%)	M	58.0	43.6	34.7	27.9	20.8	15.8	6878	***
	F	60.9	50.3	43.7	31.1	29.7	18.0	3356	***
High satisfaction	M	58.2	38.7	34.1	29.5	29.4	29.8	6865	***
(%)	F	57.5	42.2	40.3	36.6	41.6	47.7	3337	ns
Social Network/Activities									
See at least 3	M	22.1	24.8	29.0	27.2	29.7	30.6	6426	***
relatives per	F	18.9	23.7	21.1	24.1	30.4	44.9	3187	***
month (%)									
See at least 3	M	65.3	61.3	58.5	58.6	56.4	50.2	5162	***
friends per	F	71.1	62.8	67.1	63.6	52.9	49.0	2473	***
month (%)									
No hobbies (%)	M	12.4	12.9	12.7	15.0	23.0	25.4	6453	***
	F	12.5	15.4	11.3	11.9	18.3	27.5	3044	***
Social Support from Closest Person (upper third of distribution)									
Confiding/	M	31.3	33.7	28.3	28.3	34.6	26.1	5021	(*)
emotional	F	37.3	33.8	33.0	32.5	32.9	31.8	2380	ns
support (%)									
Practical support	M	41.1	40.0	37.2	33.0	36.4	29.1	5022	***
(%)	F	21.8	25.9	26.8	17.1	24.0	28.0	2384	(*)
Negative	M	25.0	28.4	31.3	30.9	38.1	39.0	5010	***
interactions	F	33.0	32.5	28.3	36.4	28.3	33.8	2379	ns
with									
confidantes									
(%)									

less control over their working lives, less varied work, and less pressure to work at a fast pace. Overall, is work satisfaction lower in the lower employment grades?

Social relationships can be described quantitatively in terms of the extent of social networks, and qualitatively in terms of the nature of the social supports they provide. More people in the lower grades report visiting relatives once a month or more; more people in the higher grades visit friends. Fewer people in the lower grades were involved in hobbies. Among men, fewer in the lower grades have a friend in whom they can confide, fewer receive practical support, and more report negative reactions from persons close to them. The patterns were less clear among women.

More people in the lower grades reported two or more from a list of eight potentially stressful life events in the previous year, as well as difficulties with bills or money in general.

Table 6-5 Continued.

	Sex	Employment Grade+						Total Sample	Test for Trend
		1	2	3	4	5	6		
Events and Difficulties									
Two or more	M	29.6	31.6	35.1	37.9	39.9	41.9	6758	***
major life	F	41.1	43.6	35.5	42.8	46.5	49.2	3247	***
events (%)									
Sometimes lack	M	7.0	12.6	21.5	26.4	34.4	37.2	4977	***
enough money	F	7.7	6.9	9.6	13.2	24.4	34.4	2282	***
(%)									
Some difficulty	M	11.0	16.2	22.8	24.7	29.6	29.6	5167	***
paying bills	F	15.2	13.2	11.8	15.7	18.1	26.9	2490	***
(%)									
Other									
Type A (defined	M	51.3	40.2	36.9	27.8	20.4	12.8	6729	***
as upper third)	F	62.6	54.6	44.0	39.0	29.0	17.6	3228	***
(%)									
Hostility score	M	9.7	10.2	10.9	11.3	12.7	14.7	4266	***
	F	9.5	9.5	9.4	10.1	10.4	12.3	1772	***
Believe one can	M	71.6	72.2	70.8	66.8	65.5	52.4	5136	***
reduce risk of	F	58.1	61.6	69.7	68.4	65.0	53.7	2487	***
heart attack									
(%)									

a. Age-adjusted figures.

+*Grade categories*
Grade 1 - Unified Grades 1–6
Grade 2 - Unified Grade 7
Grade 3 - Senior Executive Officer ⎫
Grade 4 - Higher Executive Officer ⎬ and professional equivalents
Grade 5 - Executive Officer ⎭
Grade 6 - Clerical Officer / Office Support

P-values
ns P >0.10
(*) 0.05 < P ≤0.10
* 0.01 < P ≤0.05
** 0.001 < P ≤0.01
*** P ≤0.001

Note: Scores have been calculated for the whole sample and the percent show the proportion of subjects in the highest third of each score.

Source: Marmot et al., 1991.

The Type-A behavior pattern is more common among the higher-grade participants, despite their lower rate of heart disease. It has been suggested that the component of Type-A behavior most responsible for the link to CHD risk is hostility, and the lower grades score higher on the Cook-Medley Hostility Scale.

As a measure of perceived control over their health, fewer in the lower grades reported believing that it is possible to reduce the risk of heart attack.

These findings offer a wealth of potential explanations for social inequalities in health, in conjunction with other evidence on psychosocial factors. Three important hypotheses focus on job strain, low social supports, and low control. There is a large body of evidence linking high psychological demands and low control at work to cardiovascular and other diseases (Karasek and Theorell, 1990). The relative disadvantage of the lower grades with respect to control could be a factor in their higher rates of disease (Marmot and Theorell, 1988). Similarly, evidence of meager social supports in the lower grades suggests a further contributing factor to the gradient in ill health (Berkman, 1984; House et al., 1988). Syme has suggested that increasing lack of control may help account for the increasing health disadvantage as one descends the social scale (Syme, 1989): poverty, whatever else it consists of, means lack of control.

The same mechanisms may explain international differences in health. Why have life expectancies in Central and Eastern Europe fallen behind those of the West? It cannot be solely a matter of capitalism versus communism. In the early postwar years, life expectancy in Austria and Czechoslovakia—one capitalist and the other communist—was roughly the same. Later Czechoslovakia fell behind, as did Hungary and the other countries of Eastern Europe. We have argued that this phenomenon was in some way related to the relative failure of their economies compared to the success of Western Europe. This mechanism might operate in all the ways discussed above, including psychosocial factors. Once the basic material conditions of subsistence are met, people's expectations about what is necessary to provide a reasonable standard of living rises. An economy that fails to deliver an improved standard of living, in line with people's expectations, may lead to widespread feelings of lack of control. Perceived lack of control may in turn translate into adverse health behaviors such as smoking and obesity, and it may also affect health by more direct stress pathways.

A Unifying Explanation for Social Inequalities in Health?

The rationale for research on inequalities in health is ultimately to determine whether they can be reduced. One approach to this problem is political: if we reduce social inequalities, inequalities in health will shrink. This may or may not be the case. Better understanding of the links between social position and health is needed. We have argued that a combination of factors may account for inequalities in health both within and between countries. Much progress has been made in sorting through potential explanations. A unifying explanation exists only to the extent that social position is related to a number of such factors: differences in early life experience, behavior, material conditions and psychosocial factors. Investigations typically focus on only one of these issues and fail to explore the other factors, making interpretation difficult. The challenge for researchers is to develop a methodology for exploring interactions between influences on health throughout the life span. Only then will it be possible to assess the relative importance of the various potential explanations for socioeconomic differentials in health, which is crucial in planning strategies to counter them.

References

Antonovsky, A. 1989. Social inequalities in health: A complementary perspective. In J. Fox (ed.), *Health Inequalities in European Countries*, pp. 386–397. Aldershot, U. K.: Gower.

Baker, D., and R. Illsley. 1990. Trends in inequalities in health in Europe. *Int. J. Health Sci.* 1–2:89–111.

Barker, D.J.P. 1989. The intrauterine and early postnatal origins of cardiovascular disease and chronic bronchitis. *J. Epidemiol. Community Health* 43:237–240.

Barker, D. J. 1990. The fetal and infant origins of adult disease. *Br. Med. J.* 301:1111.

Ben-Shlomo, Y., and G. Davey Smith. 1991. Deprivation in infancy or adult life: Which is more important for mortality risk? *Lancet* 337:530–543.

Berkman, L. F. 1984. Assessing the physical health effects of social networks and social support. In L. Breslow, J. E. Fielding, and L. B. Lave (eds.), *Annual Review of Public Health*, 5th ed, pp. 413–432. Palo Alto, CA: Annual Reviews.

Berkman, L. F., and S. L. Syme. 1979. Social networks, host resistance and mortality: A nine-year follow-up of Alameda County residents. *Am. J. Epidemiol.* 109:186–204.

Black, D., J. N. Morris, C. Smith, P. Townsend, and M. Whitehead. 1988. *Inequalities in Health: The Black Report; The Health Divide.* London: Penguin Group.

Blane, D., G. Davey Smith, and M. Bartley. 1992a. Social selection: What does it contribute to social class differences in health? *Social Health Illness* (in press).

Blane D., M. Bartley, and G. Davey Smith. 1992b. Disease aetiology and socio-economic mortality differentials. Paper presented to the International Congress of Behavioral Medicine, Hamburg.

Blaxter, M. 1991. Fifty years on-inequalities in health. In M. Murphy, and T. Hobcraft (eds.), *Fifty Years On; Population Research in Britain*, pp. 69–94. Cambridge, U. K.: Cambridge University Press.

Bunker, J. P., D. S. Gomby, and B.H. Kehrer. (eds.). 1989. *Pathways to Health—The Role of Social Factors.* Menlo Park, CA: The Henry J Kaiser Family Foundation.

Carstairs, V. and R. Morris. 1991. *Deprivation and Health in Scotland.* Aberdeen: Aberdeen University Press.

Cassel, J. C. 1976. The contribution of the social environment to host resistance. *Am. J. Epidemiol.* 104:107–123.

Chadwick, E. 1965. *Report on the Sanitary Condition of the Labouring Population of Great Britain, 1842.* Edinburgh: Edinburgh University Press.

Culyer, A. J., and A. Wagstaff. 1991. *Need, Equality and Social Justice. Need, Equity and Equality in Health and Health Care.* Rotterdam: Institute for Medical Technology Assessment, Erasmus University.

Davey Smith, G., M. J. Shipley, and G. Rose. 1990. Magnitude and causes of socioeconomic differentials in mortality: Further evidence from the Whitehall Study. *J. Epidemiol. Community Health* 44:265–270.

Davey Smith, G., D. Leon, M.J. Shipley, and G. Rose. 1991. Socioeconomic differentials in cancer among men. *Int. J. Epidemiol.* 20:339–345.

Davey Smith, G., and M. J. Shipley. 1991. Confounding of occupation and smoking: Its magnitude and consequences. *Soc. Sci. Med.* 32:1297–1300.

Eames, M., Y. Ben Shlomo, and M.G. Marmot. 1993. Social deprivation and premature mortality: Regional comparison across England. *Br. Med. J.* 307:1097–1102.

Elford, J., P. Whincup, and A. G. Shaper. 1991. Early life experience and adult cardiovascular disease: Longitudinal and case-control studies. *Int. J. Epidemiol.* 20:833–844.

Feachem, R.G.A., J. Kjellstrom, C.J.L. Murray, M. Over, and M. A. Phillips. 1992. *The Health of Adults in the Developing World.* New York: Oxford University Press.

Feldman, J. J., D. M. Makuc, J. C. Kleinman, and J. Cornoni-Huntley. 1989. National trends in educational differentials in mortality. *Am. J. Epidemiol.* 129:919–933.

Fox, J. (ed.). 1989. *Health Inequalities in European Countries.* Aldershot, U.K.: Gower

Fox, A. J., P. O. Goldblatt, and D. R. Jones. 1985. Social class mortality differentials: Artefact, selection or life circumstances? *J. Epidemiol. Community Health* 39:1–8.

Goldblatt, P. 1989. Mortality by social class. *Population Trends* 56:6–15.

Goldblatt, P. 1990. Mortality and alternative social classifications. In P. Goldblatt (ed.), *Mortality and Social Organisation*, series 65, no. 6. pp. 163–192. London: Her Majesty's Stationary Office.

Haan, M., G. A. Kaplan, and T. Camacho. 1987. Poverty and health: Prospective evidence from the Alameda County study. *Am. J. Epidemiol.* 125:989–998.

House, J. S., K. R. Landis, and D. Umberson. 1988. Social relationships and health. *Science* 241:540–545.

Illsley, R. 1955. Social class selection and class differences in relation to still-births and infant deaths. *Br. Med. J.* 2:1520–1524.

Illsley, R. 1986. Occupational class, selection and the production of inequalities in health. *Quart. J. Soc. Affairs* 2:151–165.

Illsley, R., and J. Le Grand. 1987. The measurement of inequality in health. In A. Williams (ed.), *Economics and Health*. London: Macmillan.

Karasek, R., and T. Theorell. 1990. *Healthy Work: Stress, Productivity, and the Reconstruction of Working Life*. New York: Basic Books.

Kitagawa, E., and P. M. Hauser. 1973. *Differential Mortality in the United States. A Study in Socioeconomic Epidemiology*. Cambridge MA: Harvard University Press.

Kogevinas, M., M. G. Marmot, A.J. Fox, and P.O. Goldblatt. 1991. Socioeconomic differences in cancer survival. *J. Epidemiol. Community Health* 45:216–219.

Krzyzanowski, M., and M. Wysocki. 1986. The relation of thirteen-year mortality to ventilatory impairment and other respiratory symptoms: The Cracow Study. *Int. J. Epidemiol.* 15:56–64.

Le Grand, J. 1989. An international comparison of distribution of ages-at-death. In J. Fox (ed.), *Health Inequalities in European Countries*. Aldershot U.K.: Gower. pp. 75–91.

Leclerc, A. 1984. Les inegalites sociales devant la mort en Grande-Bretagne et en France. *Soc. Sci. Med.* 19:479–487.

Leclerc, A. 1989. Differential mortality by cause of death: Comparison between selected European countries. In J. Fox (ed.), *Health Inequalities in European Countries*, pp. 92–108. Aldershot, U.K.: Gower.

Leon, D., and R. G. Wilkinson. 1989. Inequalities in prognosis: socio-economic differences in cancer and heart disease survival. In J. Fox (ed.), *Health Inequalities in European Countries*, pp. 250–279. Aldershot, U.K.: Gower.

Lundberg, O. 1991. Childhood living conditions, health status and social mobility: A contribution to the health selection debate. *European Sociological Review* 7:149–162.

M'Gonigle, G.C.M., and J. Kirby. 1937. *Poverty and Public Health*. London: Golantz.

Mackenbach, J. P., K. Stronks, and A.E. Kunst. 1989. The contribution of medical care to inequalities in health: Differences between socio-economic groups in decline of mortality from conditions amenable to medical intervention. *Soc. Sci. Med.* 29:369–376.

Mackenbach, J. P., and A. E. Kunst. 1992. *Socio-economic Determinants of Regional Mortality Patterns in the Netherlands*. Liege, Belgium: International Union for the Scientific Study of Population.

Marmot, M. 1989. Comments on future research on social inequalities. In J. Bunker, D. Gomby, and B. Kehrer (eds.), *Pathways to Health—the Role of Social Factors*, pp. 244–250. Menlo Park, CA. The Henry J Kaiser Family Foundation.

Marmot, M. G. 1992. Coronary heart disease: Rise and fall of a modern epidemic. In M. G. Marmot, and P. Elliott (eds.), *Coronary Heart Disease Epidemiology*, pp. 3–19. Oxford: Oxford University Press.

Marmot, M. G., and G. Davey Smith. 1989. Why are the Japanese living longer? *Br. Med. J.* 299:1547–1551.

Marmot, M. G., and M. E. McDowall. 1986. Mortality decline and widening social inequalities. *Lancet* 1:274–276.

Marmot, M. G., and T. Theorell. 1988. Social class and cardiovascular disease: The contribution of work. *Int. J. Health Serv.* 18:659–674.

Marmot, M. G., G. Rose, M. Shipley, and P.J.S. Hamilton. 1978a. Employment grade and coronary heart disease in British civil servants. *J. Epidemiol. Community Health* 32:244–249.

Marmot, M. G., M. M. Adelstein, N. Robinson, and G.A. Rose. 1978b. Changing social class distribution of heart disease. *Br. Med. J.* 2:1109–1112.

Marmot, M. G., M. G. Shipley, and G. Rose. 1984a. Inequalities in death—specific explanations or a general pattern? *Lancet* 1:1003–1006.

Marmot, M. G., A. M. Adelstein, and L. Bulusu. 1984b. Lessons from the study of immigrant mortality. *Lancet* 1:1455–1458.

Marmot, M. G., M. Kogevinas, and M. A. Elston. 1987. Social/economic status and disease. *Annu. Rev. Public Health* 8:111–137.

Marmot, M. G., G. Davey Smith, S. Stansfeld, C. Patel, F. North, J. Head, I. White, E.J. Brunner, and A. Feeney. 1991. Health inequalities among British civil servants: the Whitehall II Study. *Lancet* 337:1387–1393.

McKeown, T. 1979. *The Role of Medicine.* Oxford: Basil Blackwell.

MONICA, The principle investigators of the MONICA project. 1987. WHO MONICA Project: geographic variation in mortality from cardiovascular diseases. *World Health Stat. Q.* 40:171–184.

Moser, K., H. Pugh, and P. Goldblatt. 1990. Mortality and the social classification of women. In P. Goldblatt (ed.), *Mortality and Social Organisation,* series 65, no. 6, pp. 145–162. London: Her Majesty's Stationery Office.

Office of Population Censuses and Surveys. 1978. *Occupational Mortality 1970–1972.* London: Her Majesty's Stationery Office.

Office of Population Censuses and Surveys. 1986. *Occupational Mortality 1979–1980, 1982–1983.* London: Her Majesty's Stationery Office.

Osler, W. 1910. The Lumleian lectures on angina pectoris. *Lancet* 1:697–839.

Pamuk, E. R. 1985. Social class inequality in mortality from 1921 to 1972 in England and Wales. *Population Studies* 39:17–31.

Power, C., O. Manor, A. J. Fox, and K. Fogelman. 1990. Health in childhood and social inequalities in health in young adults. *J. Royal Statist. Soc.,* series A, 153:17–28.

Power, C., O. Manor, and J. Fox. 1991. *Health and class: The Early Years.* London: Chapman & Hall.

Rose, G. 1992. *The Strategy of Preventive Medicine.* Oxford: Oxford University Press.

Sarvotham, S. G., and J.N. Berry. 1968. Prevalence of coronary heart disease in an urban population in northern India. *Circulation* 37:939–953.

Secretary of the State for Health. 1992. *Health of the Nation.* London: Her Majesty's Stationery Office.

Sorlie, P. D., M. R. Garcia-Palmieri. 1990. Educational status and coronary heart disease in Puerto Rico: The Puerto Rico Heart Health Program. *Int. J. Epidemiol.* 19:59–65.

Stevenson, T.H.C. 1928. The vital statistics of wealth and poverty (report of a paper to Royal Statistical Society). *Br. Med. J.* 1:354.

Strong, P. M. 1990. Black on class and mortality: theory, method and history. *J. Public Health Med.* 12:168–180.

Susser, M., and Z. Stein. 1962. Civilisation and peptic ulcer. *Lancet* 1:115–119.

Syme, S. L. 1989. Control and health: A personal perspective. In A. Steptoe, and A. Appels (eds.), *Stress, Personal Control and Health*, pp. 3–18. New York: John Wiley & Sons.

Thom, J. 1989. International mortality from heart disease: Rates and trends. *Int. J. Epidemiol.* 18:S20–S28.

Townsend, P., P. Phillimore, and A. Beattie. 1988. *Health and Deprivation: Inequality in the North.* London: Crom Helm.

Uemura, K., and Z. Pisa. 1988. Trends in cardiovascular disease mortality in industrialised countries since 1950. *World Health Statist. Q.* 41:155–178.

Vagero, D., and O. Lundberg. 1989. Health inequalities in Britain and Sweden. *Lancet* 2:35–36.

Vagero, D., and O. Lundberg. 1992. *Socio-economic Mortality Differentials—Towards an Explanation. Evidence from New Swedish Studies.* Liege, Belgium: International Union for the Scientific Study of Population.

Valkonen, T. 1989. Adult mortality and level of education: A comparison of six countries. In J. Fox (ed.), *Health Inequalities in European Countries*, pp. 142–162. Aldershot, U.K.: Gower.

Valkonen, T., T. Martelin, and A. Rimpela. 1990. *Socio-economic Mortality Differences in Finland 1971-85.* Helsinki: Central Statistical Office in Finland.

Wadsworth, M.E.J. 1986. Serious illness in childhood and its association with later-life achievement. In R. G. Wilkinson (ed.), *Class and Health*, pp. 50–74. London: Tavistock Publications.

Wadsworth, M.E.J. 1991. *The Imprint of Time.* Oxford: Clarendon Press.

West, P. 1991. Rethinking the health selection explanation for health inequalities. *Soc. Sci. Med.* 32:373–384.

Wilkinson, R. G. (ed.). 1986a. *Class and Health Research and Longitudinal Data.* London: Tavistock Publications.

Wilkinson, R. G. 1986b. Income and mortality. In R. G. Wilkinson (ed.), *Class and Health*, pp. 88–114. London: Tavistock Publications.

Wilkinson, R. G. 1986c. Socio-economic differences in mortality: Interpreting the data on their size and trends. In R. G. Wilkinson (ed.), *Class and Health*, pp. 1–20. London: Tavistock Publications.

Wilkinson, R. G. 1992. Income distribution and life expectancy. *Br. Med. J.* 304:165–168.

Wong, S. L., and S.P.B. Donnan. 1992. Influence of socioeconomic status on cardiovascular diseases in Hong Kong. *J. Epidemiol. Community Health* 46:148–150.

World Bank. 1991. *World Development Report 1991.* Oxford: Oxford University Press.

World Bank. 1992. *World Development Report 1992. Development and the Environment.* New York: Oxford University Press.

World Health Organisation. 1986. *Health for All 2000.* Copenhagen: World Health Organisation, Regional Office for Europe.

7

Political Economy and Health

M. HARVEY BRENNER

The political economy—the national economy, in interaction with government policies—influences a nation's health through the mechanisms of production, distribution, and consumption. The main links between the economy and health are economic growth and instability (especially recession), economic inequality (including inequality due to structural changes), production processes and consumption of goods that are harmful to health, high-risk social-interaction patterns disproportionately prevalent in the lower socioeconomic strata, and health-care utilization. This analysis will emphasize three elements of political economy crucial to health: (1) the national economic context of growth, business cycles, and social stratification, (2) the processes of production, distribution, and consumption, and (3) government policies.

Economic growth—the creation of wealth and elevation of the national living standard—has overwhelmingly beneficial effects on health, especially in reduction in acute infectious diseases and occupational injuries as causes of death. The main material benefits of economic growth are better nutrition; better housing; more advanced sanitary, industrial, and traffic engineering; and better health care. The psychological benefits include security from catastrophic economic loss and career damage; decline in the prevalence of physically exhausting and hazardous work; improved quality of life for the ill, disabled, and frail; and a sense of control, confidence, and hope for the future.

Also an outcome of economic growth, however, is the rise of chronic diseases in the industrialized world brought about by increases in consumption of harmful substances, shifts in dietary consumption patterns, sedentary lifestyles, and chemical production. Government policies—for example, regulating or discouraging high-risk consumption and production, providing support for the economically vulnerable, promoting productivity, and cushioning the adverse effects of structural change and recession—are the most effective mechanisms in industrialized societies for moderating the health-damaging effects of economic trends.

Thus the nearly exclusive emphasis in the field of health economics on health policy, and more particularly on health-care financing, ignores those policies that most profoundly influence a nation's health, and shape the overall political economy and its components, including real family income, per capita wage rates, unemployment rates, business-failure rates, consumption patterns (based partly on income availability), and specific sources of industrial toxicity. Thus, a society-and-health perspective should not only be concerned with the regulation of occupational and environmental exposures, food quality, and traffic safety, but it needs to view industrial, economic, and social welfare policies as the essential levers for improving health.

Political Economy and Health

If we can show that specific macroeconomic indicators and aggregate patterns of consumption and production are the main determinants of trends in population health, then those policies designed and implemented to influence these indicators must be acknowledged as the main policy sources of a nation's health. This chapter will argue that the backbone of a nation's health is its overall wealth production and the productivity of its technology and labor force.

A secondary determinant of population health is the relative stability of economic growth. The quasi-cyclical economic changes that accompany variations in the business cycle, especially as they affect unemployment and business failure, represent profound shocks to the population's economic, physical, and mental health. The damaging effects of these changes persist for at least a decade.

A third determining factor is the extent of economic inequality—that is, the degree of unequal distribution of wealth and of unequal consumption of the commodities and services that represent the products of economic growth. Economic inequality is heavily influenced by the cyclical nature of economic growth, especially the unemployment rate, although such factors as government-financed income supplementation and investment in "human capital," education, and health care play a substantial role. Economic inequality is mitigated to varying degrees by government-based programs, including education, and income supplementation for the elderly, unemployed, and impoverished.

Long-term economic growth has traditionally been assumed to promote increased economic equality (that is, income). In the last 15 years, however, this fundamental assumption has been undermined in the United States by the uncoupling of wage rates from real per capita income, so that economic growth has not lead to less income inequality. Long-term decline in high- to medium-wage manufacturing jobs and a substantial increase during the 1980s in new jobs characterized by substandard wages, benefits, and tenure appears to be largely responsible. This decline has resulted from increasing pressures for the replacement of labor by high-technology machinery, and by heightened investment in overseas plants where wage rates and benefits are substantially lower, unionization is weak, and occupational and environmental regulations are minimal.

It is the overall wealth of a society that enables it to invest in occupationally and environmentally safer production processes and products. Similarly, the extent to which a firm is willing to introduce safer—and more expensive—equipment and products depends on whether such changes will threaten its economic survival. And the extent to which industry and the general public can be persuaded to replace standard but high-risk commodities with safer products partly depends on the magnitude of the financial losses that would be incurred by industry. Such losses are minimized in periods of high economic growth. Finally, the extent of investment in basic research depends on the financial health of government and industry.

This chapter will test an empirical version of this formulation, the economic-change model of population health, using U.S. mortality data for the period 1950–1988.[1] The premises of a national-level, or macro, formulation of this type are considerably strengthened and validated if we can specify the individual-level or micro theoretical components of the model and secure corroborating evidence at the micro level. The fundamental micro-level hypothesis supporting this model views changes in socioeconomic status (SES) as a byproduct of market forces, economic policy, and social-welfare policy. Changes in SES in turn influence virtually all morbidity and mortality patterns, through several mechanisms: alterations in the material standard of living; changes in consumption patterns (which amount to changes in the person-specific biochemical environment); and changes in psychophysiology involving threats to self-esteem, personal security, autonomy or sense of control, achievement and creativity, strength of social relations, and identity with social groups.

It is crucial to demonstrate the key link between national economic change and mortality is SES because the most pervasive and historically important relationship in epidemiology is between SES and morbidity and mortality rates. This relation has traditionally been demonstrated using ranked occupational differences. More recently, education and, especially, income have been used as measures of SES, and both demonstrate an inverse relation to mortality rates. A vast epidemiologic literature has also accumulated on the significant and consistent relationship between unemployment and elevated morbidity and mortality rates.

In sum, the relations between SES and health at the national level show a high degree of explanatory power, statistical significance, and robustness. They also show little tendency to change from one 15-year period to another. This consistency over time makes for a high degree of predictability, and lends considerable support to the enactment of policy interventions, designed to improve economic well-being, that are the principal sources of improvement in the population's health.

After a discussion of the multiple links between SES and health, we will consider

---

1. This model, which has been under development for many years, has benefited from both methodological and substantive critiques of its earlier versions. A principal innovation has been the use of the Shiller procedure for the estimation of the cumulative relations of economic and epidemiologic risk factors that affect mortality patterns.

SES as a set of intervening variables that act as the link between changes in the national economy and population health. We will then consider the economic-change model of population health, along with empirical data on the capacity of the model to explain changes in mortality rates.

Mechanisms Linking Economic Position and Health

Socioeconomic Status as an Intervening Variable

It is widely recognized that the performance of the economy has a profound impact on a nation's health. As the standard of living increases over time, life expectancy normally increases and age-specific illness rates from most causes decline. We also have very clear evidence of the inverse relationship between socioeconomic status and illness and mortality. Indeed, SES is the most powerful and consistent epidemiological risk factor.

Changes in population SES in turn depend almost entirely on national economic changes, which are a product of market forces and public policy, that is, the political economy. Market forces consist of the following: (1) technological changes, dependent on investment in research and development and in new technology; (2) productivity changes, based largely on technological change and investments in "human capital" and infrastructure; (3) structural changes in industry and the labor force, lately involving large-scale decline in manufacturing employment and an upsurge in relatively low-wage service employment; and (4) international competition in manufacturing, finances, and exports. The most influential but routine policy changes are those undertaken to influence the national economy and the welfare of vulnerable or dependent populations: monetary policy; fiscal policy, including defense, education and infrastructural expenditure; employment retraining and compensation; taxation, minimum-wage policy, and social-security and welfare policy. Other policy changes are based on political movements dealing with the rights of specific social groups, such as women, the elderly, and ethnic and racial groups.

Health research has typically treated the role of SES in two ways. First, SES is treated as a proxy for other epidemiological risks, such as excessive consumption of alcohol, tobacco, and fats or exposure to environmental toxins, whose association with measures of SES is taken as incidental. Or, alternatively, SES confounds (or disturbs) estimation of the "pure" statistical impact of such risk factors on health. In other words, SES is not understood as a major variable, with its own specific but profound impact on health. Third, in a more sophisticated fashion, SES is viewed as a causal precursor of a set of epidemiological risks but rarely as a variable that has origins in economic, political, and cultural change.

This chapter proposes a fourth, more dynamic view of the role of socioeconomic status, placing it in an intermediate position between macroeconomics changes and health: that is, SES is a dependent as well as an independent variable. In a technical sense, therefore, SES is an intervening variable between the macro economy and the major risks to health. It is important to note however, that SES is simultaneously an interacting variable. In this case, SES interacts with changes in culture, technology, and government policies in ways that modify, but have tended to reinforce, health inequalities.

Direct SES-Health Mechanisms

The mechanisms that link SES to health, can be classified as material, psychophysiological, and biochemical risk factors. These mechanisms are both direct and indirect (interactive) in nature. The most direct involve material factors dependent on income and wealth: nutrition, sanitation, housing, industrial engineering, transportation, primary education, health care. They are especially pertinent to infectious diseases, infant and child mortality, and injuries.

Among psychophysiological mechanisms, which influence the chronic diseases (cardiovascular, immune, metabolic) and those that involve mental health (depression, accidents, intentional injury), three broad types can be said to be direct in their effects. The most general involves the self-valuation of the person in terms of the individual's overall status and role (Linton, 1936; Parsons and Shils, 1951), that is, economic position (occupation) and social contribution (content of work and achievement). Individuals are judged against others and against the value standards of their society; Weber (1946) called this "status honor." A person's own judgment of intrinsic self-worth is not idiosyncratic but reflects that of the surrounding society (Cooley, 1902; Mead, 1934). As William James (1890) was the first to point out, public esteem is translated into self-esteem on the part of the individual. Negative self-esteem is closely related to the feelings of shame (Erikson, 1963), stigma (Goffman, 1959) and, most important, deprivation (of social importance). It is thus interpreted as a loss of "what might have been."

A second psychophysiological dimension of socioeconomic status is market position (Weber, 1947), or the ability to obtain income and wealth and thus to consume. Market position is manifested in the use of socially valued goods, services, and symbols that signify comfort, pleasure, intellectual stimulation, and participation in cultural life. From a psychological viewpoint, lack of access to desired consumption generates chronic stress, frustration, and tension, and ultimately profound deprivation.

A third psychophysiological dimension of socioeconomic status is the broad system of incentives and rewards that accompany status and role (occupation and performance) (cf. Davis and Moore, 1945). In addition to income, the rewards of assumed productivity include authority, skill and/or knowledge, access to social networks, and job and income security (cf. Weber 1947; Dahrendorf, 1959; Treiman, 1977), all of which represent basic resources with which the physical and social environment can be influenced. From a psychological standpoint, these resources contribute to a "sense of mastery" of potential life problems, or assurance of lack of vulnerability to stress or threat.

Interactive Mechanism I: Economy and SES

Let us now look at the interactions between various attributes of SES and changes in the social environment. The most important of these interactions links individual economic circumstances—especially change of job or income and work stress—to the fate of one's employer. It is the firm's capacity to survive and thrive in the competitive economic environment that determines its ability to offer employment, wages, and benefits, not to mention safe and pleasant working conditions.

In recessionary periods, strong firms with significant working capital, whose losses in sales are not substantial, usually retain their employees without adversely altering wages or working conditions. The reverse is true of the weak firm in a poor market position. According to the new ecological school of organizational demography, the environment of such a firm's employees depends largely on how well the firm manages its position in the competitive marketplace (Hannan, 1979; Nielson, 1980). When market competition creates a threat of layoffs or acceptance of adverse working conditions, the question that arises is who is to bear the brunt of those threats. In this situation, status within the firm is paramount. Socioeconomic status within the firm involves bureaucratic authority (Weber, 1947), that is, the authority attached to one's formal work position. It is this source of authority that has been hypothesized as the core of SES, or of social class (Dahrendorf, 1959; Blauner, 1972; Orum, 1978). Authority in the firm determines who is to steer it, who is sufficiently valuable to be retained in difficult times, who will be promoted in times of growth, and who will be harmed or benefited by investments in new technology.

The extent to which an individual will experience economic stress thus depends on the interaction of "demands" and "control" factors (Karasek and Theorell, 1990). Demands on the employer reflect the firm's ability to manage its economic environment, while control depends entirely on the firm's authority structure. Thus, the incidence of significant economic stresses depends largely on the economic conditions affecting one's industry and one's firm, and the responses of the firm's authority structure. Those stresses then filter down to the lower SES strata of the firm, where they stimulate individual coping strategies.

Interactive Mechanism II: "Lifestyle" and SES

Richard Doll (1987) explains patterns of change in the major causes of death since the early 1900s by applying classic "epidemic" models. According to Doll, the relevant health-risk behaviors have tended toward epidemic rises, peaks, and declines for two separate reasons. First, increased personal disposable income made items that had been relative luxuries (alcohol, tobacco, fat- and protein-rich foods) considerably more accessible to middle- and lower-income groups. Second, the diffusion of these new patterns of consumption throughout society (Hamblin et al., 1973; Burt, 1978) resembles an exponential function that approaches an asymptote. Subsequent decline in epidemic risk factors is promoted by health messages in the mass media, which report the latest findings on the health risks of various forms of consumption and exposure.

The evidence is strong that such "epidemic" changes in patterns of health-risk behaviors distribute themselves differentially among socioeconomic groups (Morris, 1979). Indeed, the rate of diffusion of common risk factors is so highly related to social class that epidemiologists are often content ot explain the entire SES health relationship by invoking this differential distribution (see Morris, 1979). Diffusion theory (Rogers and Shoemaker 1971) and social-marketing theory (Manoff, 1985) provide relatively clear-cut explanations of how the diffusion of risk factors interacts with socioeconomic level. Initially, the most highly educated individuals (those whose exposure to new information is greatest, and whose social status and wealth also tend to be high) are the first to procure goods newly available on the market. Gradually the rest of society becomes aware of their availability, and (as long as there are continual gains in real disposable income) "catches up" with the innovative leaders (Rogers and Shoemaker, 1971). The retrograde component of the diffusion curve is set in motion only after considerable investment in research on the health implications of the new patterns of consumption and exposure. The time lag between research investment and initial findings is lengthy: because 10–30 years of cumulative exposure is often required for a risk factor to take effect, a generation or more can pass before solid scientific evidence emerges of health-damaging effects.

Thus decades may pass before awareness of the risks to health of given consumption behaviors is diffused throughout the social-economic structure. The retrograde diffusion process may require another generation and may again proceed at different rates depending on social status, education, and income (McQuail, 1988). Income is especially relevant to the capacity to purchase substitutes for risk-laden consumer items. This argument has been used to explain the shift in coronary heart-disease mortality in Britain from an initially higher–SES based mortality rate to the reverse (Marmot et al., 1978, 1987). It can also be applied to any health-risk behavior in which individual choices of consumption items are relevant.

Interactive Mechanism III: Chemical Toxins and SES

Toxic residues of chemical production are a prime source of carcinogenicity and respiratory disease. Exposure to such residues is of two types: direct occupational exposure of employees in firms that produce or use such chemicals, and exposure of the general population to a contaminated environment.

Interaction with SES is substantial in both cases. Within a high-risk firm, lower-SES employees will experience the most exposure (Registrar General, 1976) because those in authority will leave the handling of dangerous materials and equipment to those who are not in a position to refuse. In general, high-risk firms, with relatively poor security measures and the least-sophisticated equipment, are found in the poorer subgroup of the segmented labor market (Doeringer and Piore, 1971; Edwards, 1975), and their employees are likely to be those with the least skills and education; these individuals also earn the lowest wages and benefits, and (in the United States) have the least adequate health-care coverage.

The relative lack of authority and, thus, heightened vulnerability of lower-SES employees is compounded by their limited knowledge of occupational health risks and tendency to assume that, in any event, they cannot alter their work situation. These sources of occupational vulnerability are exacerbated by the relative lack of political influence of lower-SES groups on the development of occupational safety and health codes.

Place of residence is also a key risk factor in exposure to chemical carcinogens (Epstein and Swartz, 1981). Here again, the relative lack of political influence of lower-SES groups makes them especially vulnerable, as do the financial and discriminatory components in "choice" of place of residence. Obviously, the families with the fewest resources are not in a position to insist on environmentally healthy neighborhoods.

Alternative Explanations For Differences In Individual SES?

Origins of SES for Individuals

Economics and sociology offer four alternative explanations of differences in socioeconomic attainment: these are referred to as (1) institutional determinants, (2) human capital, (3) statistical discrimination and (4) status attainment.

The institutional determinants of individuals' SES are the differential rates of growth (and sometimes decline) of different industries, which therefore offer differential opportunities for advancement. Of particular importance in the literature is the small firm, in the poorly capitalized sector of the "segmented labor market," that offers inferior wages, benefits, and working conditions (Doeringer and Piore, 1971; Edwards, 1975). This segment of the labor market is subject to high failure rates and high unemployment rates, and is obviously highly sensitive to national, regional, and even international business conditions. The literature on institutional determinants makes clear that the basic structure of SES for a nation, and thus the parameters of socioeconomic attainment for the individual, are highly dependent on macroeconomic conditions.

Human capital signifies the skill level and productive capacity of the workforce, and thus its occupational abilities and earning capacity. The human-capital school of thought maintains that investment in education and training, by the individual and by society, is crucial to advances in SES (Becker, 1964; Thurow, 1969). Development of human capital requires both institutional structures (e.g., social investments in science and/or knowledge development, educational organizations, and manpower) and, on the part of the individual, sufficient income, leisure, and willingness to forego employment opportunities. Clearly, human-capital investments depend, foremost, on national economic growth and per capita disposable income.

The statistical-discrimination approach posits that, beyond skill and appropriate credentialing, "ascriptive" (Parsons, 1951) aspects of social status (sex, race/ethnicity, age, religion, national origin, region of origin) play a part in determining occupation, job position, and earnings (Coleman, 1974; Thurow, 1987). Over the long term, however, "universalistic" (i.e., objective) and formalized standards increasingly dominate hiring practices, work authority, and incentive and reward systems. This tendency is due to the increasing formalization ("bureaucratization") and professionalization of work, and to increasing requirements for formal training and certification (as suggested by the human-capital school).

The status-attainment approach to differences in SES (e.g., Blau and Duncan, 1967; Sewell and Hauser, 1972; Treiman and Terell, 1975; Featherman and Hauser, 1975) views socialization in childhood as a crucial determinant of future occupation and living standards. This outlook views the family subculture, particularly the occupation of the father (and, increasingly, the mother), as a powerful influence on future socioeconomic status. The SES of family of origin is thus a conservative force, tending to preserve the stability of the social-stratification system.

In sum, leaving aside issues of family and poor socialization, theoretical explanations of differential socioeconomic status focus on economic development and change, emphasizing the mechanisms of industrial development, human-capital formation, and formalization of occupational requirements. One might also add social-welfare payment mechanisms to support the incomes of lower socioeconomic groups, and government policies favoring progressive income taxation and labor-management wage-benefit negotiations.

Effects of Economic Change on Socioeconomic Status

Changes in the overall socioeconomic level, i.e., the standard of living, and structure (industrial and occupational) of a population are largely dependent on its rate of economic productivity, which in turn largely reflects technological developments (Krugman, 1991; Griliches, 1988; Kendrick, 1980, 1984). The degree of income inequality is related, over time, to several phenomena: the unemployment rate as an indicator of macroeconomic fluctuations (Dunlop, 1938; Menderhausen, 1946; Budd and Whiteman, 1978; Nolan, 1987; Podgursky and Swaim, 1987a, b); differential rates of development (and decline) of specific industries and regions (Kendrick, 1983; Harrison et al., 1986); union activity (Economic Policy Council, 1983; Weisskopf et al., 1983; Freeman and Medoff, 1984; Marshall, 1986); and policies on investments in human capital, infrastructure, and support of vulnerable and dependent groups (Kuttner, 1986; Anderson, 1986). Of lesser significance to income inequality are birth-cohort size (Dooley and Gottschalk, 1984) and such attributes of firms as size, market concentration, and capital to labor ratios (Hodson, 1983). Genetically based ability and aspects of family background are potentially important, but do not appear to influence the SES structure over time. Income discrimination based on race, ethnicity, sex and age, though subject to political change, can alter the structure of economic inequality.

Feedback Mechanisms

While relations between measures of SES and health have proven consistent and powerful, causation has not been well delineated, often because its direction is incompletely specified. Reverse causation is logically possible: genetic and biological (that is, intrauterine) factors could account for differing intellectual abilities and functional capacities (thus affecting SES), and for differing morbidity and mortality rates. A substantial research literature stresses the impact of illness, disability, and addictions on reduced functional capacity, including work productivity (Rice, 1966; Luft, 1978; Manning et al., 1982). The possibility of reverse, or lack of, causation even applies to the impact of unemployment on health and mortality. It is plausible, for example, that even in a recession those most likely to be laid off are the least psychologically or physically healthy, who function most poorly. In the short term and certainly in the long term, this group might plausibly have higher mortality and morbidity rates than the employed, apart from any effects of unemployment itself. It is undoubtedly true that illness can lead to declines in economic functioning and thus in occupational level and income.

To the degree that either of these reverse-causation arguments is accurate, economic and social policy intended to improve health would clearly be ineffectual. When the SES-health relation is indirectly measured, however, and given a general ecological expression in which the subjects are unable to influence the economic environment, the relation persists. It thus becomes difficult to argue that the causal direction is reverse. At the macro level, several additional observations make reverse causation unlikely.

First, changes in the overall economy are unlikely to be influenced by the activities of seriously ill individuals. (One could even argue that the death of the very ill contributes to the economy by freeing up resources.) There is a mass of literature on the factors that normally influence economic growth and economic cycles, and mortality patterns (especially in industrialized countries) are not among them. Second, economic changes precede changes in mortality patterns: both short-term and long-term relationships are identifiable between changes in the economy and changes in mortality. Third, relations at the macro level are in accord with similar relations at the micro level, and with theoretical explanations of mortality patterns both in the social sciences and in psychophysiology.

A more plausible explanation is a straightforward feedback mechanism. Thus (1) low SES involves higher incidence of illness and/or disability due to inequalities in the distribution of material, biochemical, and psychosocial benefits and risks. In turn (2) serious illness and/or disability adversely affects employment possibilities, earnings, and productivity. This feedback effect may explain how recessions engender latent increases in mortality rates due to chronic disease: namely, downward social mobility is accelerated and reinforced by chronically compromised health.

Macroeconomic Determinants of Social Stratification

Long-Term Growth of the Economy

The distribution of jobs (i.e., the distribution of skilled and semi-skilled manufacturing versus customer-service and sales jobs), which depends on the level of technology prevailing in the economy, and the pay levels associated with the status of those jobs, are widely agreed to be the major determinants of income inequality. As Shorrocks (1987) puts it: "Job distribution, together with customary wage and salary differentials, . . . is the principal determinant of earnings inequality. Personal characteristics appear to be important only because they are used by firms to ration entry into the more attractive jobs."[2]

Long-term income inequality is accounted for by factors of economic growth, demography, and education. Kuznets (1955), whose work addressed the relation between economic growth and income dispersion within countries, found an increase in inequalities at the early stage of industrialization, in conjunction with large-scale movement out of agriculture into the modernizing sector. As the modernizing sector becomes dominant, inequalities decrease. Williamson and Lindert (1980) found evidence of this pattern in the United States: relative wage equality prior to 1816; striking increases in inequality in 1816–1856 and 1899–1916; and secular declines in inequality between 1929 and the Korean War.

The Impact of Recession and Unemployment

The business cycle, and specifically the unemployment rate, is the second macroeconomic influence on income inequalities. Inequalities widen as the business cycle contracts, specifically as unemployment rates grow. Kuznets (1953) found a tendency in the interwar period (1919–1939), for overall inequality to move inversely with the business cycle, the upper-income group gaining at the expense of the vast majority (probably no less than 85–90 percent) of wage-earners in periods of economic downturn (Kuznets, 1953, pp. 57–58). An earlier study (Menderhausen, 1946), found a similar pattern during the Great Depression (1929–1933).

---

2. On the issue of wage levels conventionally linked to social status of occupations, Phelps Brown (1987) states: "People insist on the maintenance of customary relations. They require that relative pay conform with status. That the laborer's rate stood at two-thirds of the craftsman's in the building industry of Southern England over more than six centuries . . . can be attributed only to convention. If women's rates had been simply proportioned to productivity, it is hard to account for their relative rise when the rule of 'equal pay for equal work' was enforced in the UK and the Netherlands . . . These observations are all consistent with differences of pay being set to match accepted gradations of status."

The pattern of increasing inequality in recessions and narrowing inequality in subsequent recoveries has persisted in a less extreme form in the postwar period, according to annual data from the U.S. Bureau of the Census.

Post-1970s Structural and Demographic Shifts

Income inequality in the United States, continued to shrink from the end of World War II until the late 1970s and early 1980s, when inequality began to increase again. This trend continues in the present (Levy, 1987; Maxwell, 1989; Winnick, 1989; U.S. Congress House of Representatives, 1989; Phillips, 1990; Ryscavage and Henle, 1990). For the first time in American history in fact, the economic expansion of the 1980s was accompanied by deterioration in the standard of living for a majority of households (Sweeney and Nussbaum, 1987; Harrison and Bluestone, 1990; Litan et al., 1990).

The existence of increasing inequality and real-wage stagnation in a period of economic expansion has several linked explanations (Maxwell, 1989). First, striking increases in foreign competition and dollar devaluation since the 1970s have forced fundamental changes in the manufacturing and export-oriented industries. These changes may reflect cyclic movements intrinsic to market economies (Thurow, 1980; Feldstein, 1980), as well as a permanent structural shift from manufacturing to service employment (Bluestone and Harrison, 1982). Because the resulting slowdowns in real wages and productivity vary among industries and occupations, changes in income distribution have resulted.

Dooley and Gottschalk (1985) have shown that low-wage workers experienced below-average wage growth. Meanwhile, workers in the rapidly growing high-technology industries, a high proportion of whom are highly paid (Rosenthal, 1985), experienced gains in real income (McMahon and Tschetter, 1986). Polarization of income distribution, and potentially a decline in middle-class income, follows in turn from simultaneous growth of low-wage and high-wage employment (Harrison et al., 1986).

Maxwell's (1989) multivariate statistical analysis of U.S. income inequality in the period 1947–1985 considers these factors as well as demographic shifts and government programs. The results show that income inequality is promoted by increases in the proportion of the nonworking (dependent) population, in service-sector employment, and in the proportion of blue-collar workers. Growth in the dependency ratio and in service-oriented industrial employment increase inequality by increasing the top quintile's income share and decreasing the bottom quintile's. Industrial and demographic forces, such as changes in labor market and immigration, exert the greatest impact on the income share of the lower quintiles, particularly that of the very lowest quintile.

While Maxwell (1989) found government spending on social welfare programs only affects the top and bottom quintiles, cross-national studies do indicate that social-welfare expenditures can have a marked effect on income equality. Of 10 intensively studied Western European and North American countries (Smeeding, 1991), the Scandinavian countries and Germany show the lowest income inequalities and the United States the highest.

The Cyclical Behavior of Income Inequality

The cyclical nature of earnings distribution is a major generator of income inequality. Even if workers who lost their jobs were drawn proportionately from all wage levels, according to Menderhausen (1946), they would be pushed into zero-income or very low income positions compared to those who retained their jobs; this enlarges the income gap between the unemployed and underemployed on the one hand and those with relatively full-time employment on the other. And, in reality, all workers do not face the same probability of becoming unemployed in a recession; the incidence of unemployment is greater among the less skilled and lower paid. Thus, wage differentials can be expected to widen, partly because unemployed workers are reemployed in lower-wage jobs.

During periods of declining product demand, Oi (1962) argues the employer has an incentive to retain workers with larger investments in human capital (the more skilled and highly paid) and to lay off those with little specific training. The result is larger increases in unemployment among the unskilled, and/or widening of wage differentials.

In the same vein, Reder (1955) argues that, instead of laying off both skilled and unskilled workers in a recession, employers choose to assign their underemployed skilled workers to less skilled jobs and to concentrate layoffs among the less skilled. Employers also tighten hiring standards in recessions and relax them in subsequent expansions.

Among the many studies of the impact of macroeconomic conditions on inequality, the most consistent finding has been a significant disequalizing effect of increases in unemployment, reducing the share of total income earned by lower-SES groups.[3]

Economic Change and Health: Macro and Micro Evidence

Stable Economic Growth and Health

Having explored the relationship between SES and health, we can now ask: What, theoretically, is the importance of the economy to the nation's health? To answer this question, let us look first at the health implications of stable economic growth.

The material contribution of economic growth is the basic differentiator among societies in terms of mortality rates. It separates the high-life-expectancy countries from

---

3. Schultz (1969) initiated the econometric analysis of the topic and estimated an equation relating the inequality in the distribution as measured by the Gini coefficient to variables such as inflation, unemployment, the growth rate, and time trend. Schultz failed to identify any significant influence of macroeconomic variables on the Gini coefficient for the U.S. distribution, while the remaining, disaggregated studies, did find such effects on the distribution time series. Simulation approaches based on micro data (Mirer 1973a,b; Budd and Whiteman, 1978; Nolan, 1987), panel analysis (Gramlich, 1974) and studies specifically of poverty (e.g., Hollister and Palmer, 1972) were also able to estimate the positive relation between recession, or unemployment, and income inequality.

low, and is the prime factor in infant and child survival and infectious diseases rates. Its key elements, as we have seen, are nutrition, housing, sanitary engineering, primary education (of the mother), and primary health care, all of which require societal investments and thus sufficient national wealth. Investments in industrial design and sophisticated equipment are also necessary to prevent disability and mortality due to unintentional injuries.

Stable economic growth is the *sine qua non* of investment in knowledge development, including systematic epidemiological investigation of health-risk factors. Such investment is crucial not only to engineering and the biological and physical sciences but also to the social and economic sciences instrumental in managing the overall economy and individual firms. Joint development of the material economy and of the scientific base provides for predictability, manageability, and comprehensibility in the human and physical environments. Stable economic growth is the prerequisite for fundamental political undertakings designed to promote equality of distribution (labor-management bargaining, taxation, and social-welfare expenditures). These fundamentals contribute in turn to a human psychology of hope and confidence (control, "self-efficacy," and security).

Stable growth is critical to social integration as well. Perhaps the most significant source of social integration is the process of urbanization. The transition of the bulk of the population from rural to urban life may well have caused a basic shift in human relations, as Toennies (1952) and Durkheim (1947) have asserted. In any event, the development and maintenance of urban life has generated the formation of numberless social organizations based on interests and values. It is inaccurate to say that the advent of such formal "secondary" institutions has caused the wellsprings of primary face-to-face relations to "dry up." On the contrary, formal organizations—from workplaces to government—require primary relations *within* the groups that constitute their working parts.

The Impact of Recession and Unemployment on Health: Descriptive Epidemiology

Studies conducted over the last 20 years on the relationship of economic change to morbidity and mortality in industrialized countries represent two distinct epidemiological traditions in the mental and physical disorders. The earlier work on mental-health problems tended to emphasize the role of economic loss in stress. More recent work on physical health has made it apparent that recession itself plays a causal role. It is now recognized that loss of resources and psychological stress are not easy to isolate causally: the implication is that, in the vast majority of pathologies, including mental and physical illness and criminal aggression, some combination of resource loss and psychological stress is probably involved.

Suicide

Suicide was the first indicator of mental pathology found to increase consistently with adverse changes in the economy (Durkheim, 1951; Henry and Short, 1954; Brenner

1971b, 1980a, 1984a; Vigderhous and Fishman, 1978; Boor, 1980; Marshall and Hodge, 1981). A number of researchers have replicated these findings, attesting to the severe stress brought about by economic recession (Brenner 1976b, 1984a, b; reviewed in Platt, 1986).

Mental Health

Research on the relationship between adverse economic changes and increases in mental-hospital admissions has demonstrated that the relationship can be measured consistently over time (Dayton, 1940; Pugh and MacMahon, 1962; Brenner, 1973a). The first of these studies dealt with Massachusetts during the 1930s, the second with the United States as a whole during the Depression, and the third with New York State in the period 1841–1967. During each recession since 1841, first admissions and readmissions to mental hospitals increased substantially. Cyclical change in the economy was the single most important factor affecting trends in admission. The New York State study has been replicated for the entire United States and for each state in the periods 1936–1970 and 1950–1980, with nearly identical results (Brenner, 1976b, 1984a).

Numerous epidemiological studies on the relation of unemployment to mental health have found symptoms of psychological disorder to be consistently associated with unemployment (Ferman and Gardner, 1979; Dooley and Catalano, 1984; Elder and Capri, 1988; Forcier, 1988; Kessler et al., 1988; Penkower et al., 1988; Warr et al., 1988; Hamilton et al., 1990).

The relation of criminal aggression—especially homicide, crimes known to the police, arrest rates, and imprisonment, particularly for violent crimes but also for all crimes against persons and property—to economic recession and especially unemployment has been observed for decades (Brenner 1976a, b, 1980a, b, 1984a).

Alcohol Abuse

The findings on alcohol abuse are consistent with a hypothesis of increased mental disorder precipitated by social-psychological stress during economic recession. Increases in mortality rates due to cirrhosis of the liver are positively related, over time, to consumption increases with distilled spirits (rather than wine or beer), and such consumption increases with cyclic declines in the national economy. Cirrhosis mortality itself increases substantially 1–2 years after national economic recession. Because it takes a long time to acquire chronic cirrhosis of the liver, it is clear that the short-term economic trauma had not initiated the cirrhotic condition, but that, once morbidity was present, economic recession tended to hasten mortality (Brenner, 1975).

Other findings underline the relationship between increased consumption of distilled spirits and declines in the national economy. Admissions to mental hospitals for psychosis related to alcoholism and other alcohol-related mental disorders showed substantial and stable increases during economic recessions during the period 1921–1968. Similarly, arrests for drunkenness in Massachusetts increased with adverse changes in the national economy over the period 1915–1968; the arrests lagged 2 years behind fluctuations in the economy. Finally, arrest rates for driving while intoxicated were found to increase substantially during national economic recessions (Brenner, 1975).

Heart Disease

Early, empirical research on heart-disease incidence and mortality clearly demonstrated that fluctuations in heart-disease mortality rates were inversely related to the employment rate in New York State in 1915–1967. Mortality from coronary-artery disease was found to be related to fluctuations in the unemployment rate for the United States as a whole in the period 1930–1960. Both studies found that mortality peaked at least 2–3 years after economic recessions (Brenner, 1971a, b).

Subsequent studies of the relationship between national economic indicators and cardiovascular-renal disease hypothesized that these illnesses are characterized by significant psychophysiological factors involving hypertension and serum-cholesterol levels. Cardiovascular-renal diseases account for approximately 60 percent of all mortality in many industrialized nations. An examination of U.S. data for 1914–1968, by race, sex, and 10-year age groups, found a consistent relationship between national economic fluctuations, measured by per capita income or employment rates, and mortality rates due to cardiovascular renal disease. For cardiovascular-renal diseases in general, the peak lagged behind economic recessions by 3–6 years, depending on age; the peak for chronic nephritis lagged from 0 to 2 years; for cerebrovascular diseases, the lag ranged from 6 to 9 years (Brenner, 1971a, b).

Infant Mortality

The infant-mortality rate has long been recognized as one of the most sensitive indicators of the general socioeconomic level of a nation. The relationship between the economy, and infant, fetal, and maternal mortality has thus been extensively examined. In all industrialized countries for which data are available, industrial growth is inversely related to the long-term trend in infant-mortality rates (Susser et al., 1985). However, a society's adaptation to economic change is less a matter of the level of economic growth than of whether that growth is relatively smooth or unstable.

An investigation of the relationship between economic instability and mortality in infants under 1 year of age found fetal and infant mortality to increase sharply in response to economic recession, with a peak lag of 0–2 years (Brenner, 1973b). This relation has been demonstrated for the United States in 1936–1974 and 1950–1980 (Brenner 1976a, b, 1984a), the United Kingdom (Brenner, 1979, 1983), and Sweden (Brenner, 1987b). The relationship between economic fluctuations and trends in infant-mortality rates has historically been an important component of the relationship between low socioeconomic status and increased infant mortality; that is, the impact of economic shock, such as on infant mortality, is greater for lower–SES groups. The influence of economic instability, especially recession, on infant mortality trends has grown since 1950, perhaps because of a relative decline in the beneficial impact of secular economic growth in an economy that is already highly developed.

Overall Mortality

The influence of economic change on overall (non-cause) mortality rates has been studied for several decades. The principal long-term declines in overall mortality, as well as age-specific mortality for all age groups, are associated with long-term improvements in the national economy, especially real per capita incomes. The business cycle is heavily influential in the short- to medium-term fluctuations in mortality rates. Such variables as unemployment and business-failure rates are typically associated with increases in mortality two to three years following the lowest point in the business cycle and extending for at least the next 10 to 15 years. The relationships have been most fully explored with data for the United States, United Kingdom, and Sweden (Brenner, 1976a, 1979, 1980b, c, 1984a, 1987b, c, 1991, 1993). Middle-aged mortality rates have also been examined from this viewpoint in at least 10 additional countries (Brenner, 1989).

These types of relationships for overall mortality—with long-term trends inversely related to economic growth and short- to medium-term fluctuations significantly associated with economic cycles—have also been observed for the principal cardiovascular diseases, even when the models included controls for tobacco, fat, and alcohol consumption patterns (Brenner, 1976b, 1984a, 1987a, b, c; Brenner and Mooney, 1982).

Microepidemiological Research on Unemployment

Unexpected large-scale increases in unemployment rates in European countries that have occurred since the 1973 oil crisis and which continue to the present day have interested epidemiological researchers working at the individual level in prospective studies of morbidity and mortality. A classic study by Moser, Fox, and Jones (1984) examined a nationwide sample of employed and unemployed British men in 1971 to see whether an impact on mortality in 1982 could be discerned. They found not only that the unemployed men had substantially higher standardized mortality ratios (SMRs), after controlling for social-class differences in mortality, but that the wives of these men (who were not themselves unemployed) also showed significantly elevated SMRs. Similar studies in the United States (Sorlie and Rogot, 1990), Denmark (Iversen et al., 1987), Sweden (Stefansson, 1991), and Finland (Martkainen, 1990) found significantly elevated SMRs a decade after the unemployment event; those who were not seeking work or were otherwise outside the labor force tended to show the highest mortality rates.

Studies of psychiatric and somatic morbidity in Germany (reviewed by Schwefel, 1986), the United Kingdom (Jackson and Warr, 1987), Norway (Westin et al., 1989; Westin, 1990), the United States (Linn et al., 1985), and Denmark (Iversen et al., 1989) have repeatedly confirmed the importance of unemployment as a prospective risk factor in physical and mental illness. These studies have taken care to separate out the effects of social selection, which can be especially pernicious in unemployment-health studies because seriously ill and disabled individuals are highly vulnerable to job loss.

While there has been remarkable consistency in the findings of individual-level epi-demiological studies, studies of the relation between unemployment and subsequent morbidity and mortality at the national level have not been as consistent. Macro-level suicide and mental-health studies have tended to confirm the generally adverse impact of unemployment, but the results of studies of overall and chronic-disease mortality have been more mixed (Forbes and McGregor, 1987). Whenever controls for tradi-tional risk factors (alcohol, tobacco, fat consumption) have been used, however, the re-sults have uniformly shown elevated mortality rates following recessions, peaking after approximately 2–3 years (Brenner, 1971a, b, 1980a, 1984b, 1987a), and fre-quently extending as long as 10–15 years (Brenner, 1976a, b, 1984b, 1989). The over-all length of the lags is similar to those found in longitudinal epidemiological studies involving traditional risk factors, and may in fact reflect the interaction of recession and downward mobility with those risk factors. If so, the interaction of unemployment with "lifestyle" and toxicological risks may be similar to the well-documented inverse relation of SES with these risk factors.

Mechanisms Linking Recession and Health

Economic recession engenders damage to health by means of at least six mechanisms: (1) reduced financial access to health care, resulting in underutilization; (2) psy-chophysiological reactions to stress and loss; (3) damage to social relations and sources of social support; (4) maladaptive coping mechanisms involving high-risk con-sumption patterns; (5) less thorough and frequent maintenance of manufacturing plants and reduced investment in modernization, with a consequent effect on health and safety; (6) increased work stress during the economic recovery as firms that lost heav-ily during the recession take on more work but do not yet hire additional workers, due to a capital shortfall and uncertainty about the stability of the recovery.

First, the lack of health insurance and relative poverty of workers in the "secondary" labor market and of people outside the labor force contribute to comparatively low uti-lization rates of inpatient, ambulatory-curative, and preventive health services, espe-cially among the very young and the elderly (Ford and Marlis, 1990; Rowland, 1990; Whitman et al., 1991; Ahern and McCoy, 1992; Kirkman and Kronenfeld, 1992). Even people who have health insurance are typically required to make copayments so that there is significantly lower utilization of these types of services (Shapiro et al., 1986; Anderson et al., 1991).

Second, psychophysiological coping reactions to stress and loss are known to be highly varied. They include a compromised immune system, which is less able to resist infection and malignancy (Bartrop et al., 1977; Eysenck et al., 1991); effects on the cardiovascular system (Grossarth-Maricek and Eysenck, 1991; Goldstein and Niaura, 1992; Niaura and Goldstein, 1992), including hypertension (Pickering et al., 1991; Schnall et al., 1992), myocardial infarction, angina, and acute cholesterol response (Muldoon et al., 1992); peptic ulcer (Anda, 1992); asthma (Isenberg et al., 1992); dis-orders of the central nervous system such as migraine, anxiety, and psychotic and adjustment disorders (American Psychiatric Association, 1987); and emotional reactions, especially depression (Paykel et al., 1969; Brown et al, 1973; Brown and Harris, 1978), aggression (Dollard et al., 1939; Miller, 1941; Berkowitz, 1962), and somatization (American Psychiatric Association, 1987).

Third, the ties of family and friendship and peer relations among coworkers have been found to moderate the impact of stress and loss (Brenner and Starrin, 1988; Turner et al., 1990). However, depressive or aggressive reactions to loss and stress can damage social networks by alienating close associates and discouraging them from providing further social support. Indeed, the impact of depression, aggression, or general tension can bring about divorce, and separation or destruction of friendship networks (Liker and Elder, 1983; Coyne et al., 1987; Krantz and Moos, 1987; Rath et al., 1989; Dew and Bromet, 1991; Rook et al., 1991).

Damage to social relations can also result directly from changes in population dynamics during and after economic recessions. According to the push-pull theory of migration, regional (and international) migration is characterized by movement away from areas of meager employment or career prospects to those that offer economic opportunity. This important demographic mechanism comes forcefully into play following nationwide recessions, when people move away from areas (or industries) that have not yet experienced economic recovery and/or expansion to those that have. Such migration therefore peaks at the high point of business cycles. This migration pattern calls for the migrating worker to adapt to a new social setting (Cassel and Tyroler, 1961; Syme et al., 1965; Marmot and Syme, 1976) and overcome social isolation. It also means that the family members and friends left behind will experience loss and long-term deprivation. Furthermore, the communities left behind will suffer a loss of population, and ultimately of economic viability; meanwhile, if migration is substantial, the regions (usually urban) and firms that receive it will also experience problems of adjustment, including weaker social ties among the local (nonmigrant) population.

Relations among different social classes and ethnic groups can suffer considerably under conditions of economic decline (Van Hook, 1990), a phenomenon that lends support to the hypotheses of "frustration-aggression" and scapegoating (Dollard et al., 1939; Miller, 1941; Berkowitz, 1962). This correlation appears to be confirmed by repeated instances of serious ethnic and civil conflict during and after periods of national economic adversity. The related assumption of a strong connection between national economic adversity and changes of government has nearly evolved to the status of a formal theory, in which "political cycles" are a central concept.

Fourth, many social scientists assume that maladaptive responses to chronic stress and adverse life events include adoption of unhealthy consumption patterns. Alcohol (Pearlin and Radabaugh, 1976) in particular has been cited as a maladaptive tool for management of stress and depression, as have tobacco and other addictive substances (Lee et al., 1991; Serxner et al., 1991). Alterations in diet, especially increases in fat and sugar consumption, are also often assumed to be coping devices (Schlundt et al., 1990).

Fifth, minimizing health risks due to occupational and chemical environmental hazards (Susser, 1985) requires considerable investment in equipment maintenance, waste disposal, and substitution of nontoxic substances for traditional ones. Substantial health risks, therefore, accompany the depletion of investment capital, which can reduce compliance with the regulations of occupational and environmental safety agencies (Leigh, 1989).

Finally, the impact of recession and economic instability on a firm's efforts to survive may be the source of severe work stresses related to serious illness and premature mortality. During a recession, anxieties over potential job loss and threats to career and financial solvency pervade the firm (e.g., Kasl and Cobb, 1982). Recessional stresses are also likely to diminish worker autonomy, due to decreased managerial tolerance for error while the firm struggles for survival. This situation is compounded by damage to social relations (and thus social support) among workers when every worker is worried about job security and no one wants to be linked to those whose jobs are to be terminated (House et al., 1988). More influential, however, in a financially damaged firm is the perpetuation of work stress well into the period of national recovery and expansion. Such a firm will have experienced a shrinkage of working capital and will have an especially difficult time knowing when to hire in the face of growing market demand, a phenomenon known as "the signal extraction problem" (Attfield and Duck, 1985). This difficulty will result in acute and chronic shortages of staff and an extraordinary emphasis on high employee productivity. The result for employees is a situation of "high demands/low control," which has been shown to be related to cardiovascular disease and overall mortality risks (Karasek and Theorell, 1990).

The Initial 2- to 3-Year Lag of Mortality Following Economic Recessions

The initial elevation of overall mortality rates, including the major causes of death, occurs at approximately two to three years following the recession. This point of elevated mortality is then typically followed by continually heightened mortality rates for at least the next decade. Both of these phenomena are related to the initial impact of the recession.

The basis of the 2- to 3-year lag is as follows. The recession itself is the first phase of loss; the individual's response to unemployment is mental depression and probably the beginnings of other serious physiological disturbances related to chronic diseases. This is a phase of cataclysmic stress, affecting large numbers of people (thus equated with a "disaster") such that the loss of job and income is part of a national or regional phenomenon. These conditions foster social support for the affected individual.

This first phase, however, is not the critical point in the "stressful life event" associated with recession. The most important issue is whether the individual will recover his or her economic and social status, or will undergo a permanent loss. This is decided mainly during the economic recovery. At the peak of the business cycle, occurring about 2–3 years after the recession, a social distance has arisen between individuals who have not recovered and those who have. Since the highest level of employment occurs at this point, the individual who has not economically reintegrated will lose much of the social support received during the recession itself. Also at the peak of the business cycle, the economy is beginning to slow at a time of considerable overoptimism about the economic future. This is a time of great frustration, when it becomes clear that heightened expectations will be unfulfilled—which is especially acute for the individual who has not yet fully recovered from the effects of the preceding recession, but is still desperately hoping to do so.

Thus, at the peak of the business cycle, three states prevail: a maximum economic inequality between those who have recovered from the recession and those who have not; uncertainty about the economic future; and frustration over the failure to achieve the hoped for continuing recovery. All of these are particularly acute in those who suffered loss of employment and income during the preceding recession.

Macroeconomic Change and Mortality: The Economic-Change Model of Population Health

As we have seen, mortality rates in many Western industrialized societies are typically related inversely to economic growth for the population as a whole and for nearly all age groups. Also, short- to medium-term increases in mortality rates tend to be inversely related to economic recessions, with an average lag of 2–3 years; this early peak heralds the start of a long-term effect of recession, lasting 10–15 years. Epidemiological evidence based on individual-level research, and extrapolation from it to national levels via epidemic models (Doll, 1987) and diffusion theory (Rogers and Shoemaker, 1971), support the view that the major consumption-and-production risk factors (alcohol, tobacco, fats, chemical production) account for much of the hyperbolic shape of mortality trends since the Second World War. Finally, national policies providing for transfer payments (especially those for Old Age, Survivors, Disability and Health Insurance (OASDHI), education and welfare) and health-care expenditures tend to significantly modify mortality trends.

The "economic-change model of population health" helps to organize the empirical data expressing these and other variables in such a way that they can be used jointly to account for changes in mortality patterns. The economic change model (e.g., Brenner 1984a, b) includes measures of the following concepts: economic growth, economic instability (including recession), economic inequality, maladaptive responses to economic growth (excessive consumption of alcohol, tobacco, fat), chemical production, social-isolation measures such as divorce rates, and random "shocks" not predictable by other factors in the model (epidemics, abrupt population movements, military conflict, and high-impact medical technology). The final output of an analysis using this model will bring together, in the same multivariate equation, variables expressing each (or at least several) of these benefit and risk factors; relations for each variable will then cover a distributed-lag period involving at least a decade.

We begin the analysis by identifying the simplest short-term relationships for a single variable; we then examine the cumulative impact of the same variable over multiple years (distributed lag), and finally show the relations of multiple variables in a "full" time-series multiple-regression model.

The Box-Jenkins technique (Box and Jenkins, 1982) of time-series analysis, using autoregressive and moving-average terms to fit (and thereby forecast) basic trends and cycles in mortality, is useful for analyzing short-term relations. Our analysis asks, for example, whether changes in the unemployment rate, as a basic cyclic economic indicator, will help explain changes in mortality trends after the autoregressive and moving-average components of these trends have been accounted for. Previous research indicates that mortality from all causes and from major chronic diseases reaches a first peak of increase approximately 2–3 years following the bottom of a recession, as measured by the highest point in the unemployment rate (e.g., Brenner 1971a, b, 1980a, 1984b, 1987a). This is apparent in our analysis of age-adjusted mortality, both total mortality and mortality for specific sex-race groupings (see Table 7–1). For white males, a significant positive relationship between the unemployment rate and mortality is observed after a 2-year lag. For white females and nonwhite males and females, the positive relations for unemployment can be seen at 2 and 3 years.

Because, on average, economic cycles tend to be 4–5 years in length (Mitchell, 1951), this classic 2- to 3-year lag in mortality after the peak in the unemployment rate means that the first peak in mortality following recession approximately coincides with the subsequent peak in the business cycle—that is, the peak of "recovery" or "expansion." Given this observation, one should also note that the zero-lag relationship between unemployment and mortality rates is actually inverse. The *first* peak in the lagged mortality rate at 2–3 years after recession is not accidental: the delayed impact of economic distress interacts with chronic-disease mortality in such a way that the first wave of increased mortality peaks at about the same time as growth in the economic cycle. The explanation for this phenomenon involves three different populations that experience considerable loss due to recession.

The first population will have experienced loss of employment and income during the recession, and these losses may have been compounded by illness. Illness, in turn, reduces the likelihood of rapid reentry into the labor force, and substantially decreases productivity if reemployed. Over time, therefore, this population will at least remain at a lower economic level than prior to the recession, and may have a permanently decreased economic status. Meanwhile, with the subsequent expansion of employment and income, the bulk of the population will have found its economic position significantly advanced. Between the bottom of the recession and the peak of the upturn, therefore, the differences in economic position between the majority and this minority (as a specific cohort) will reach a maximum of inequality. The minority population's ensuing relative deprivation and social isolation will then expose it to its highest risk of psychological distress during the entire economic cycle.

A second population seriously harmed by recession consists of employees of firms in vulnerable industries. As we have seen, these firms frequently have difficulty adjusting to the subsequent economic upturn, due to a severe shortage of capital and the "signal-extraction problem." These difficulties result in minimal hiring despite increased market demand. Understaffing then calls for high productivity from existing employ-

Table 7-1 Box-Jenkins Model of Short-Term Time-Series Relations Between Unemployment Rate and Age-Adjusted Mortality Rate, by Race, United States 1947–1988

(Second Differences, 2- and 3-Year Lags)[a]

Variable	Lag (Years)	Coefficient	Standard Error	T Statistic
White Males				
Unemployment Rate	2	.443E-01	.151E-01	2.935
AR	1	−.525	.148	−3.542
MA	1	−.514	.163	−3.156
RBAR Sq. .592;				
Q(18) = 4.714				
White Females				
Unemployment Rate	2	.171E-01	.929	1.836
AR	1	−.915	.139	−6.563
AR	2	−.491	.139	−3.529
RBAR Sq. .480;				
Q(18) = 13.353				
Unemployment Rate	3	.165E-01	.933E-02	1.778
AR	1	−.824	.133	−6.154
AR	2	−.535	.139	−3.841
RBAR Sq. .485;				
Q(18) = 15.489				
Nonwhite Males				
Unemployment Rate	2	.733E-01	.387E-01	1.896
AR	1	−.734	.143	−5.139
AR	2	−.398	.149	−2.673
RBAR Sq. .387;				
Q(18) = 17.051				
Unemployment Rate	3	.980E-01	.326E-01	3.004
AR	1	−.774	.130	−5.957
AR	2	−.548	.130	−4.215
RBAR Sq. .447;				
Q(18) = 12.386				
Nonwhite Females				
Unemployment Rate	2	.593E-01	.259E-01	2.291
AR	1	−.751	.150	−5.012
AR	2	−.357	.151	−2.365
RBAR Sq. .322;				
Q(18) = 15.328				
Unemployment Rate	3	.706E-01	.243E-01	2.906
AR	1	−.744	.146	−5.102
AR	2	−.449	.149	−3.011
REAR Sq. .370;				
Q(18) = 10.771				

a. For white males, only the 2-year lag model.

Abbreviations: AR, autoregression term; MA, moving average; E−01, exponent to the power −.01 (e.g., .443 E−01 = .0443); RBAR Sq., adjusted coefficient of determination (i.e. adjusted explanation of variance); Q, measure of autocorrelation of residuals used in Box-Jenkins model.

Sources: Mortality data from the National Center for Health Statistics; employment data from the U.S. Bureau of Labor Statistics.

ees—a classic case of the "high-demand/low-control" situation that is gaining attention in the literature on work stress and cardiovascular disease (Karasek and Theorell, 1990). This situation would also lead to higher accident rates and, in some groups (especially the ill and impaired), feelings of hopelessness-helplessness prompted by inability to cope with severe work demands.

A third population combines features of the first two. This population loses employment and income during a recession, and is rehired possibly at a lower socioeconomic level only after economic recovery and often by firms that themselves suffered serious financial reverses during the recession. This population too may carry an additional burden of illness. That illness may have been further exacerbated in the case of the United States by loss of access to health care due to loss of income or insurance during the recession. When this ill population finds new employment during a recovery, it probably enters the economy at a time when demand for labor is high and work pressures are therefore extreme. This group, grateful to have found employment, is desperate to retain that employment despite the conflict between work pressure and illness. But if work pressure exacerbates the illness (such as cardiovascular symptoms), the individual will either be forced to quit or to work at a less intensive pace despite the requirements of the firm. In either case, inability to function "adequately" in the face of such pressure could lead to a sense of dejection and ultimately hopelessness. There is evidence that a psychological state of hopelessness-helplessness is an important factor in fatality due to chronic disease (Karasek and Theorell, 1990).

It is only the first peak in mortality, however, that occurs 2–3 years after recession. Mortality rates lag behind such economic indices as unemployment and business-failure rates by 10–15 years. To demonstrate this relationship, let us look again at the unemployment rate in its distributed-lag relation to mortality for the total population (see Tables 7–2 and 7–3). As these distributed-lag equations show, the basic cumulative temporal pattern can be measured over 2–13 years. The Shiller distributed-lag technique (Shiller, 1973) is used because it eliminates the need for a mathematically rigid functional form (as compared to the polynomial distributed lag), and because the curve-fitting method for the full distributed lag requires the expenditure of only one degree of freedom. The resulting relations, modeled in second differences (rate of change), can also be transformed to first differences (annual changes) and levels, with all variables retaining statistical significance (see Table 7–3). The statistical relationships originally modeled with both independent and dependent variables in second difference form indicate that the level of mortality rates is influenced by the level of cyclical and structural changes in the national economy.

The addition to this equation of the unemployment rate at zero-lag results in a significant distributed-lag relationship, but no longer a significant zero-lag relationship. This finding further confirms the view that, in chronic-disease mortality and in mortality from all causes, the basic short-term relation between unemployment and mortality rates peaks at a 2- to 3-year lag.

Now let us look at whether the relationship between unemployment and mortality-rate changes is still apparent after we control for the influences of other economic vari-

Table 7-2 Time-Series Regression Equation Showing Relations Between Economic and Consumption Variables and Age-Adjusted Mortality Rates for the United States, 1950–1988

(Second Differences, Shiller Distributed Lag)

Order	Economic Change	Lag (Years	Coefficient	Standard Error	T Statistic
		1950–1988			
1	Unemployment rate	2–13	.290	.569E.01	5.094
2	Per capita real disposable income	2–14	−.294E-02	.475E-03	−6.183
3	Per capita fat consumption	0–14	.152E-02	.255E-03	5.979
4	RHO		−.628	.131	−4.784

RBAR Sq. .885
Durbin-Watson 1.941
F Chow (3, 31) = .111

1950–1968

Order	Economic Change	Lag (Years	Coefficient	Standard Error	T Statistic
1	Unemployment rate	2–13	.240	.793E-01	3.031
2	Per capita real disposable income	2–14	−.327E-02	.662E-03	−4.941
3	Per capita fat consumption	0–14	.209E-02	.414E-03	5.044
4	RHO		−.497	.270	−1.842

1969–1988

Order	Economic Change	Lag (Years	Coefficient	Standard Error	T Statistic
1	Unemployment rate	2–13	.263	.121E-01	2.168
2	Per capita real disposable income	2–14	−.305E-02	.642E-03	−4.749
3	Per capita fat consumption	0–14	.106E-02	.246E-03	3.052
4	RHO		−.822	.138	−5.965

Abbreviations: RHO, autocorrelation term; RBAR Sq., adjusted coefficient of determination (adjusted explanation of variance); Durbin-Watson, measure of autocorrelation among regression residuals; F Chow, F statistic for the Chow test of lack of equivalence of regression coefficients between the first (1950–1968) and second (1969–1988) halves of the period over which the regression equation is calculated; E−01, E−02, etc, exponents to the power −.01, −.001, etc (see footnote to Table 7-1).

Sources: U.S. Government data: unemployment rates, *Handbook of Labour Statistics;* per capita real disposable income, Bureau of Economic Analysis; fat consumption, Agricultural Statistics.

ables (such as per capita disposable income) and high-risk consumption and production factors.

First, we can observe the relation between unemployment and mortality rates, in two- or three-variable distributed lag models, including the long-term cumulative relation between per capita disposable income and a single biochemical risk factor such as fat consumption per capita (see Table 7–4).

Second, the Shiller distributed-lag procedure enables us to estimate the simultaneous impact of several predictors, including unemployment and wage rates, social-welfare and health-care expenditures, and consumption and production risk factors. These variables are entered into a step-wise multiple-regression time-series equation, again with

Table 7-3 Time-Series Regression Equation Showing Relations Between Economic and Consumption Variables and Age-Adjusted Mortality Rates[a] United States, 1950–1988

(First Differences, Shiller Distributed Lag)

Order	Economic Change	Lag (Years)	Coefficient	Standard Error	T Statistic
1	Trend	0	−.559	.194E-02	−2.877
2	Unemployment rate	2–13	.294	.797E-01	3.687
3	Per capita real disposable income	2–14	−.295E-02	.485E-03	−6.078
4	Per capita fat consumption	0–14	.149E-02	.343E-03	4.343
5	RHO		.548	.150	3.668

RBAR Sq. .650
Durbin-Watson 2.553
F(4, 34) = 38.800

Level Equation (Shiller Distributed Lag)

Order	Economic Change	Lag (Years)	Coefficient	Standard Error	T Statistic
1	Trend	0	−.250	.726E.01	−3.440
2	Trend square	0	.354E-02	.124E-02	2.832
3	Unemployment rate	2–13	.273	.790E-01	3.463
2	Per capita real disposable income	2–14	−.159E-02	.387E-03	−4.098
3	Per capita fat consumption	0–14	.130E-02	.127E-03	10.225
4	RHO		−.914	.104	−8.795

RBAR Sq. .998
Durbin-Watson 1.889
F (5, 33) = 701.490

a. These models are algebraically transformed from the second-difference model in Table 7-2.

Abbreviations: See Tables 7-1 and 7-2.

Sources: As in Table 7-2.

a hypothesized lag of approximately 0–14 years. For total mortality rates and for the sex-race breakdown, the basic relationship can be initially estimated in second differences. (The reason for the initial second-difference modeling is that it permits necessary controls for multicollinearity, long-term linear, and quadratic trends.) It is also feasible to observe each of these sets of multivariate relations in first-difference and in level (undifferenced) form.

In the case of the level relationships, we hypothesize that the principal long-term linear trend is central both to the rate of productivity that gives rise to the standard of living and to the production of scientific knowledge, which ultimately leads to the diminution in consumption and production of factors found to be health risks. We suggest that the "factor" behind this trend is long-term investment in research and development, financed by both private sources and government. We do not yet understand, however, the empirical basis of the (relatively weak) quadratic trend that appears to increase the mortality rate. Apart from these two long-term trends, the remainder of the model remains intact, with its full set of benefit and risk factors, each variable showing statistical significance.

Table 7-4 Time-Series Regression Equation Showing Relations Between National Economic Changes and Age-Adjusted Mortality Rates[a] United States, 1950–1988

Order	Economic Changes	Lag (Years)	Coefficient	Standard Error	T Statistic
Economy					
4	Per capita real disposable income	1–14	−.841E-02	.346E-03	−24.303
7	Annual change in wage rate	1–12	−.361E-01	.593E-02	−6.090
9	Unemployment rate	0–10	.982E-01	.234E-01	4.193
11	Business-failure rate	1–7	.102E-01	.193	5.293
Policy					
14	Health Expenditures as a proportion of GNP	0–8	−24.298	11.660	−2.083
Consumption					
10	Per capita fat consumption	0–14	.203E-02	.252E-03	8.075
12	Per capita cigarette consumption	2–10	.778E-03	.240E-03	3.244
5	Per capita spirits consumption	0–13	7.648	.391	19.585
6	Per capita energy consumption	0–8	.120E-01	.575E-02	4.651
Production					
8	Per capita chemical production	0–11	.796E-01	120E-01	6.614
1	Constant		19.182	3.917	4.897
2	Linear trend		429.776	35.290	−12.178
3	Trend sq.		.206E-01	.158E-02	−13.022
13	Marriage rate	0–9	−.350	.329E-01	−10.621

RBAR Sq. .99947
Durbin-Watson 1.840
$F_{(14, 25)} = 33914.5$

a. These relations between *levels* of mortality (rates) and levels of economic and social variables were originally estimated in second differences, and are easily transformable algebraically into first differences (annual changes) as well.

Abbreviations: See Tables 7-1 and 7-2.

Sources: U.S. Government data: per capita disposable income, Bureau of Economic Analysis; unemployment rates, *Handbook of Labour Statistics;* business-failure rates and health expenditures, Historical Statistics of the U.S.—Statistical Abstracts; cigarette and spirits consumption, Statistical Abstracts of the U.S.

When this method of applying (1) Box-Jenkins, (2) single-variable distributed-lag, and (3) multivariate distributed-lag approaches was used to analyze overall mortality by age, sex, and major cause of death (total cardiovascular disease, coronary heart disease, malignancies, cirrhosis, suicide, and homicide) the overall findings were as follows:

1. Economic growth, as measured by real per capita disposable income (and/or by real wage rates), is inversely related to overall (and chronic-disease) mortality rates over at least 1–14 years.
2. Economic recession, as measured by the unemployment rate, and/or by the business-failure rate, i.e., bankruptcy, is positively related to mortality over 0–10 and 1–7 years, respectively. The initial peak of this relation is an elevated mortality rate 2–3 years after the recession's peak.

3. During the recessional year itself, however, overall mortality declines, followed by a sharp increase (with no lag) during the initial year of recovery. Important exceptions include suicide, homicide, and other mental-health indices and infant mortality, whose positive relation to unemployment rates *begins* at the zero year.
4. Rates of consumption of fats, cigarettes, and alcohol are positively related to total cardiovascular and cancer mortality-rate increases over at least 0–14 years.
5. Chemical production is related to increased overall mortality, and specifically to that due to malignancies, over at least 0–14 years.
6. Social-welfare and health-care expenditures per capita are inversely related to overall mortality rates over at least 0–8 years. These relations are statistically significant only after the variables representing economic change and high-risk consumption patterns are held constant.

These findings have been replicated in analyses in other countries and over different time periods.

Conclusion

The mechanisms that link SES to health also link changes in SES to changes in health. Thus, stable and equitably distributed economic growth brings about material gains (improved nutrition, sanitation, injury control, health-care technology, and access to health care), and increased potential for control of biochemical risks as a result of investments in health sciences and public education. Psychologically, stable economic growth increases self-esteem (via achievement), security, mastery, and social integration. Recession brings about the opposite effects—notably psychophysiological reactions to economic threats and losses and increased inequality—and tends to increase work stress in firms that have experienced severe economic loss.

During the recovery phase of the business cycle, illness induced by the stresses of recession may prevent reintegration of recession-displaced workers. This lack of economic recovery may be the greatest source of recession-induced health problems in some populations, combining as it does absolute loss, downward mobility, relative deprivation in relation to the majority, and probable loss of social support from peers. In combination with family instability, this set of circumstances serves to elevate the mortality rate over at least a decade following recession.

While the economy is instrumental in advancing the population's health, it is clear from the findings of this study that it does not do so through market factors alone. Market forces, in fact, often generate considerable morbidity and mortality by promoting high-risk consumption and production. Investment in the health sciences, public-health knowledge, and regulation are crucial to counterbalance these tendencies.

Trends in economic productivity and inequality have been adverse for at least the last decade and a half. Action is obviously needed to remedy the short- and long-term problems of the U.S. economy—especially relatively low investment, wage stagnation, and poverty. Perhaps debate on economic and social-welfare policy would become more pointed if it were clearly understood that the health and life expectancy of the nation are at stake.

References

Ahern, M., and H. V. McCoy. 1992. Emergency room admissions: Changes during the financial tightening of the 1980s. *Inquiry* 29:67–79.

American Psychiatric Association. 1987. *Diagnostic and Statistical Manual of Mental Disorders* (3rd edition), *DSM-III-R*. Washington, DC: American Psychiatric Association.

Anda, R. F. 1992. Self-perceived stress and the risk of peptic ulcer disease: A longitudinal study of U.S. adults. *Arch. Intern. Med.* 152:829–33.

Anderson, B. 1986. In D. R. Obey and P. Sarbanes (eds.), *The Changing American Economy*, pp. 147–155, New York, NY: Basil Blackwell.

Anderson, G. M., R. Brook, and A. Williams. 1991. A comparison of cost-sharing versus free care in children: Effects on the demand for office-based medical care. *Med. Care.* 29:890–898.

Attfield, C. L., and N. W. Duck. 1985. *Rational Expectation in Macroeconomics: An Introduction to Theory and Evidence*, pp. 42–43. Oxford: Basil Blackwell,

Bartrop, R. W., E. Lockhurst, L. Lazarus, L. G. Kilon, and R. Penney. 1977. Depressed lymphocyte function after bereavement. *Lancet* 1:834–836.

Becker, G. S. 1964. *Human Capital*. New York: National Bureau of Economic Research.

Berkowitz, L. 1962. *Aggression: A Social Psychological Analysis*. New York: McGraw-Hill.

Blau, P., and O. Duncan. 1967. *The American Occupational Structure*. New York: Wiley.

Blauner, R. 1972. *Internal Colonialism*. Berkeley, CA: University of California Press.

Bluestone, B., and B. Harrison. 1982. *The De-Industrialization of America*. New York: Basic Books.

Boor, M. 1980. Relationships between unemployment rates and suicide rates in eight countries, 1962–1976. *Psychol. Rep.* 47:1095–1101.

Box, G., and G. Jenkins. 1982. *Time Series Analysis: Forecasting and Control*. San Francisco: Holden Day.

Brenner, M. H. 1971a. Economic changes and heart disease mortality *Am. J. Public Health* 61:606–611.

Brenner, M. H. 1971b. *Time Series Analysis of the Relationships Between Selected Economic and Social Indicators,* Vol. 1 and 2. Springfield, VA: National Technical Information Service.

Brenner, M. H. 1973a. *Mental Illness and the Economy*. Cambridge: Harvard University Press.

Brenner, M. H. 1973b. Fetal, infant, and maternal mortality during periods of economic instability. *Int. J. Health Serv.* 3:145–159.

Brenner, M. H. 1975. Trends in alcohol consumption and associated illnesses: Some effects of economic changes. *Am. J. Public Health* 65:1279–1292.

Brenner, M. H. 1976a. Effects of the economy on criminal behavior and the administration of criminal justice in the United States, Canada, England and Wales, and Scotland. In *Economic Crises and Crime: Correlations and the State of the Economy, Deviance and the Control of Deviance*, pp. 26–28. Rome: United Nations Social Defense Research Institute.

Brenner, M. H. 1976b. *Estimating the Social Costs of National Economic Policy: Implications for Mental and Physical Health and Criminal Aggression.* U.S. Congress, Joint Economic Committee. Washington DC: Government Printing Office.

Brenner, M. H. 1979. Mortality and the national economy: A review and the experience of England and Wales, 1936–1976. *Lancet* 2:568–573.

Brenner, M. H. 1980a. Impact of social and industrial changes on psychopathology: A view of stress from the standpoint of macro societal trends. In L. Levi (ed.), *Society, Stress and Disease: Working Life* Vol. 4, pp. 249–260. Oxford: Oxford University Press.

Brenner, M. H. 1980b. Industrialization and economic growth: Estimates of their effect on the health of populations. In M. H. Brenner, A. Mooney, and T. J. Nagy (eds.), *Assessing the Contributions of the Social Sciences to Health* (AAAS Symposium 26), pp. 65–115. Boulder, CO: Westview Press.

Brenner, M. H. 1980c. Importance of the economy to the nation's health. In L. Eisenberg and A. Kleinman (eds.), *The Relevance of Social Science for Medicine*, pp. 371–398. Dordrecht, Holland: Reidel.

Brenner, M. H. 1983. Mortality and economic instability: Detailed analyses for Britain and comparative analysis for selected industrialized countries. *Int. J. Health Serv.* 13:563–620.

Brenner, M. H. 1984a. *Estimating the Effects of Economic Change on National Health and Social Well-Being.* U.S. Congress, Joint Economic Committee. Washington, DC: Government Printing Office.

Brenner, M. H. 1984b. Economic change and the suicide rate: A population model including loss, separation, illness, and alcohol consumption. In American College of Psychiatrists, *Stress in Health and Disease*, pp. 160–185. New York: Brunner Mazel.

Brenner, M. H. 1987a. Economic change, alcohol consumption, and heart disease mortality in nine industrialized countries. *Soc. Sci. Med.* 25:119–131.

Brenner, M. H. 1987b. Relation of economic change to Swedish health and social well-being, 1950–1980. *Soc. Sci. Med.* 25:183–195.

Brenner, M. H. 1987c. Economic instability, unemployment rates, behavioral risks, and mortality rates in Scotland, 1953–1983. *Int. J. Health Serv.* 17:475–484.

Brenner, M. H. 1989. Economic change and mortality in first world countries: Post war to mid 1980s. In R. Veenhoven (ed.), *Did the Crisis Really Hurt?*, pp. 174–220. Rotterdam: University of Rotterdam.

Brenner, M. H. 1991. Health, productivity and the economic environment: The dynamic role of socioeconomic status. In G.M. Greene and F. Baker (eds.), *Health and Productivity*, pp. 241–255. New York: Oxford University Press.

Brenner, M. H. 1993. Health and the national economy. In A. Sorkin, P. C. Huang, R. S. Lin, and L. E. Chow (eds.), *Research in Human Capital and Development*, Vol. 7, pp. 369–391. Greenwich, CT: JAI Press.

Brenner, M. H., and A. Mooney. 1982. Economic change and sex-specific cardiovascular mortality in Britain 1955–1976. *Soc. Sci. Med.* 16:431–442.

Brenner, S. O., and B. Starrin. 1988. Unemployment and health in Sweden: Public issues and private troubles. *Journal of Social Issues* 44:125–140.

Brown, G. W., and T. Harris. 1978. *Social Origins of Depression. A Study of Psychiatric Disorder in Women.* New York: Free Press.

Brown G. W., F. Sklair, T. O. Harris, and J.L.T. Birley. 1973. Life events and psychiatric disorders, 1. Some methodological issues. *Psychol. Med.* 3:74–87.

Budd, E. C., and T. C. Whiteman. 1978. Macroeconomic fluctuations and the size distribution of income and earnings in the United States. In Z. Griliches, W. Krelle, H.-J. Krupp, and O. Kyn (eds.), *Income Distribution and Economic Inequality*, pp. 11–27. New York: Wiley.

Burt, R. S. 1978. Applied network analysis: An overview. *Sociological Methods and Research* 7:123–130.

Cassel, J., and H. A. Tyroler. 1961. Epidemiological studies of culture change, I. Health status and recency of industrialization. *Arch. Environ. Health* 3:25–33.

Coleman, J. S. 1974. *Power and the Structure of Society.* New York: W.W. Norton.

Cooley, C. 1902. *Introduction to Sociology.* New York: Wiley.

Coyne, J. C., R.C. Kessler, M. Tal, J. Turnbull, C. B. Wortman, and J.F. Greden. 1987. Living with a depressed person. *J. Consult. Clin. Psychol.* 55:347–352.

Dahrendorf, R. 1959. *Class and Class Conflict in Industrial Society.* Stanford, CA: Stanford University Press.

Davis, K., and W. E. Moore. 1945. Some principles of stratification. *Am. Soc. Rev.* 10:242–249.

Dayton, N. A. 1940. *New Facts on Mental Disorders.* Springfield, IL: Charles C. Thomas.

Dew, M. A., and E. J. Bromet. 1991. Effects of depression on social support in a community sample of women. In J. Eckenrode (ed.), *The Social Context of Coping,* pp. 189–211. New York: Plenum Press.

Doeringer, R., and C. Piore. 1971. *Internal Labor Markets and Manpower Analysis.* Lexington, MA: D.C. Heath.

Doll, R. 1987. Major epidemics of the 20th century: From coronary thrombosis to AIDS. *J. R. Stat. Soc.* 150:373–395.

Dollard, J., L. W. Doob, N. E. Miller. 1939. *Frustration and Aggression.* New Haven, CT: Yale University Press.

Dooley, D., and R. Catalano. 1984. The epidemiology of economic stress. *Am. J. Community Psychol.* 12:387–409.

Dooley, M. D., and P. Gottschalk. 1984. Earnings inequality among males in the U.S.: Trends and the effect of labor force growth. *Journal of Political Economy* 92:59–89.

Dooley, M. D., and P. Gottschalk. 1985. The increasing proportion of men with low earnings in the U.S. *Demography* 22:25–34.

Dunlop, J. T. 1938. The movement of real and money wage rates. *Economic Journal* 48:413–434.

Durkheim, E. 1951. *Suicide.* Glencoe, IL: Free Press.

Durkheim, E. 1947. *The Division of Labor in Society* (translated by George Simpson). Glencoe, IL: Free Press.

Economic Policy Council. 1983. United Nations Association, *The Productivity Problem: U.S. Labor-Management Relations.* New York: United Nations.

Edwards, R. 1975. The social relations of production in the firm and labor market structure. In R. C. Edwards, M. Reich, and D.M. Gordon (eds.), *Labor Market Segmentation,* pp. 1–26. Lexington, MA: D.C. Heath.

Elder, G. and A. Capri. 1988. Economic stress in lives: Developmental perspectives. *J. Social Issues* 44:25–46.

Epstein, S. S., and J. Swartz. 1981. Fallacies of lifestyle cancer theories. *Nature* 289:127–130.

Erikson, E. 1963. *Childhood and Society.* New York: Academic Books.

Eysenck, H. J., R. Grossarth-Maticek, and B. Everitt. 1991. Personality, stress, smoking, and genetic predisposition as synergistic risk factors for cancer and coronary heart disease. *Integr. Physiol. Behav. Sci.* 26:309–322.

Featherman, D., and P. Hauser. 1975. *Opportunity and Change.* New York: Basic Books.

Feldstein, M. 1980. *The American Economy in Transition.* Chicago: University of Chicago Press.

Ferman, L., and J. Gardner. 1979. Economic deprivation, social mobility, and mental health. In L. Ferman and J. Gordus (eds.), *Mental Health and the Economy,* pp. 193–224. Kalamazoo, MI: WE Upjohn Institute for Employment Research.

Forbes, J. F., and A. McGregor. 1987. Male unemployment and cause-specific mortality in postwar Scotland. *Int. J. Health Serv.* 17:233–240.

Forcier, M. 1988. Unemployment and alcohol abuse: A review. *J. Occup. Med.* 30:246–261.

Ford, M., and M. Marlis. 1990. Preventive health services: A call for action. The Pepper Commission Supplement to the Final Report. Sept 1990, p. 69. Washington, DC: U.S. Government Printing Office.

Freeman, R. B., and J. L. Medoff. 1984. *What Do Unions Do?* New York: Basic Books.

Goffman, E. 1959. *Stigma*. Glencoe, IL: Free Press.

Goldstein, M. G., and R. Niaura. 1992. Psychological factors affecting physical condition cardiovascular disease. Literature review, part I: Coronary artery disease and sudden death. *Psychosomatics* 33:134–145.

Gramlich, E. M. 1974. The distributional effects of higher unemployment. *Brookings Papers on Economic Activity* 2:293–342.

Griliches, Z. 1988. *Technology, Education and Productivity*. New York: Basil Blackwell.

Grossarth-Maricek, R., and H. J. Eysenck. 1991. Personality, stress, and motivational factors in drinking as determinants of risk for cancer and coronary heart disease. *Psychol. Rep.* 69:1027–1043.

Hamblin, R., R. Jacobsen, and J. Miller. 1973. *A Mathematical Theory of Social Change*. New York: Wiley.

Hamilton, V., C. Broman, W. Hoffman, and D. Renner. 1990. Hard times and vulnerable people: Initial effects of plant closing on autoworkers' mental health. *J. Health Soc. Behav.* 31:123–140.

Hannan, M. T. 1979. *National Development and the World System*. Chicago: University of Chicago Press.

Harrison, B., and B. Bluestone. 1990. *The Great U-Turn: Corporate Restructuring and the Polarizing of America*. New York: Basic Books.

Harrison, B., C. Tilly, and B. Bluestone. 1986. Rising inequality. In D.R. Obey, and P. Sarbanes (eds.), *The Changing American Economy*, pp. 111–134. New York: Basil Blackwell.

Henry, A. F., and T. F. Short. 1954. *Suicide and Homicide: Some Economic, Sociological and Psychological Aspects of Aggression*. Glencoe, IL: Free Press.

Hodson, R. 1983. *Workers' Earnings and Corporate Economic Structure*. New York: Academic Press.

Hollister, B., and J. L. Palmer. 1972. The impact of inflation on the poor. In K. E. Boulding and M. Pfaff (eds.), *Redistribution to the Rich and the Poor*, pp. 240–270. Belmont, CA: Wadsworth.

House, J. S., K. R. Landis, and D. Umberson. 1988. Social relationships and health. *Science* 241:540–544.

Isenberg, S. A., P. M. Lehrer, and S. Hochron. 1992. The effects of suggestion and emotional arousal on pulmonary function in asthma: A review and a hypothesis regarding vagal mediation. *Psychosom. Med.* 54:192–216.

Iversen, L., O. Andersen, P. K. Andersen, K. Christoffersen, and N. Keiding. 1987. Unemployment and mortality in Denmark, 1970–1980. *Br. Med. J. Clin. Res.* 295:879–884.

Iversen, L., S. Sabroe, and M. I. Damsgaard. 1989. Hospital admissions before and after shipyard closure. *B.M.J.* 299:1073–1076.

Jackson, P. R., and P. Warr. 1987. Mental health of unemployed men in different parts of England and Wales. *B.M.J.* 295:525.

James, W. 1890. *The Principles of Psychology*. New York: Holt.

Karasek, R., and T. Theorell. 1990. *Healthy Work: Stress, Productivity, and the Reconstruction of Working Life*. New York: Basic Books.

Kasl, S. V., and S. Cobb. 1982. Variability of stress effects among men experiencing job loss. In L. Goldberger and S. Breznitz (eds.), *Handbook of Stress—Theoretical and Clinical Aspects*, pp. 445–465. New York: Free Press.

Kendrick, J. W. 1980. *Productivity in the U.S.: Trends and Cycles*. Baltimore: Johns Hopkins University Press.

Kendrick, J. W. 1983. *Interindustry Differences in Productivity Growth*. Washington, DC: AEI Studies.

Kendrick, J. W. 1984. *International Comparisons of Productivity and Causes of the Slowdown.* Cambridge, MA: Ballinger.

Kessler, R., J. Turner, and J. House. 1988. Effects of unemployment on health in a community survey: Main, modifying and mediating effects. *Journal of Social Issues* 44:69–86.

Kirkman, L. B., and J. J. Kronenfeld. 1992. Access to cancer screening services for women. *Am. J. Public Health* 82:733–735.

Krantz, S. E., and R. H. Moos. 1987. Functioning and life context among spouses of remitted and non-remitted depressed patients. *J. Consult. Clin. Psychol.* 55:353–360.

Krugman, P. 1991. *The Age of Diminished Expectations: U.S. Economic Policy in the 1990s.* Cambridge: MIT Press.

Kuttner, R. 1986. Renewing opportunity. In D.R. Obey and P. Sarbanes (eds.), *The Changing American Economy*, pp. 135–146. New York: Basil Blackwell.

Kuznets, S. 1953. *Shares of Upper Income Groups in Income and Savings.* New York: National Bureau of Economic Research.

Kuznets, S. 1955. Economic growth and income inequality. *American Economic Review* 45:1–28.

Lee, A. J., L. K. Crombie, W.C. Smith, H. D. Tunstall-Pedoe. 1991. Cigarette smoking and employment status. *Soc. Sci. Med.* 33:1309–1312.

Leigh, J. P. 1989. Firm size and occupational injury and illness incidence rates in manufacturing industries. *J. Community Health* 14:44–52.

Levy, F. 1987. *Dollars and Dreams: The Changing American Income Distribution.* New York: Russell Sage Foundation.

Liker, J. K., and G. H. Elder, Jr. 1983. Economic hardship and marital relations in the 1930s. *Am. Soc. Rev.* 48:343–359.

Linn, M. W., R. Sandifer, and S. Stein. 1985. Effects of unemployment on mental and physical health. *Am. J. Public Health* 75:502–506.

Linton, R. 1936. *The Study of Culture.* New York: Appleton.

Litan, R. E., R. Z. Lawrence, and C. Schultze (eds.). 1988. *American Living Standards: Threats and Challenges.* Washington, DC: The Brookings Institution.

Luft, H. S. 1978. *Poverty and Health Economic Causes and Consequences of Health Problems.* Cambridge, MA: Ballinger.

McMahon, P. J., and J. H. Tschetter. 1986. The declining middle class: A further analysis. *Monthly Labor Review* 109:22–27.

McQuail, D. 1988. *Mass Communication Theory—An Introduction*, 2nd edn. Beverly Hills, CA: Sage.

Manoff, R. K. 1985. *Social Marketing: New Imperative for Public Health.* New York: Praeger.

Manning, G.W., I.P. Newhouse, and J. E. Ware. 1982. The status of health in demand estimation: Or beyond excellent, good, fair and poor. In V. R. Fuchs (ed.), *Economic Aspects of Health*, pp. 143–184. Chicago: University of Chicago Press.

Marmot, M. G., M. Kogenvinas, and M.A. Elston. 1987. Social/economic status and disease. *Annu. Rev. Public Health* 8:111–135.

Marmot, M. G., A. M. Adelstein, N. Robinson, and G.A. Rose. 1978. Changing social-class distribution of heart disease. *B.M.J.* 2:1109–1112.

Marmot, M. G., and S. L. Syme. 1976. Acculturation and coronary heart disease. *Am. J. Epidemiol.* 104:225–247.

Marshall, J. R., and R. W. Hodge. 1981. Durkheim and Pierce on suicide and economic change. *Social Science Research* 10:101–114.

Marshall, R. 1986. Working smarter. In D.R. Obey and P. Sarbanes (eds.), *The Changing American Economy*, pp. 180–202. New York: Basil Blackwell.

Martikainen, P. T. 1990. Unemployment and mortality among Finnish men, 1981–1985. *B.M.J.* 301:407–411.

Maxwell, N. L. 1989. Demographic and economic determinants of United States income inequality. *Social Science Quarterly* 70:245–264.

Mead, G. 1934. *Mind, Self and Society*. New York: Vantage Press.

Menderhausen, H. 1946. *Changes in Income Distribution During the Great Depression, NBER Conference on Research in Income and Wealth*. New York: ARNO Press.

Miller, N. E. 1941. The frustration-aggression hypothesis. *Psychol. Rev.* 48:337–342.

Mirer, T. 1973a. The distributional impact of the 1970 recession. *Review of Economics and Statistics* 55:214–224.

Mirer, T. 1973b. The effects of macroeconomic fluctuations on the distribution of income. *Review of Income and Wealth Series* 19:385–405.

Mitchell, W. C. 1951. *What Happens During Business Cycles*. New York: National Bureau of Economic Research.

Morris, J. N. 1979. Social inequalities undiminished. *Lancet* 1:87–90.

Moser, K. A., A. J. Fox, and D. R. Jones. 1984. Unemployment and mortality in the OPCS longitudinal study. *Lancet* 2:1324–1329.

Muldoon, M. P., E. A. Bachen, S. B. Manuck, S. R. Waldstein, P. L. Bricker, and J. A. Bennett. 1992. Acute cholesterol responses to mental stress and change in posture. *Arch. Intern. Med.* 152:775–780.

Niaura, R., and M. G. Goldstein. 1992. Psychological factors affecting physical condition. Cardiovascular disease literature review, II. Coronary artery disease and sudden death and hypertension. *Psychosomatics* 33:146–155.

Nielson, F. 1980. The Flemish movement in Belgium after World War II. A dynamic analysis. *Am. Soc. Rev.* 45:76–94.

Nolan, B. 1987. *Income Distribution and the Macroeconomy*. Cambridge, U.K.: Cambridge University Press.

Oi, W. 1962. Labor as a quasi-fixed factor. *Journal of Political Economy* 70:538–555.

Orum, A. M. 1978. *Introduction to Political Sociology: The Social Anatomy of the Body Politic*. Englewood Cliffs, NJ: Prentice-Hall.

Parsons, T. 1951. *The Social System*. Glencoe, IL: Free Press.

Parsons, T., and E. A. Shils (eds.). 1951. *Toward a General Theory of Action*. Cambridge: Harvard University Press.

Paykel, E. S., J. K. Myers, M. N. Dienelt, G. L. Klerman, J. J. Lindenthal, and M. P. Pepper. 1969. Life events and depression: A controlled study. *Arch. Gen. Psychiatry* 21:753–760.

Pearlin, L. I., and C. Radabaugh. 1976. Economic strains and the coping function of alcohol. *Am. J. Soc.* 1982:652–663.

Penkower, L., E. Bromet, and M. Dew. 1988. Husbands' layoff and wives' mental health: A prospective analysis. *Arch. Gen. Psychiatry* 45:994–1000.

Phelps Brown, H. 1987. Inequality of pay. In J. Eatwell, M. Milgate, and P. Newman (eds.), *The New Palgrave: A Dictionary of Economics*, Vol. 2, pp. 827–828. New York: Stockton Press.

Phillips, K. 1990. *The Politics of Rich and Poor*. New York: Random House.

Pickering, T., P. L. Schnall, J. E. Schwartz, and C. F. Pieper. 1991. Can behavioral factors produce a sustained elevation of blood pressure? Some observations and a hypothesis. *J Hypertens Suppl* 9:S66–S68.

Platt, S. 1986. Parasuicide and unemployment. *Br. J. Psychiatry* 149:401–405.

Podgursky, M. and P. Swaim. 1987a. Job displacement and earnings loss: Evidence from the displaced worker survey. In *Industrial and Labor Relations Review* 41:17–29.

Podgursky, M., and P. Swaim. 1987b. Duration of joblessness following displacement. *Industrial Relations* 26:213–226.

Pugh, T. F., and B. MacMahon. 1962. *Epidemiological Findings in the United States Mental Hospital Data*. Boston: Little Brown.

Rath, G. D., L. G. Jarratt, and G. Leonardson. 1989. Rates of domestic violence against adult women by men partners. *J. Am. Board Fam. Pract.* 2:227–233.

Reder, M. 1955. The theory of occupational wage differentials. *American Economic Review* 45:833–852.

Registrar General. 1976. *Occupational Mortality: The Registrar General's Decennial Supplement for England and Wales, 1970–1972*. London: Her Majesty's Stationery Office.

Rice, D. P. 1966. *Estimating the Cost of Illness*. Washington, DC: U.S. Government Printing Office.

Rogers, E. M., and F. F. Shoemaker. 1971. *Communication of Innovations: A Cross Cultural Approach,* 2nd edn. New York: Free Press.

Rook, K., D. Dooley, and R. Catalano. 1991. Stress transmission: The effect of husbands' job stressors on the emotional health of their wives. *J. Marriage Fam.* 53:165–177.

Rosenthal, N. 1985. The shrinking middle class: Myth or reality? *Monthly Labor Review* 108(March):3–10.

Rowland, D. 1990. Fewer resources, greater burdens: Medical care coverage for low-income elderly people. In The Pepper Commission, *A Call for Action: Supplement to the Final Report*, Sept 1990, pp. 137–138. Washington, DC: Government Printing Office.

Ryscavage, P., and P. Henle. 1990. Earnings inequality accelerates in the 1980s. *Monthly Labor Review* 113:3–16.

Schlundt, D. G., J. O. Hill, I. Sbrocco, J. Pope-Cordle, and I. Kasser. 1990. Obesity: A biogenetic or biobehavioral problem. *Intern. Obesity* 14:815–828.

Schnall, P. L., P. A. Landsbergis, C. F. Pieper, J. Schwartz, D. Dietz, W. Gerin, Y. Schlussel, K. Warren, and T. Pickering. 1992. The impact of anticipation of job loss on psychological distress and worksite blood pressure. *Am. J. Ind. Med.* 21:417–432.

Schultz, T. P. 1969. Secular trends and cyclical behavior of income distribution in the United States: 1944–1965, In L. Soltow (ed.), *Six Papers on the Size Distribution of Wealth and Income*. New York: Columbia University Press.

Schwefel, D. 1986. Unemployment, health and health services in German speaking countries. *Soc. Sci. Med.* 22:409–430.

Serxner, S., R. Catalamo, D. Dooley, and S. Mishra. 1991. Tobacco use: Selection, stress or culture. *J. Occup. Med.* 33:1035–1039.

Sewell, W., and R. Hauser. 1972. Causes and consequences of higher education: Models of the status attainment process. *American Journal of Agricultural Economics* 54:851–861.

Shapiro, M. F., J. E. Ware, Jr., and C. D. Sherbourne. 1986. Effects of cost sharing on seeking care for serious and minor symptoms. Results of a randomized controlled trial. *Ann. Intern. Med.* 102:246–251.

Shiller, R. J. 1973. A distributed lag estimator derived from smoothness priors. *Econometrica* 411:775–788.

Shorrocks, A. F. 1987. Inequality between persons. In J. Eatwell, M. Milgate, and P. Newman (eds.), *The New Palgrave: A Dictionary of Economics*, vol. 2, p. 821. New York: Stockton Press.

Smeeding, T. M. 1991. Cross-national comparisons of inequality and poverty position. In L. Osberg (ed.), *Economic Inequality and Poverty: International Perspectives*, pp. 39–59. Armonk, NY: M.E. Sharpe.

Sorlie, P., and E. Rogot. 1990. Mortality by employment status in the National Longitudinal Mortality Study. *Am. J. Epidemiol.* 132:983–992.

Stefansson, C. G. 1991. Long-term unemployment and mortality in Sweden, 1980–1986. *Soc. Sci. Med.* 32:419–423.

Susser, D. I. 1985. Union carbide and the community surrounding it: The case of a community in Puerto Rico. *Int. J. Health Serv.* 15:561–583.

Susser, M., W. Watson, and K. Hopper. 1985. *Sociology in Medicine*, 3rd ed. New York: Oxford University Press.

Sweeney, J., and K. Nussbaum. 1987. *Solutions for the New Work Force: Policies for a New Social Contract.* Cabin John, MD: Seven Locks.

Syme, S. L., N. O. Borhani, and R. W. Buechley. 1965. Cultural mobility and coronary heart disease in an urban area. *Am. J. Epidemiol.* 82:334–346.

Thurow, L. 1969. *Poverty and Discrimination.* Washington, DC: Brookings Institution.

Thurow, L. 1980. *The Zero-Sum Society.* New York: Basic Books.

Thurow, L. 1987. A surge in inequality. *Sci. Am.* 256:30–37.

Toennies, F. 1952. *Community and Society* (translated by C. P. Loomis). East Lansing, MI: Michigan State University Press.

Treiman, D., and K. Terell. 1975. Sex and the process of status attainment: A comparison of working women and men. *Am. Soc. Rev.* 40:174–200.

Treiman, D. J. 1977. *Occupational Prestige in Comparative Perspective.* New York: Academic Press.

Turner, J. B., R. C. Kessler, and J. S. House. 1990. Factors facilitating adjustment to unemployment. *Am. J. Community Psychol.* 19:521–542.

U.S. Congress. House of Representatives. Committee on Ways and Means. 1989. *Background Material and Data on Programs Within the Jurisdiction of the Committee on Ways and Means.* Washington, DC: Government Printing Office.

Van Hook, M. 1990. Family response to the farm crisis: A study in coping. *Social Work* 35:425–431.

Vigderhous, G., and G. Fishman. 1978. The impact of unemployment and familial integration on changing suicide rates in the U.S.A., 1920–1969. *Social Psychiatry* 13:239–248.

Warr, P., P. Jackson, and M. Banks. 1988. Unemployment and mental health: Some British studies. *J. Soc. Issues* 44:47–68.

Weber, M. 1946. *Essays in Sociology* (translated by H. H. Gerth and C. W. Mills). New York: Oxford University Press.

Weber, M. 1947. *The Theory of Social and Economic Organization* (translated by A. M. Henderson and T. Parsons). New York: Oxford University Press.

Weisskopf, T., S. Bowles, and D. Gordon. 1983. Hearts and minds: A social model of U.S. productivity growth. *Brookings Papers on Economic Activity* 2:381–450.

Westin, S. 1990. The structure of a factory closure: Individual responses to job-loss and unemployment in a 10-year controlled follow-up study. *Soc. Sci. Med.* 31:1301–1311.

Westin, S., J. J. Schlesselman, and M. Korper. 1989. Long-term effects of a factory closure: Unemployment and disability during ten year's follow-up. *J. Clin. Epidemiol.* 42:435–441.

Whitman, S., D. Ansell, L. Lacey, E. H. Chen, N. Ebie, J. Dell, and C. W. Phillips. 1991. Patterns of breast and cervical cancer screening at three public health centers in an inner-city urban area. *Am. J. Public Health* 81:1651–1653.

Williamson, J. G., and P. H. Lindert. 1980. *American Inequality: A Macroeconomic History.* New York: Academic Press.

Winnink, A. J. 1989. *Toward Two Societies: The Changing Distributions of Income and Wealth in the U.S. Since 1960.* New York: Praeger.

8

Class, Work, and Health

JEFFREY V. JOHNSON and ELLEN M. HALL

The inquiry into the interconnections of work, social class, and human well-being have been a basic theme in social science since the advent of the industrial revolution in the nineteenth century. Interpreting these complex interrelationships remains a challenge, however.

The association between lower social class position and adverse physical and mental health (Hollingshead and Redlich, 1958; Dohrenwend and Dohrenwend, 1969) has been reported in the United States (Antonovsky, 1967, 1968; Kitagawa and Hauser, 1973; Haan et al., 1987, 1989; Williams, 1990), in Great Britain (Marmot et al., 1984, 1987, 1991; Marmot and McDowall, 1986; Carr-Hill, 1989, Smith, 1990) and in Scandinavia (Vagero and Lundberg, 1989; Vagero, 1991).

Social class is a powerful determinant of a multitude of factors that affect health: access to social resources, such as medical care and adequate housing; the nature of the physical and urban environment; and individual resources, such as income and education, that reflect differential opportunities. Exposure to hazards and stresses of daily life are also differentially distributed along social-class lines. Those at the lower end of the social-class hierarchy are more likely to be exposed to chemical and physical hazards in their work, to be threatened with unemployment, and to have to contend with a deteriorating urban physical and social environment. Indeed, it has been suggested that lower social-class position is characterized by meager social and individual resources in combination with high levels of daily stress, and that it is this imbalance, or strain, that ultimately explains the higher morbidity and mortality rates of less-advantaged social-class groups (Haan et al., 1989).

It can be argued that social class is the primary determinant of exposure to adverse factors; however, the mechanisms by which class might influence health remain underspecified. Biomedical researchers commonly employ three measures of social status that have been found to be predictive of adverse health outcomes: income, education, and occupation, or combinations of these demographic factors. Relying on such indicators, however, creates the danger of reducing class differences in health status to differences in the characteristics of individuals. In what sense is social class really an "individual" risk factor at all? Modern epidemiology directs its attention largely to elucidating risk factors that influence disease processes in individual organisms. This way of conceptualizing the problem makes it difficult to envision emergent levels of reality beyond that of the individual, such as those of the social group, the community, and the class structure of the society itself. Yet as Syme (1991, p. 23) has pointed out:

> Population groups often have a characteristic pattern of disease over time, even though individuals come and go from these groups. If groups have different rates of disease over time, there may be something about the groups that either promotes or discourages disease among individuals in those groups.

Perhaps it would be simpler if the components of class could be ascribed to individual characteristics, such as literacy, previous training or job occupancy, and experience. But if that were the case, why would it be that one's chances of surviving birth, the length of one's life, the amount of money one has, the ability to provide a college education for one's children, safety at home and at work, access to health care, the cause of one's death, and a multitude of other factors are distributed along class lines? Access to the goods and services our society offers is sometimes attributed to hard work or worthiness, but an examination of these ideas indicates that good luck and hard work are necessary but not sufficient for success. It is hard work to be a miner, for instance, but such work rarely yields lavish rewards.

If we are indeed interested in the link between society and health, our research focus must shift from the properties of individuals to the nature of the social-class structure itself. This will not be easy, as Marshall Becker has recently suggested (Becker, 1993, pp. 4–5):

> To turn our attention beyond the individual—to recognize the social and economic determinants of disease, health, and "wellness"—is complex and threatening. Doing something about poverty, racism, unemployment, inequitable access to education and other resources and quality of environment involves notions of planned social and economic change, alterations not likely to be achieved by lowering the public's cholesterol levels.

The need for a deeper understanding of class is also evident in psychosocial research on the work environment. Conceptual models have been developed that examine the relationship of work-organization factors (such as control over the work process, social support in the work setting and production demands) to chronic-disease mortality and morbidity (Alfredsson et al., 1982, 1985; Baker, 1985; Johnson and Hall, 1988; Karasek and Theorell, 1990; Syme, 1991; Johnson and Johansson, 1991). With a few notable exceptions (Laurell, 1979; Navarro, 1982; Marmot and Theorell, 1988;

Karasek, 1991), however, this work has been done without reference to an underlying theory of class formation. Indeed, although the study of work organization and research on social class are two of the most promising subjects for research in social epidemiology, a tendency has emerged to juxtapose their effects on health: One position argues that the association between work characteristics and health is due not to the adverse aspects of work exposure *per se* but to the concomitant exposures associated with lower social-class status (Albright et al., 1992). Another perspective holds that since work-organization exposures vary as a function of social class, they are in fact important mediators, or proximate causal mechanisms, that contribute to an explanation of the class-and-health relationship (Marmot and Theorell, 1988). We will argue that the realities of class and work are inextricably linked together in the lives of human populations and that it is unnecessary and even undesirable to attempt to distinguish conceptually between class and work. What is needed instead is a theoretical framework that clarifies the linkages among class, work, and health. To this end, we will explore certain theoretical issues pertaining to the concept of class and its relationship to theories of work and the labor process. We will then review current thinking on the relationship between work and health, including both biomedical and sociological theories, and will propose a way to look into the possibility of class-determined exposure ecologies.

Class as a Relational Concept

Although the concept of class has been explored in depth by sociologists and political economists (Granovetter and Tilly, 1988), controversy about what class is and is not persists in the theoretically oriented sociological literature. It is beyond the scope of this chapter to review all aspects of this debate (Halaby and Weakliem, 1993; Wright, 1993). Nevertheless, it is important that our analysis of the relationship between class and work and the examination of class differences in health-related research be informed by this discussion (Braverman, 1974, Edwards, 1979; Zimbalist, 1979; Giddens and Held, 1982; Wright and Singelmann, 1982; Wright, 1989).

The classical approaches to conceptualizing social class originated with Marx and Weber. An overly simplified treatment of Weber's theories has led to the prevailing view that class can be understood as a social-status gradient, and that no fundamental discontinuities exist between levels except with regard to access to social resources and/or prestige (Nam and Powers, 1983). The concept of socioeconomic status, frequently encountered in the epidemiological literature, is one expression of this interpretation. A structural orientation such as that of Marx, by contrast, views class as a fundamental social category that defines individuals' basic relationship to their work, their general material existence, and their relationships with members of other class groups (Laurell, 1979). As Therborn (1982, p. 235) points out: "The Weberian question for determining what class A belongs to is: *How much does he have* (i.e., of market resources)? Whereas Marx asks: *What does he do?* What is his position in the process of production?"

Individuals' relationships to the social organization of production not only define their experience of working life but also determine their social community, their financial and residential resources, their cultural experiences, their health-related behavior, and even the life-course opportunities open to them and their children. One's relationship to work and the labor process is critical not only as a source of job-related exposure *per se* but also because it is so central to class definition. By contrast, the relationship to production does not play such a key role in a status hierarchy, such as SES, that is based on access to general marketplace resources and the perceived social status associated with what one possesses (Giddens, 1973). Some authors argue that the terms *social class* and *social stratification* though used interchangeably, are indeed quite different. For example, Kohn and Slomczynski (1990, p. 2) make the following distinction:

> By social classes, we refer to groups defined in terms of their relationship to ownership and control over the means of production and of their control over the labor power of others. By social stratification, we mean the hierarchical ordering of society in terms of power, privilege and prestige.

Although information about knowledge of individuals' occupation, education, and income may be somewhat useful in classifying them within a particular class, our understanding of how class is related to health and well-being should be based on a more considered view of the essential social processes embodied in the concept. One advantage of a structural Marxist perspective, where class is rooted in the labor process, is that it focuses attention on the qualitative essence of class relationships—in other words, on relations of exploitation: of domination and subordination. Although these social processes are particularly evident in the workplace, domination and subordination are certainly not restricted to working life; they are the essence of inequality in the social organization of gender and race as well. The exercise of power by a dominant group over a subordinate group for purposes of relative material, social, or emotional advantage is the social kernel of exploitation.

Class is a relational and dialectical social process that changes over time, and that involves active strategies on the part of both dominant and subordinate groups. As a process, we would argue, it is best examined along a number of dimensions. We will propose five bipolar concepts that might be usefully employed as theoretical guides in the study of class, work, and health. We see these concepts as overlapping with regard to the exercise of power and the potential for freedom and control:

1. Domination and subordination
2. Freedom and alienation
3. Control and resistance
4. Core and marginality
5. Visible and invisible labor

Domination and Subordination

With respect to how work is organized, those in the upper levels of the professional and managerial hierarchy enjoy ample financial remuneration. They also have the right to exercise authority over others, to expect obedience and even subservience, and to enjoy prominent social position, the privileges of voluntary action and association, and the many ineffables of an affluent lifestyle.

While a great deal can be said about the values and behaviors that contribute to class differences, we will argue that the hierarchical structure of domination and subordination in the organization of work and of society—not an individual's income, education or occupation *per se*—is the bedrock of class difference.

The theoretical works of Marx (1974a, b) are the traditional starting point for thinking and research in this area. Marx believed that the underlying dynamic of social change throughout human history had been a struggle for power between a dominant class and a subordinate class. In his view, the ability of industrial capitalism to harness and transform the natural environment by organizing the human and material resources necessary for industrial manufacture resulted in a fundamental contradiction: that the production process was socially and collectively realized, but privately owned. Therefore, although industrial capitalism was constructing the material basis for human freedom, the accompanying process of domination and exploitation resulted in widespread alienation in the working population.

Freedom and Alienation

Only human beings, according to Marx, are capable of complex and deliberate activity uniting conceptualization and execution. This human capacity for free labor, although potentially realizable under capitalism, is in Marx's view realized only for those who own and control the means of production. The human tragedy of capital, for Marx, is that most individuals are not allowed to exercise their human capabilities. As Erich Fromm (1967, p. 50) pointed out 30 years ago:

> Marx's aim is . . . the emancipation of the human being through the restitution of the unalienated and hence free activity of all men, and a society in which man, not the production of things, is the aim, in which man ceases to be 'a crippled monstrosity' and becomes a fully developed human being.

Alienation is the emotional and instrumental isolation of individuals from each other, from their work, and from the larger society. Alienation is an outcome of work and lives that do not call forth the full human capacity for thought, skilled execution, and cooperative relationships. In modern industrial sociology, Marx's concept of alienation is often interpreted narrowly as a set of attitudes or subjective responses, including powerlessness, normlessness, rootlessness, a sense of not belonging or of having no meaningful role in the production process or the larger society. For Marx, however, alienation also involved a series of structural separations or cleavages: workers are disconnected from ownership of the work process, from decisions about what is produced and how, from each other through competition for employment, and consequently from themselves through the disparity between their potential for free activity and their actual experience in the labor process. In other words, Marx viewed alienation as a fundamental objective consequence of the social relations of production and class inequalities in power (Schweitzer and Geyer, 1989).

Alienation is likely to result when the limits imposed on human autonomy, control, and collectivity are so constraining that the only remaining response is to withhold effort, affect (caring, dedication, and the like) and attention. Active resistance to forestall alienation can even be a creative act: "I am not just a machine, because I can exercise my will to resist as a Luddite." Even in the most difficult situations, such as war, concentration camps, and prisons, alienation can generate stunningly creative acts of resistance. At the other extreme, the occurrence of alienation in privileged occupations such as medicine and law demonstrates that alienation has to do with meaningfulness, hope, and efficacy as well as with control.

Control and Resistance

Control over the work process decreases as a function of class, such that even talking on the job, moving freely, and attending to the call of nature must be permitted and cannot be assumed. Thus subordination can be defined in terms of decision-making authority and control over one's time, activities, and resources. Seen in terms of class distinctions, one's degree of control affects one's ability to determine a life course, extent of occupational selection, possibilities for mobility, and even use of leisure time.

One example of a structural and class-oriented perspective on alienation that focuses on loss of control is the work of Braverman (1974) on the historical process of "deskilling" within the industrial labor force. Braverman describes the corporate strategy known as scientific management, developed in the latter part of the nineteenth century by the industrial designer Frederick Winslow Taylor, as consisting of three basic principles:

1. Disassociation of the work process from the skills of workers
2. Separation of conception from execution
3. Use of the resulting monopoly over knowledge to control each step of the work process and its mode of execution

Braverman views Taylorism as a manifestation of a deeper process, built into capitalism, that involves the replacement of skilled workers by machines, the division and subdivision of jobs and allocation of any remaining skilled jobs to a few specialized workers, and the fragmentation of the remaining semiskilled and unskilled tasks.

There is still debate about how widely Taylorism has been diffused, and whether or not the countervailing impact of reskilling in the context of flexible manufacturing methods will eventually create a more highly qualified labor force (see Wright, 1985; Zuboff, 1988; Karasek and Theorell, 1990.) Sociologists of work have shown work fragmentation and the hierarchical centralization of control to have been a prevailing tendency for at least the last century (Montgomery, 1979; Edwards, 1979; Wright and Singelmann, 1982). Nevertheless, Braverman's work has been criticized for being too one-sided–specifically, for implying that deskilling is an immutable social process, unalterable by social forces (Thompson, 1983; Stark, 1980), and for ignoring worker resistance. An alternative position emphasizes the potential of individuals and groups acting as agents to shape the structures of their daily lives. Georg Lukacs' useful distinction between the objective and subjective aspects of class identity "class-in-itself" (class as object) and "class-for-itself" (class as subject) (Gouldner, 1980)—allows us to differentiate between the objective structure of class relations and the willingness and ability of a class or a portion of a class to organize and act in its own interest.

It is a comment on the nature of our species that the very idea of freedom itself has grown out of the experience of slavery (Patterson, 1991). Where there is exploitation and domination, there will be resistance, often invisible and informal (Scott, 1990). As Scott (1990, p. xii) notes: "Every subordinate group creates, out of its ordeal, a 'hidden transcript' that represents a critique of power spoken behind the back of the dominant." This concept is well expressed by an old Ethiopian proverb: "When the great lord passes, the wise peasant bows deeply and silently farts." Power relations are always a two-way proposition, and those in subordinate positions often translate their knowledge of the day-to-day practical realities of their situation into a degree of individual and collective control (Giddens, 1973).

The work of Pierre Bourdieu, a French sociologist, has been influential in reintroducing the concept that human beings are agents as opposed to "epi-phenomena of structure" (Bourdieu, 1990, p. 9). Human beings do not simply adapt to social rules, according to Bourdieu; through experience, they put into practice a "generative habitus," which Bourdieu describes as a "feel for the game" that enables "an infinite number of 'moves' to be made adapted to the infinite number of possible situations which no rule, however complex, can foresee." Another way of thinking about the habitus is as a set of survival strategies that evolves in the course of an individual's contact with the social structure. Although Bourdieu emphasizes the creative, inventive, and active aspects of the habitus, as a "system of acquired dispositions" it is grounded in class experience. And, though not a necessary product of social structure, the "system of social conditions" provides the context that makes a particular way of doing things possible (Bourdieu, 1984). Later we will examine two class-based forms of habitus that we consider of particular relevance to the study of work and health.

The remaining two conceptual polarities, core/marginality and visible/invisible labor, serve in our view to condition and shape the dynamics of domination, alienation and resistance.

Core and Marginality

Certain macro-level factors, such as broad economic trends and historicity, influence the social structure in such a way that those in core industries will enjoy greater resources and continuity in their working life and class experience than those at the periphery. Mobility and discontinuity are characteristic of the peripheral sectors of the labor market, as are greater risk for unemployment (marginality of labor force) and less generous benefits. To a considerable degree, these trends cut across class and occupation. The nature of work, career opportunities, and organizational structure have been shown to differ in industries whose market concentration, capital intensity, and productive capacity differ (Gordon et al., 1982; Kalleberg, 1983). Research performed in the United States, Japan, and Europe indicates that the core set of large industrial firms is characterized by a high proportion of unionized workers, stable employment and regulated working conditions. Peripheral firms, by contrast, tend to be smaller, less unionized, and economically dependent on larger firms, and to offer much less job security, lower wages, and less favorable working conditions (Kallberg and Sorensen, 1979; Wanner and Lewis, 1983). When compared with their class counterparts in core industries, those in all class positions within peripheral industrial organizations would be considered disadvantaged with respect to most aspects of working life.

Gender and race/ethnicity are aspects of the marginality phenomenon. Women, immigrants, and minorities often function as a surplus labor pool that is tapped in times of economic growth and/or emergency (e.g., during wars). Even with steady growth in overall labor force participation, these groups often rotate in and out of the labor force, with economic (and family) cycles. Furthermore, a high level of segregation in activities is evident. Women tend to perform service and caring work, for instance, and immigrants often perform menial and manual labor, or operate small businesses.

Visible and Invisible Labor

"Visible" labor is paid labor, leading to the production of goods and services. Most thinking on the issue of work concentrates on the conditions and results of visible labor. Many women motivated by a set of biological, social, and emotional imperatives, also pursue "invisible" labor in the home. Such work is invisible because it has not always been considered work; many a woman has said, "I don't work; I'm just a housewife." Such labors entail no direct payments, no protective legislation, and no Social Security, and social regard for such work is low.

The invisible work of women is ancient and universal. Although technology, social policies, and birth control have modified the relative effort involved in bearing children, caring for the home, maintaining social connections, preparing food, making clothes, and so forth, the fundamental nature of the activities that constitute "women's work" has changed very little. The invisible work of women involves not merely hours of activity but also complex socio-emotional efforts of long duration, evident in such expressions as "You never stop being a mother." Caring for home and family involves repetition, but never closure; the same daily chores and obligations keep recurring.

Invisible employment has generally been segregated from the larger economic and institutional spheres of effort and money transactions. While indirect relationships to the larger economy exist (notably through advertising of products used in the home), the actual work is performed in isolation. In short, household workers are visible as consumers, and the home is widely acknowledged as a marketplace; but they are not publicly regarded as workers, and the home is not regarded as a workplace.

In a sense, employed women are straddling pre- and postindustrial social structures. Although appliances and the like have changed the amount of physical labor involved in cleaning and cooking, studies suggest that the amount of time devoted to these activities has not changed (Cowan, 1983). The amount of time spent on housework has actually increased in the middle and affluent classes, according to Cowan, because few people now have servants. She asserts that contemporary women of all but the wealthiest classes spend about the same amount of time on housework as did poorer women in 1912. During the preindustrial era, most people worked as part of a family unit, and expended the bulk of their effort on producing enough to feed and clothe the family. This largely agrarian existence did not lend itself to larger social and economic involvements. Arlie Hochschild (1989) characterizes the housewife as a peasant, because her work is low-status and isolated from the "more important" world of paid labor and because it is a last bastion of an older craft-based form of production. It is not surprising, then, that conflicts arise between the values and behaviors embedded in the two worlds of visible and invisible labor. (See Hall, 1989, 1990, 1992, for a fuller discussion of these concepts.)

The Class Basis of Work Exposures

Having examined the overarching mechanisms of social class, let us turn to the nature of work within class society, and how differential work exposures might contribute to inequalities in health.

Class differences in exposure can be approached from two conceptually distinct orientations: typological and dimensional. The differences between these two models have recently been discussed in an exchange between Halaby and Weakliem (1993) and Erik Olin Wright (1993) on the effects of social-class position on earnings. The dimensional model of class focuses on aspects of jobs, such as control and authority, that are empirically overlapping and potentially scalable across class groups. The advantage of a dimensional approach is that it "deconstructs the underlying structure" of class (Halaby and Weakliem, 1993, p. 29) into a parsimonious set of key variables, such as authority and control. The typological approach uses the ownership and authority components of jobs to locate them in a system of "discrete, nominal class categories" (Halaby and Weakliem, 1993, p. 17). Wright (1993, p. 32) advances two arguments for considering class as a typology:

> First, . . . these nominal categories correspond to qualitatively distinct causal mechanisms. Second, because these causal mechanisms are imbedded in a structure of social relations, categorically defined classes are particularly useful for explaining class conflict.

We will employ a combined model with both categorical and dimensional elements in our discussion of the relationships among class, work, and health. We will first discuss the dimensional approach by looking at models that have been generalized across class groups, focusing specifically on control over the work process.

Class Dimensionality in Exposure: The Case of Work Control

A substantial literature indicates that work control varies systematically as a function of social class (Kohn, 1969; Marmot and Theorell, 1988; Karasek and Theorell, 1990). The structural origin of this variation is suggested by our earlier discussion of deskilling. Subjugation to the tenets of Taylorization and the experience of alienation are not restricted to manual workers, and appear to be encroaching on nonmanual workers as well. Case studies have documented the adverse effects of work fragmentation and deskilling on computer programmers (de Kadt, 1979) and clerical workers (Glenn and Feldberg, 1979). Our own research on physicians indicates that, even in this highly privileged occupational group, there is considerable variation in the degree of work control across different practice settings, and that physicians with low levels of control and social support experience increases in prospectively measured mental and physical distress.

Early work on the limits of human adaptation treat overload and underload as essentially class-neutral, investigating the conditions of under- and overstimulation, lack of control, and mental strain without reference to macro-level social structure (Frankenhaeuser and Gardell, 1976; Frankenhauser, 1980, 1991). Attention to control over the work process first emerged in the late 1960s in the collaborative work of the Swedish researchers Gardell and Frankenhaeuser (Gardell and Frankenhaeuser, 1976; Gardell, 1977, 1981); Gardell's findings about the relationship between organizational characteristics and mental health, and Frankenhaeuser's findings concerning physiological responses to under- and overload were merged, resulting in a new synthesis. The terms *under-* and *overload* were more broadly defined to signify mechanized, alienating work and hectic, strenuous work, respectively. In both cases, it was lack of control over the work process that determined whether the demands of the job were experienced as stressful.

These concepts have been refined and modeled more completely in Karasek and Theorell's demand-control formulation (Karasek, 1976, 1979, 1991; Karasek et al., 1981). Karasek predicted that biologically aversive strain will occur when the psychological demands of a job exceed the available resources for control over task content. Many studies supportive of this theory have demonstrated that workers in jobs characterized by high demands and low control report greater depression and anxiety, and are at increased risk of developing and dying from cardiovascular disease. (Karasek, 1979, 1991; Karasek et al., 1981; Alfredsson et al., 1982; Theorell et al., 1984, 1985; Baker, 1985; Karasek and Theorell, 1990; Schnall et al., 1990; Theorell, 1992; Schnall, 1994).

Implicit in Karasek's model are two important findings. The first is a learning-generalization process, whereby what is learned in the course of working is applied in other spheres of life as well (Karasek and Theorell, 1989). Theorell et al. (1984) suggest that the psychosocial work environment influences an individual's overall life strategy, self-efficacy, and self-esteem. One implication for cardiovascular health is that certain kinds of work, such as monotonous jobs, may tend to produce a fatalistic attitude toward life: "If life is meaningless, why make the effort to stop smoking or to adopt a more healthy lifestyle?" Second, this formulation provides a means by which all work, regardless of specific features, can be evaluated or ranked in terms of structural factors. (Such an examination of the research hypothesis would be extremely difficult, for example, using only Type-A behavior, or person-environment-fit theories.)

It has also recently become possible to use the demand-control formulation to evaluate individual-level changes in behavior or risk. Theorell and colleagues (1988) report that 28-year-old men who had shown a propensity to blood-pressure elevation earlier in life, and who worked in high-strain occupations, exhibited much more marked blood-pressure elevations at work than other men in the same age group. Another longitudinal study by Theorell and colleagues evaluated the health of working men and women in six service occupations (Theorell et al., 1988; Theorell, 1992), and found a strong association between increasing job strain and increasing blood pressure at work. These observations point to the possibility of a direct relationship between the psychosocial work environment and risk of heart disease (Johnson, 1991).

We (Johnson and Hall, 1993) have developed and tested an expanded version of Karasek and Theorell's formulation to determine whether social support from workmates is another structural factor that moderates the impact of job demands. We found that social isolation at work functions as an independent risk factor: when coupled with lack of control and high demands, it substantially increases cardiovascular prevalence risk. We have used our demand-control-support model to define a specific risk group, which we call the "high iso-strain" group (Johnson et al., 1989). This indicator—a multiplicative combination of the standardized demand, control and support scales—was then used to examine whether individuals whose work is high-strain and socially isolated developed cardiovascular disease at an earlier age than those with more positive working conditions. When considering class differences, two findings are notable: male manual workers are much more likely to be exposed to high iso-strain conditions than are male nonmanual workers, and they are likely to be more adversely affected by this exposure. In a prospective study of cardiovascular mortality among 4235 blue-collar Swedish men, we found an age-adjusted relative risk of 2.54 (95 percent confidence interval 1.06–6.28) for those with high iso-strain, whereas the relative risk for white-collar (n = 2984) workers in the high iso-strain groups was only 1.31 (95 percent confidence interval 0.58–2.96). This observation underscores our earlier findings that the demand-control model works very well for blue-collar men but is less predictive for white-collar men and for women (Johnson and Hall, 1988; Hall, 1990). More recently we have examined the effects of demands, control, and support over the entire working life of a large cohort study of 25,000 Swedish men and women. Exposure to low control jobs over a period of 25 years was associated with nearly a two-fold risk of CHD mortality during a 14 year follow-up period, even after adjusting for a number of cardiovascular disease risk factors, such as smoking, exercise, physical demands of the job, as well as social class position and educational attainment (Johnson et al, 1991; Johnson and Stewart, 1993).

The demand-control model, though developed to be generalizable across class strata has served to make specific class-oriented predictions with regard to ill health. It is important to note that its introduction to the field of psychosocial work environment research has helped correct the "received" assumption of the 1960s that job stress was primarily a problem of the upper-level business executive with too many responsibilities. It identified the highly Taylorized and deskilled high-demand and low-control quadrant of the manual and service-sector work force as the most highly stressed, and as the group at highest risk for chronic illnesses.

Class Specificity in Work Exposure

Let us now turn to exposures that are specific to particular social-class categories. In discussing differences in occupational conditions across social-class groups, we will use the most obvious class-based occupational distinction (which echoes the earliest division of the industrial revolution): between manual and nonmanual workers. Although the differences between the work environments of manual and nonmanual workers may be less vast than they were when Marx distinguished between mental and physical production, this distinction continues to capture a fundamental aspect of class difference, as Braverman's discussion of the separation of conception from execution in twentieth century industrial manufacture attests. Although the manual/nonmanual dichotomy does not encompass the dimensional complexity discussed earlier, we agree with Kohn and Slomczynski (1990), Gagliani (1981), Vanneman and Pampel (1977), Carchedi (1975, 1987), and Poulantzas (1975) that this distinction remains an important aspect of class structure.

The continuing value of these simple categories is due, in part, to the cultural differences ascribed to "blue-collar" and "white-collar" worlds. Although what we understand as social class may be partially measured by examining the differential distribution of certain structural dimensions, such as work control, this approach does not sufficiently address those aspects of class that are cultural expressions of the "habitus."

After entering the labor market, individuals are socialized into class-based cultures that exist both within the workplace and extra-occupationally. The workplace is a primary institution for adult socialization, and new forms of learning and adaptation occur as a result of socialization processes in adulthood (Kohn, 1969; Karasek, 1976;

Frese, 1982; Gardell, 1982a, b; Kohn and Schooler, 1983; Kohn and Slomczynski, 1990). Contrary to the conventional view that individuals cease to learn after about age 18, the work environment can be a source of an adult-learning template. One's interactions with other adults, can transmit a workplace-based system of norms and values.

What defines class-based cultural systems? Income, place of residence, leading a white- or blue-collar life, and behaviors, habits, and emotions that are occupationally related and extend into nonworking life are all part of occupational culture. Most readers can accurately describe the neighborhoods and eating, working, and leisure-time habits of accountants, bus drivers, construction workers, physicians.

Age and education level at entry into the labor market also vary by class, as does the typical duration of reward cycles. For academics and business people, the period of apprenticeship and training can be quite lengthy, and such individuals typically do not reap high rewards until middle age or later. By contrast, many blue-collar workers enter the job market immediately after leaving high school and hold the same job at approximately the same pay and skill level throughout their working lives.

The marked cultural differences we find in different class groups may largely be a consequence of the pronounced disparity in the nature of the material environment within which each class group constructs its characteristic "habitus." We will turn now to a discussion of several specific ways in which work exposure and culture differs by class.

Manual Workers: Exposure and Resistance

A major factor that distinguishes manual workers from nonmanual workers is exposure to job hazards (Weeks et al., 1991). Beginning in the late 1960s, epidemiological studies of work focused on chemical and physical hazards. Mounting evidence showed that premature morbidity and mortality among certain occupational groups was a result of workplace hazards. In both Europe and the United States, workers, health activists, and unions entered into scientific and political debates, and even undertook strikes and media campaigns, to underscore the message that "your job is dangerous to your health." The resulting scientific and political movement began by addressing the most hazardous (and easily documented) conditions, such as those experienced by miners and chemical and steel workers, and later moved onto less easily documented concerns, such as the impacts of noise and radiation, and thence to more widespread but harder to measure problems such as job stress.

These initiatives, coupled with environmental activism, raised concern about the distribution of environmental and occupational toxins by class. Many groups began to question whether there was equity in the distribution of adverse occupational exposures leading to disease. In the mid-1970s the National Institutes of Health (Mason et al., 1975) published a series of cancer atlases, in which the relationship between occupational and environmental pollution and increased rates of particular cancers was addressed and linked to industrial processes. During the same period the American Public Health Association (1975) documented the distribution of the major diseases, and found that race and class were both important determinants.

An important component of these social concerns of the 1970s was volitionality in exposure. While those who smoke and drink are presumed to be exposing themselves voluntarily to health hazards (a proposition that might be questioned), those who work or live in environments polluted by asbestos, chlorinated hydrocarbons, or mercury are viewed by law, social convention, and science as having little recourse. What can individuals do to end such exposure, should they wish to maintain their livelihood and/or residency?

The question "Why must some people sacrifice their health and well-being as a requirement of working?"—a question that is central to any real concern with occupation and health—represents a serious social lacuna. Even the most hard-nosed proponents of "take responsibility for your health" will admit that options for worried workers are paltry in the current system, with its emphasis on individual-level solutions to health problems. To return to our primary argument, economically necessitated subordination can explain why people would expose themselves to toxic substances 8 hours a day. One cannot imagine a Wall Street lawyer or even a company clerk accepting the heat, noise, and toxicity that accompany the manufacture of rubber, garbage collection, or foundry work, or life next to Love Canal or Three Mile Island. Yet others are forced to accept such conditions as part of their life in the manual working class.

It is widely acknowledged that manual work is often monotonous, dirty, and difficult. That a further price of subordination is the necessity of accepting danger, harm, and even death is unspoken but socially accepted. It is noteworthy that as one descends the national and international hierarchy of social class, the dangers and the toxicity of working life increase. Many fear that U.S. companies will relocate in less-developed countries, where lack of workplace regulation permits exposing workers more cavalierly to hazardous conditions.

Given that individual coal miners or chemical workers can do virtually nothing about the respirable particles and danger in their work environment, the alternative to lack of individual-level control is collective response. Historically, in fact, citizens' groups and trade unions have been the means by which such problems have been addressed and even changed. Although our research has focused on psychosocial conditions, the physical hazards of work (including shift work, toxic exposure, high noise levels and the like) are a central component of the work, class, and health relationship.

Formal and informal collective mobilization and active resistance is frequently considered within the manual working class to be a legitimate mechanism for contending with a hazardous work environment. By contrast, collective activity is considerably less evident in the white-collar work force. While lack of individual control, marginality, danger, and subordination may reside most unambiguously in the working class, collectivity may represent a significant compensating or controlling mechanism for addressing these problems.

In earlier work, we have suggested that the concept of social support should be broadened to encompass the capabilities inherent in a social group to alter the nature of its environment (Johnson, 1989a, b, 1991; Johnson and Hall, 1993). Among many manual and service sector employees when individual-level control over one's task or one's career is limited, social and collective alliances become vitally important. For many manual workers, the quiet, endless desperation associated with working is partially ameliorated by relationships with fellow workers. What is created in such situations is inadequately characterized as "social support"; it is more satisfactorily viewed as a culture of solidarity (Fantasia, 1988). Through such groups, which share common work experiences, workers collectively create a habitus, a strategy for surviving on the job (Gryzb, 1981). The concept of "the workers' collectivity," originated by the Norwegian sociologist Sverre Lysgaard, synthesizes the cultural and political aspects of this survival strategy (1961). According to Lysgaard (1961), Gardell (1982a, b), and others (Aronsson, 1991; Frese, 1989; Laurell, 1979), the workers' collectivity arises as a group response to the demands of the production system, whose performance pressures are beyond the capacity of any individual worker to modify. The collectivity serves to preserve the interests of both the individual and the group by establishing a counterauthority to that of management. Historical sociologists suggest that the elimination of collective control has been a relatively consistent tendency of scientific management since the late nineteenth century (Braverman, 1974; Edwards, 1979; Montgomery, 1979; Noble, 1979, 1984; Zimbalist, 1979; Gryzb, 1981; Thompson, 1983). Taylor and his successors understood that job design and technology could be used to desocialize workers through social isolation, job fragmentation, and the dissolution of informal work groups. This strategy has, in fact, been successful at many workplaces in preventing workers from exercising collective control and receiving social support.

Lysgaard has identified three prerequisites for the formation of the workers' collectivity: (1) spacial proximity is a precondition for social interaction; (2) jointly experienced problems create a common frame of reference; and (3) occupying equivalent positions encourages the formation of a collective identity.

The workers' collectivity is class-based in part because these preconditions are more likely to prevail among lower-level industrial and service-sector employees than among administrative or professional personnel. Yet even when Lysgaard's preconditions exist, collective entities do not always emerge. Group formation is influenced by a number of factors, including the size of the workplace, the duration of the employment cycle, the nature of the production process, and the stability of the enterprise. In some jobs, the structural preconditions for collectivity simply do not exist. In machine-paced assembly-line jobs, for instance, high noise levels, lack of physical proximity, rotating shifts, piece-rate payment systems, and company policies that prohibit talking can effectively prevent social interaction (House, 1981a).

Nonmanual Workers: Immersion in the Work Role

A factor that distinguishes different class groups but appears rarely in the literature is work obsession. Although several researchers have informally discussed and even tentatively investigated organizational culture (Frost et al., 1985) and its connection with

Type-A behavior, it is possible to postulate a more subjective and more global phenomenon relevant to stress and eventual ill-health that involves an overinvolvement in
the work role (Schaef and Fassel, 1990). The value of working hard is communicated
initially within the family, and later reinforced by school, peers, and social norms. Beliefs and assumptions about what constitutes an appropriate amount of effort begin to
develop early in life and are reinforced when a person enters the labor market. Many
academics and business people, for example, heard in youth, "If it's worth doing, it's
worth doing well" and "Hard work never hurt anyone." Many white-collar workers are
socialized, even when very young, to maximize effort to achieve goals. By contrast, an
alternative perspective suggests that repose and play—not hard work—are more natural and common conditions for humans and other primates (Eyer and Sterling, 1977).
As noted recently in *The Overworked American* (Schor, 1991), in materially poor cultures (such as the !Kung) and in earlier eras (such as the medieval and ancient periods),
material goods and services were meager, as was effort. But time—for everything from
caring for children to spirituality—was abundant (Lee, 1979).

   With the advent of the industrial era, the experience of time was separated from the
experience of life. That is, time as measured by clocks became the basis for measuring
activities. The clock became a means of subdividing the day into a span governed by
one's employer and a span that is free and private. The price of material progress, at
least according to Schor (1991), has been not simply an increase in the amount of time
spent working but also a form of psychic imprisonment by the organization of time.
Adults' lives are now almost completely consumed by the lengthening workday (calculated by Schor to be about twice as long as it was in the seventeenth century).

   Generally, though not universally, the compulsion to work, the drive to dedicate the
bulk of one's creativity and energy to paid employment increases as the social regard
and competition elicited by the job increase. Physicians and business executives, who
occupy the top of the social ladder and receive the highest disposable income, typically
have the least free time. As this passage from *A Passion For Excellence* (Peters and
Austin, 1985) suggests, the work culture of such people can make cruel demands:

> Even a pocket of excellence can fill your life like a wall-to-wall revolution. We have found
> that the majority of passionate activists who hammer away at the old boundaries have
> given up family vacation, little league games, birthday dinners, evenings, weekends and
> lunch hours, gardening, reading, movies and most other pastimes. We have a number of
> friends whose marriages or partnerships crumbled under the weight of their devotion to a
> dream. There are more newly single parents than we expected among our colleagues. We
> are frequently asked if it is possible to 'have it all'—a full and satisfying personal life and a
> full and satisfying hard-working professional life. The answer is no.

Among the impacts of work obsession, according to Schor, are "child neglect, marital
distress, sleep deprivation and stress-related illness" (Schor, 1991 p. 13). As one might
expect, the health consequences of such punishing and obsessional attitudes tend toward psychiatric, psychosomatic, and cardiovascular symptoms rather than injuries,

strains or cancers. Characteristic styles of coping tend toward reliance on one's own resources and dominating the environment rather than dependence on other people. Such personality traits as "hardiness" may in fact be most relevant in the upper-level nonmanual strata, where success and failure are largely determined by individual efforts.

The Type-A pattern of cardiovascular risk behavior, and its related burden of anger and hostility, may be related to work obsession. As various authors have noted (Eyer, 1975; Marmot and Syme, 1976), a competitive, hard-driving style, accompanied by an internalized sense of time urgency, can be viewed as a behavioral adaptation to the demands of the white-collar workplace. Henry (1986) suggests that the Type-A behavior pattern fostered in the workplace is destructive to the successful maintenance of marital relationships and other forms of social intimacy, particularly for men. Eyer (1975) asks "What would happen to the productivity of modern firms if Type-A behavior was somehow eliminated?" In the Whitehall study of British civil servants, Type-A behavior was found to be more prevalent at higher levels (Marmot et al., 1991). Similarly, the Framingham data (Kannel and Eaker, 1986) indicate that it is a coronary heart disease risk factor for coronary heart disease in nonmanual but not manual workers. Among manual workers, whose work involves greater dependency on collective relationships, such individualistic and competitive behavior may actually impede survival. In other words, Type-A behavior may be expected and reinforced in nonmanual, white-collar work while collective behavior is reinforced in manual, blue-collar work.

It is important to emphasize, however, that those most likely to become overly identified with their work role continue to be in a relatively advantaged position compared to their manual working class counterparts. Their working lives are richer, in terms of both the substantive complexity of the task structure itself and the rewards associated with their occupational position—greater power, social prestige, income, as well as improved health and longevity.

We conclude this chapter with a brief discussion of several practical and conceptual problems that are currently hindering our ability to examine the linkages between class, work, and health.

Substantive Challenges to the Study of Work, Class, and Health

The development of a societally oriented social epidemiology faces three substantive and methodological challenges: (1) the difficulty of examining causal sequences or pathways, (2) the interpenetration of different levels of analysis, and (3) the question of combined exposures.

Causal Pathways

The biomedical bias is to identify the primary cause most proximate to the cellular pathophysiological process. For example, lung cancer is caused by the effects of smoke inhalation on the lungs, through particulate deposition. Taking one step back for a broader perspective, one might examine psychological traits related to smoking and the inability to stop. Most research stops here, at the individual level. Other research, including our own, has examined the relationship of work and social structures to health behaviors such as smoking and sedentary leisure time (Green and Johnson, 1990; Johansson et al., 1991). As noted earlier, the nature of one's daily work life may influence these behaviors, perhaps via mechanisms that operate psychologically and socially. Individuals who enjoy substantial work control may experience, in Kohn's (Kohn, 1969; Kohn and Schooler, 1983) terms, a "learning-generalization effect" that enhances their general sense of mastery over their own situations.

Taking one more step back, we can observe that the potential to control one's own environment is differentially distributed along class lines. People with power exercise control over those who lack power. Superimposed on the labor process is a system of social stratification that simultaneously shapes individuals' coping repertoires and the nature of their work environments. Meanwhile, class-based experiences in the home and in the educational system inculcate certain beliefs, attitudes, and psychological structures.

"What causes a certain person to smoke?" becomes a very different question if we approach it in terms of a causal sequence of socially structured life circumstances that are differentially distributed throughout the society. Proximate causes, such as biomedical factors and health behaviors, are more readily and precisely measured. Therefore they are more likely to explain variance in health outcomes than more distal measures, such as those related to class of origin or work environment. Causal chains that are socially determined often unfold over the life span, and, particularly with reference to social-class factors, may include an intergenerational component. Period and cohort effects (such as changes in the labor process, war, and economic depression) must also be considered as manifestations of class experience in the lives of individuals of different ages. To examine the relationship between social inequalities and health adequately, we must replace our dependence on causally naive analytic models and research designs, with methods that do justice to the complexity of the relationship between human biography and social structure. The rich theoretical tradition in the sociology of social structure and personality (Kohn, 1969; House, 1981b; Kohn and Slomczynski, 1990; Williams, 1990) provides a model illustration of a research program grounded in a substantive theory process and using sophisticated comparative designs and causal analytic methods.

Emergent Levels of Analysis

As we have noted in earlier work, individual-based analysis faces a "decomposability" problem (Johnson, 1989a, b,), in that many social and organizational-level phenomena cannot be decomposed to an individual level. For example, the collective forms of organization that evolve in particular work settings represent an emergent reality over and above that of the individuals who comprise them; the collectivity influences individual perception, attitude, and behavior. By examining only individuals, one might entirely overlook the importance of this social structure.

It might be useful to expand on the traditional "macro and micro" dichotomy by adding a third "meso" level of analysis. In terms of the factors that shape work, the macro level includes such phenomena as market segmentation and historical changes in the labor process. The meso level consists of the organizational level, the organization of work, and the nature of the work process. Most research on the link between work and health operates at the micro level of analysis, where exposure to the characteristics of work occurs. Forces operating at all three levels shape individuals and their socialization and exposure processes, but individuals are most conscious of, and best able to report on, exposures occurring within their immediate range of vision.

The Problem of Combined Exposures

Bjorn Gustavsson (1991, p. 230) has described work organization as a "meta-exposure." In his words, "The way work is organized can be seen as the factor that decides exposure to *all* work environment hazards since it is the organization of work that determines who is to do what for how long."

Different patterns of work organization impose different patterns of performance demands, social support, exposure to physical demands, and/or chemical hazards. Gustavsson offers an ecological model of work, in which various features combine to create an indivisible whole. To examine exposure to only one factor is to ignore the fact that different work organizations constitute different sets of multiple factors. This problem is clearly intertwined with the issue of multiple levels of analysis noted above. The class structure is the major determinant of the ecology of exposure (Hasan, 1986), such that different class groups are "normally" exposed to different sets of interlocking risk factors.

Conclusion

Social class has a profound effect on the individual life course and work experience. Within the manual blue-collar world, physical hazards and lack of work control are key difficulties; in nonmanual, white-collar work, high performance demands and an internalized work ethic are more central. In other words, the environment itself tends to be oppressive in blue-collar work, while in white-collar work the oppression is often internalized, or even idealized as an ethic. Blue-collar work offers the compensations of collectivity and social support, while white-collar work offers social status and power.

In essence, work is a system characterized by rewards and strains, which differ fundamentally as a function of class. Future studies of work and health will benefit from greater theoretical vigor, the use of such key concepts as control, collectivity, alienation, and core/marginality, and a more explicit understanding of the interrelationships of class, culture, and work.

References

Albright, C. L., M. A. Winkleby, D. R. Ragland, J. Fisher, and S. L. Syme. 1992. Job strain and prevalence of hypertension in a biracial population of urban bus drivers. *Am. J. Public Health* 82:984–989.

Alfredsson, L., R. Karasek, and T. Theorell. 1982. Myocardial infarction risk and psychosocial work environment characteristics: An analysis of the male Swedish work force. *Soc. Sci. Med.* 16:463–467.

Alfredsson, L., L. Spetz, and T. Theorell. 1985. Type of occupation and near-future hospitalization for myocardial infarction and some other diagnoses. *Int. J. Epidemiol.* 14:378–388.

American Public Health Association. Washington, DC: American Public Health Association. 1975. *Minority Health Chart Book.*

Antonovsky, A. 1967. Social class, life expectancy and overall mortality. *Millbank Q.* 45:31–73.

Antonovsky, A. 1968. Social class and the major cardiovascular diseases. *J. Chron. Dis.* 21:65–106.

Aronsson, G. 1991. Dimensions of control as related to work organization, stress, and health. In J. V. Johnson and G. Johansson (eds.), *The Psychosocial Work Environment: Work Organization, Democratization and Health*, pp. 111–120. Amityville, NY: Baywood.

Baker, D. 1985. The study of stress at work. *Annu. Rev. Public Health* 6:367–381.

Becker, M. H. 1993. A medical sociologist looks at health promotion. *J. Health Soc. Behav.* 34:1–6.

Bourdieu, P. 1984. *Distinction: A Social Critique of the Judgement of Taste.* Cambridge, MA: Harvard University Press.

Bourdieu, P. 1990. *In Other Words: Essays Towards a Reflexive Sociology.* Stanford, CA: Stanford University Press.

Braverman, H. 1974. *Labor and Monopoly Capital.* New York: Monthly Review Press.

Carchedi, G. 1975. Reproduction of social classes at the level of production relations. *Economy and Society* 4:1–86.

Carchedi, G. 1987. *Class Analysis and Social Research.* Oxford: Basil Blackwell.

Carr-Hill, R. 1990. The measurement of inequities in health: Lessons from the British experience. *Soc. Sci. Med.* 11:393–404.

Carr-Hill, R. 1989. The inequalities in health debate: A critical review of the issues. *J. Soc. Politics* 16:509–542.

Cowan, R. S. 1983. *More Work for Mother: The Ironies of Household Technology from the Open Hearth to the Microwave.* New York: Basic Books.

Edwards, R. 1979. *The Contested Terrain.* New York: Basic Books.

de Kadt, M. 1979. Insurance: A clerical work factory. In A. Zimbalist (ed.), *Case Studies on the Labor Process*, pp. 242–256. New York: Monthly Review Press.

Dohrenwend, B. P., and B. S. Dohrenwend. 1969. *Social Status and Psychological Disorder: A Causal Inquiry.* New York: John Wiley & Sons.

Eyer, J. 1975. Hypertension as a disease of modern society. *Int. J. Health Serv.* 5:539–558.

Eyer, J. and P. Sterling. 1977. Stress-related mortality and social organization. *Rev. Radical Political Economics* 9:1–44.

Fantasia, R. 1988. *Cultures of Solidarity: Conciousness, Action, and Contemporary American Workers.* Berkeley, CA: University of California Press.

Frankenhaeuser, M. 1980. Psychoneuroendrocrine approaches to the study of stressful person-environment transactions. In H. Selye (ed.), *Selye's Guide to Stress Research*, pp. 46–70. New York: Van Nostrand Reinhold.

Frankenhaeuser, M. 1991. A biopsychosocial approach to work life issues. In J. V. Johnson and G. Johansson (eds.), *The Psychosocial Work Environment and Health: Work Organization, Democratization and Health*, pp. 49–60. Amityville, NY: Baywood.

Frankenhaeuser, M., and B. Gardell. 1976. Overload and underload in working life: Outline of a multidisciplinary approach. *J. Human Stress* 2:35–46.

Frese, M. 1982. Occupational socialization and personality development: An underemphasized research perspective in industrial psychology. *J. Occupational Psychol.* 55:209–224.

Frese, M. 1989. Theoretical models of control and health. In S. L. Sauter, J. J. Hurrell, and C. L. Cooper (eds.), *Job Control and Worker Health*, pp. 107–128. London: John Wiley & Sons.

Fromm, E. 1967. *Marx's Concept of Man.* New York: Frederick Ungar.

Frost, P. J., L. Moore, M. Louis, C. Lundberg, and J. Martin. 1985. *Organizational Culture.* Beverly Hills: Sage Publications.

Gagliani, G. 1981. How many working classes? *Am. J. Soc.* 87:259–285.

Gardell, B. 1977. Autonomy and participation at work. *Hum. Relations* 30:515–533.

Gardell, B. 1981. Psychosocial aspects of industrial production methods. In L. Levi (ed.), *Society, Stress and Disease*, Vol. 4, pp. 65–75. Oxford: Oxford University Press.

Gardell, B. 1982a. Scandinavian research on stress in working life. *Int. J. Health Serv.* 12:31–41.

Gardell, B. 1982b. Work participation and autonomy: A multilevel approach to democracy at the workplace. *Int. J. Health Serv.* 12:527–558.

Giddens, A. 1973. *The Class Structure of the Advanced Societies.* New York: Harper & Row.

Giddens, A., and D. Held (eds.). 1982. *Classes, Power, and Conflict.* Berkeley, CA: University of California Press.

Giddens, A. 1979. *Central Problems in Social Theory: Action, Structure and Contradiction in Social Analysis.* Berkeley, CA: University of California Press.

Glenn, E. N., and R. L. Feldberg. 1979. Proletarianizing clerical work: Technology and organizational control in the office. In A. Zimbalist (ed.), *Case Studies on the Labor Process*, pp. 51–72. New York: Monthly Review Press.

Gordon, D., R. Edwards, and M. Reich. 1982. *Segmented Work, Divided Workers.* New York: Cambridge University Press.

Gouldner, A. W. 1980. *The Two Marxisms: Contradiction and Anomalies in the Development Theory.* London: Macmillan.

Granovetter, M. and C. Tilly. 1988. Inequality and the labor process. In N. J. Smelser (ed.), *Handbook of Sociology,* pp. 175–221. Beverly Hills, CA: Sage.

Green, K, J.V. Johnson. 1990. The effects of psychosocial work organization on the prevalence of cigarette smoking among chemical plant employees. *Am. J. Public Health* 80:1368–1371.

Gryzb, G. J. 1981. Decollectivization and recollectivization in the workplace: The impact on informal work groups and work culture. *Econ. Industrial Democracy* 2:455–482.

Gustavsen, B. 1991. Democratizing occupational health: The Scandinavian experience of work reform. In J. V. Johnson and G. Johansson (eds.), *The Psychosocial Work Environment and Health: Work Organization, Democratization and Health,* pp. 225–239. Amityville, NY: Baywood.

Haan, M., G. Kaplan, and T. Camacho. 1987. Poverty and health: Prospective evidence from the Alameda County Study. *Am. J. Epidemiol.* 125:989–998.

Haan, M., G. Kaplan, and S. L. Syme. 1989. Socioeconomic status and health: Old observations and new thoughts. In J. P. Bubker, D. S. Comby, and B. H. Kehrer (eds.), *Pathways to Health: The Role of Social Factors*, pp. 76–135. Menlo Park, CA: Henry J. Kaiser Family Foundation.

Halaby, C. N., and D. L. Weakliem. 1993. Ownership and authority in the earnings function: Alternative specifications. *Am. Soc. Rev.* 58:16–34.

Hall, E. M. 1989. Gender, work control, and stress: A theoretical discussion and an empirical test. *Int. J. Health Serv.* 19:725–745.

Hall, E. M. 1990. *Women's Work: An Inquiry into the Health Effects of Invisible and Visible Labor*. Stockholm: Akademitryck AB. (Doctoral Dissertation published by the Karolinska Institute.)

Hall, E. M. 1992. Double exposure: The combined impact of the home and work environments on psychosomatic strain in Swedish women and men. *Int. J. Health Serv.* 22:239–260.

Hasan, J. 1986. Way-of-life, stress, and differences in morbidity between occupational classes. Paper presented at the 1986 ESR Workshop Inequalities in Health, June 1986. Tampere, Finland.

Henry, J. P. 1986. Mechanisms by which stress can lead to coronary heart disease. *Postgrad. Med. J.* 62:687–693.

Hochschild, A. (with A. Machung). 1989. *The Second Shift: Working Parents and the Revolution at Home*. New York: Viking Press.

Hollingshead, A. B., and F. C. Redlich. 1958. *Social Class and Mental Illness*. New York: Wiley & Sons.

House, J. 1981a. *Work Stress and Social Support*. Reading, MA: Addison-Wesley.

House, J. 1981b. Social structure and personality. In M. Rosenberg and R. H. Turner (eds.), *Social Psychology: Sociological Perspectives*, pp. 525–561. New York: Basic Books.

Johansson, G., J.V. Johnson, and E. M. Hall. 1991. Smoking and sedentary behavior as related to work organization. *Soc. Sci. Med.* 32:837–846.

Johnson, J. V., 1989a. Control, collectivity and the psychosocial work environment. In S. L. Sauter, J. J. Hurrell, and C. L. Cooper (eds), *Job Control and Worker Health*, p. 55–74. London: John Wiley & Sons.

Johnson, J. V., 1989b. Collective control: Strategies for survival in the workplace. *Int. J. Health Serv.* 19:469–480.

Johnson, J. V. 1991. The significance of the social and collective dimensions of the work environment for human health and well-being. In A. Enander, B. Gustavsson, J. Karlsson, B. Starrin (eds.), *Work and Welfare: Papers from the Second Karlstad Symposium on Work*, July 15, 1990, pp. 31–45. Karlstad, Sweden: University of Karlstad.

Johnson, J. V., and E. M. Hall. 1988. Job strain, workplace social support and cardiovascular disease: A cross sectional study of a random sample of the Swedish working population. *Am. J. Public Health* 78:1336–1342.

Johnson, J. V., and E. M. Hall. 1994. Social support in the work environment and cardiovascular disease. In S. Shumaker and S. Czajkowski (eds.), *Social Support and Cardiovascular Disease*, pp. 145–166. New York: Plenum Press.

Johnson, J. V., and G. Johansson (eds.) 1991. *The Psychosocial Work Environment and Health: Work Organization, Democratization and Health*. Amityville, NY: Baywood.

Johnson, J. V., and W. F. Stewart. 1993. Measuring work organization exposure over the life course with a job exposure matrix. *Scand. J. Work Environ. Health* 19:21–28.

Johnson, J. V., E. M. Hall, and T. Theorell. 1989. Combined effects of job strain and social isolation on cardiovascular disease morbidity and mortality in a random sample of the Swedish male working population. *Scand. J. Work Environ. Health* 15:271–279.

Johnson, J. V., E. M. Hall, W. Stewart, P. Fredlund, T. Theorell. 1991. Combined exposure to adverse work organization factors and cardiovascular disease: Towards a life-course perspective. In L. Fechter (ed.), *Proceedings of the Fourth International Conference on the Combined Effects of Environmental Factors*, November 17, 1990, pp.117–121. Baltimore, MD: Johns Hopkins University.

Kalleberg, A. L. 1983. Work and stratification: Structural perspectives. *Work and Occupations* 10:251–259.

Kalleberg, A. L., and A. B. Sorensen. 1979. The sociology of labor markets. *Annu. Rev. Sociol.* 5:351–379.

Kannel, W. B., and E. D. Eaker. 1986. Psychosocial and other features of coronary heart disease: Insights from the Framingham Study. *Am. Heart J.* 112:1066–1073.

Karasek, R. A. 1976. *The Impact of the Work Environment on Life Outside the Job.* Doctoral Dissertation, Massachusetts Institute of Technology. Published by the Institute for Social Research, University of Stockholm.

Karasek, R. A. 1979. Job demands, job decision latitude, and mental strain: Implications for job redesign. *Admin. Sci. Q.* 24:285–308.

Karasek, R. A., D. Baker, F. Marxer, A. Ahlbom, and T. Theorell. 1981. Job decision latitude, job demands, and cardiovascular disease: A prospective study of Swedish Men. *Am. J. Public Health* 71:694–705.

Karasek, R. 1991. The political implications of psychosocial work redesign: A model of the pyschosocial class structure. In J. V. Johnson, and G. Johansson, (eds.), *The Psychosocial Work Environment and Health: Work Organization, Democratization and Health,* pp. 163–190. Amityville, NY: Baywood.

Karasek, R., and T. Theorell. 1990. *Healthy Work: Stress, Productivity, and the Reconstruction of Working Life.* New York: Basic Books.

Karasek, R., D. Baker, F. Marxer, A. Ahlbom, and T. Theorell. 1981. Job decision latitude, job demands, and cardiovascular disease: A prospective study of Swedish men. *Am. J. Public Health* 71:694–705.

Kitagawa, E. M., and P. M. Hauser. 1973. *Differential Mortality in the United States: A Study in Socioeconomic Epidemiology.* Cambridge, MA: Harvard University Press.

Kohn, M. L. 1969. *Class and Conformity: A Study in Values.* Homewood, ILL: Dorsey.

Kohn, M. L., and C. Schooler. 1983. *Work and Personality: An Inquiry into the Impact of Social Stratification.* Norwood, NJ: Albex.

Kohn, M. L., and K. M. Slomczynski. 1990. *Social Structure and Self-Direction: A Comparative Analysis of the United States and Poland.* Oxford: Basil Blackwell.

Laurell, A. C. 1979. Work and health in Mexico. *Int. J. Health Serv.* 9:543–568.

Lee, R. B. 1979. *The !Kung San: Men, Women and Work in a Foraging Society.* Cambridge: Cambridge University Press.

Lysgaard, S. 1961. *Arbeiderkollectivet.* (Workers collectivity.) Oslo: Universitets forlaget.

Marmot, M., and S. L. Syme. 1976. Acculturation and coronary heart disease in Japanese Americans. *Am. J. Epidemiol.* 104:225–247.

Marmot, M., and M. E. McDowall. 1986. Mortality decline and widening social inequalities. *Lancet* 1:274–276.

Marmot, M., and T. Theorell. 1988. Social class and cardiovascular disease: The contribution of work. *Int. J. Health Serv.* 18:659–674.

Marmot, M., M. J. Shipley, and G. Rose. 1984. Inequalities in death—specific explanations of a general pattern? *Lancet* 1:1003–1006.

Marmot, M., M. Kogevinas, and M. A. Elston. 1987. Social-economic status and disease. *Annu. Rev. Public Health* 8:111–135.

Marmot, M., G. Davey Smith, S. Stansfeld, C. Patel, F. North, J. Head, I. White, E. Brunner, and A. Feeney. 1991. Health inequalities among British civil servants: The Whitehall II Study. *Lancet* 337:1387–1393.

Marx, K. 1974a. *Capital, Vol. 1.* Moscow: Progress.

Marx, K. 1974b. *Economic and Philosophic Manuscripts of 1844.* Moscow: Progress.

Mason, T. J., F. W. McKoy, R. Hoover, W. J. Blot, and J. F. Fraumeni. 1975. Atlas of Cancer Mortality of U.S. Counties. U.S. Department of Health, Education and Welfare. Pub No. (NIH) 75–780. Washington, D.C.: U.S. Government Printing Office.

Montgomery, D. 1979. *Workers' Control in America.* Cambridge: Cambridge University Press.

Nam, C. B., and M. G. Powers. 1983. *The Socioeconomic Approach to Status Measurement.* Houston: Cap and Gown.

Navarro, V. 1982. The labor process and health: A historical materialist interpretation. *Int. J. Health Serv.* 12:5–29.

Noble, D. 1979. Social choice in machine design: The case of automatically controlled machine tools. In A. Zimbalist (ed.), *Case Studies on the Labor Process*, pp. 18–50. New York: Monthly Review.

Noble, D. 1984. *Forces of Production: A Social History of Industrial Automation.* New York: Alfred A. Knopf.

Patterson, O. 1991. *Freedom in the Making of Western Culture.* New York: Basic Books.

Peters, T., and N. Austin. 1985. *A Passion for Excellence.* New York: Warner Books.

Poulantzas, N. 1975. *Classes in Contemporary Capitalism.* London: New Left Books.

Schaef, A. W., and D. Fassel. 1990. *The Addictive Organization.* New York: Harper & Row.

Schor, J. B. 1991. *The Overworked American: The Unexpected Decline of Leisure.* New York: Basic Books.

Schnall, P., C. Pieper, J. Schwartz, R. Karasek, Y. Schlussel, R. Devereux, A. Ganau, M. Alderman, K. Warren, and T. Pickering. 1990. The relationship between "job strain," workplace diastolic blood pressure, and left ventricular mass index: Results of a case-control study. *JAMA* 263:1929–1935.

Schnall, P. L., P. A. Landsbergis, and D. Baker. 1994. Job strain and cardiovascular disease. *Annu. Rev. Public Health* 15:381–411.

Schweitzer, D., and R. F. Geyer. 1989. *Alienation Theories and De-Alienation Strategies.* Great Britain: Science Reviews.

Scott, J. C. 1990. *Domination and the Arts of Resistance.* New Haven: Yale University Press.

Smith, G. D., M. Bartley, and D. Blane. 1990. The Black Report on Socioeconomic Inequalities in Health 10 years on. *B.M.J.* 301:18–25.

Stark, D. 1980. Class struggle and the transformation of the labour process: A relational approach. *Theory and Society* 9:89–130.

Syme, S. 1991. Social epidemiology and the work environment. In J. V. Johnson and G. Johansson (eds.), *The Psychosocial Work Environment and Health: Work Organization, Democratization and Health,* pp. 21–31. Amityville, NY: Baywood.

Theorell, T., L. Alfredsson, S. Knox, A. Perski, J. Svensson, and D. Waller. 1984. On the interplay between socioeconomic factors, personality and work environment in the pathogenesis of cardiovascular disease. *Scand. J. Work Environ. Health* 10:373–380.

Theorell, T., S. Knox, J. Svensson, and D. Waller. 1985. Blood pressure variations during a working day at age 28: Effects of different types of work and blood pressure level at age 18. *J. Hum. Stress* 11:36–41.

Theorell, T., A. Perski, T. Akerstedt, F. Sigala, G. Ahlberg-Hulten, J. Svensson, and P. Eneroth. 1988. Changes in job strain in relation to changes in physiological state. *Scand. J. Work Environ. Health* 14:189–196.

Theorell, T. The psychosocial environment, stress, and coronary heart disease. In M. Marmot, and P. Elliott (eds.), *Coronary Heart Disease Epidemiology*, pp. 256–273. Oxford: Oxford University Press.

Therborn, G. 1982. What does the ruling class do when it rules? In A. Giddens, and D. Held (eds.), *Classes, Power and Conflict: Classical and Contemporary Debates*, pp. 224–248. Berkeley: University of California Press.

Thompson, P. 1983. *The Nature of Work: An Introduction to Debates on the Labour Process.* London: Macmillan.

Vagero, D., and O. Lundberg. 1989. Health inequalities in Britain and Sweden. *Lancet* 2:35–36.

Vagero, D. 1991. Inequality in health—some theoretical and empirical problems. *Soc. Sci. Med.* 32:367–371.

Vanneman, R., and F. C. Pampel. 1977. The American perception of class and status. *Am. Soc. Rev.* 42:422–437.

Wanner, R. A., and L. S. Lewis. 1983. Economic segmentation and the course of the occupational career. *Work and Occupations* 10:307–324.

Weeks, J. L., B. S. Levy, and G. R. Wagner. 1991. *Preventing Occupational Disease and Injury.* Washington, DC: American Public Health Association.

Williams, D. R. 1990. Socioeconomic differentials in health: A review and redirection. *Soc. Psychol. Q.* 53:81–99.

Wright, E. O. 1985. *Classes.* London: Verso Editions.

Wright, E. O. 1989. *The Debate on Classes.* London: Verso Editions.

Wright, E. O. 1993. Typologies, scales and class analysis: A comment on Halaby and Weakliem's "Ownership and Authority in the Earnings Function." *Am. Soc. Rev.* 58:31–34.

Wright, E. O., and J. Singlemann. 1982. Proletarianization in the changing American class structure. *Am. J. Sociol.* 88 (Suppl.): 176–209.

Zimbalist, A. (ed.). 1979. *Case Studies on the Labor Process.* New York: Monthly Review Press.

Zuboff, S. 1988. *In the Age of the Smart Machine: The Future of Work and Power.* New York: Basic Books.

9

The Cultural Frame: Context and Meaning in the Construction of Health

ELLEN CORIN

The Cultural Frame

In Western countries, and more specifically in North America, ethnic diversity is a growing topic of concern for health planners and service providers. There is evidence that the prevalence of health problems varies among ethnic communities, but to what extent this variation is influenced by cultural features, by social status, and by differential access to economic and social resources remains unknown. Rates of utilization of health services have also been shown to vary by cultural group. Culture, therefore, has increasingly come to the fore as a potential determinant of health. What we now need is a more precise definition of "culture," as well as approaches and methods to elucidate the mechanisms through which culture could influence health and health behaviors.

Over the last two decades, epidemiological research has been increasingly concerned with the mechanisms by which key determinants of health promote health and disease. Studies of stress have focused on identifying variables (such as social support and coping strategies) that mediate the impact of stressful life conditions. Awareness that determinants of health are not randomly distributed has also led researchers to examine collective variables that describe the positions of individuals and groups within the social structure, and such "cultural" variables as beliefs, values, and lifestyles. By and large, however, these variables have been documented on an individual level, using crude indices, rather than as a collective matrix.

I will argue that a thorough consideration of the cultural dimension of determinants of health would generate more complex frameworks for understanding how the environment influences the production of health and disease. Current epidemiological research deals with complexity by means of multivariate analyses, which allow one to trace the influences of a set of variables related along hypothetical causal pathways. Considering culture as amenable to study with appropriate concepts and methods allows one to penetrate more deeply into the significance of these causal pathways, and to discover less well known mechanisms of influence. It also suggests more appropriate socially and culturally grounded strategies of action. This perspective treats culture not as a label to name the "otherness" of others, but as a way of considering ourselves and of reframing the meaning of the variables commonly used in epidemiological surveys.

"Culture" is a complex notion, and it has been defined in a number of ways. In anthropology, culture has classically been described as a shared, learned, and intergenerationally transmitted pattern of customs, beliefs, values, and behaviors. European anthropologists have tended to focus on description of social structures and institutions, kinship systems, and patterns of authority, while North American anthropologists have used a restricted notion of "culture" as an attribute of the individual and have been more interested in psychocultural phenomena (Littlewood, 1992). Around the 1970s, this first definition of culture gave way to the idea that culture is above all a system of meanings and symbols. This system shapes every area of life, defines a world view that gives meaning to personal and collective experience, and frames the way people locate themselves within the world, perceive the world, and behave in it. Every aspect of reality is seen as embedded within webs of meaning that define a certain world view and that cannot be studied or understood apart from this collective frame. Recently, anthropologists have begun to examine the relativity of their own vantage point, and the ways it influences their ethnographic descriptions (Crapanzano, 1992). They have adopted the Western mode of scientific inquiry as an object of investigation, and have denounced its embodiment in a particular, culturally relative world view and system of power relationships.

Meanwhile health and disease have become an important topic of research for anthropologists; medical anthropology is now one of the major divisions within the American Anthropological Association. This new field of study has developed three different orientations, which correspond roughly to the three approaches to culture I have just outlined.

The *biocultural approach* to health and disease concentrates on the processes by which the human body adapts to changing environmental conditions. It examines how the body has been shaped by evolution and how it is influenced by environmental stressors, as well as the way bodily processes influence people's behavior. In principle, biocultural anthropologists consider adaptation to be a dynamic, interactive, and multi-level process; they advocate interdisciplinary studies and integrative thinking (McElroy, 1990). However, most biomedical studies focus on biotic and abiotic features of the environment and do not adequately integrate the social and cultural dimensions (Wiley, 1992). Some biocultural anthropologists have even suggested that many aspects of culture could be seen as epiphenomena of evolutionary adaptation in response to microbes (Konner, 1991).

The *interpretive approach* to medical anthropology shifts the focus from disease as a biological entity to the experience of illness in a given social and cultural context. In humans, phenomena are never just phenomena; they are always imbued with meaning at the junction between the personal and collective frames. Interpretive medical anthropologists see meaning as influencing the course of disease by shaping subjective experience as well as individual and social behavior in response to disease (Good and Good, 1984; Kleinman, 1988).

Critical medical anthropology focuses on the social origins of disease and on the ways that imbalances in power relations influence health and sickness. Critical medical anthropologists aim at describing how individual activities and practices are embedded within the larger frame of a political economy. Cultures are not only webs of significance. They also shape ideologies that disguise reality and power relationships; they have to be seen as webs of mystification in an historical, economic, and political context. Critical medical anthropologists address themselves to the social production of disease and the social context of biomedicine and biomedical practice (Singer, 1990).

Despite their differences, these three approaches share certain perspectives. First, they all view culture as a pervading reality; far from dismissing it as a mere variable to be controlled for in research designs and statistical analyses, culture is conceived as a dynamic and pervasive dimension of the lived world. All conceptions of reality are filtered through the premises and postulates that constitute a particular world view and that are taken for granted by those within the cultural frame; no representation of reality, including the "scientific" one, can be taken as a pure and intrinsically valid image of reality. The concepts we use, the ways we classify things and understand the world, are not "natural"; they represent specific and always "situated" visions of a polysemous reality open to multiple interpretations. The second perspective shared by the three approaches to medical anthropology is a cross-cultural orientation. Because our culture is the context we live in, it remains very difficult to disentangle culture from "reality" as long as we remain within our cultural frame. Cross-cultural comparisons are a unique way of discovering the relativity of our concepts and theories and of challenging and enlarging our conception of reality.

The three approaches to medical anthropology differ in the emphasis on cultural phenomena in relation to health and disease. This chapter will concentrate on the second approach, the interpretive one, to show how it can be used to expand and broaden epidemiological research models. The first section will trace how a concern for meaning has emerged from within the epidemiological frame, with reference mainly to gender studies, cross-cultural studies of cardiovascular diseases, and comparative studies of schizophrenia. The second section will present examples of studies that substantiate the idea that collective meaning systems influence the process of stress in modifying what is perceived as stressor, social support, and coping. Studies of culture change and immigration will lead to a discussion of the cultural dimension of the process of adaptation so important in biocultural medical anthropology. The third section, focusing more specifically on the sociohistorical and sociostructural context of meaning, will emphasize that meanings are not only embedded within a sociocultural context but are also components of a "meaning game" molded by considerations of control and power. This section will discuss the sociopolitical challenges associated with research and interventions in the realm of health and disease.

The Contribution of Semiology

Adopting an interpretive stance toward cultural phenomena is fraught with traps and difficulties; thus one needs to rely on a theory of meaning that offers some analytical guidelines. In recent decades, intellectual and methodological developments within the sciences of meaning and interpretation, particularly semiology and hermeneutics, have had a profound influence on the development of anthropology (Marcus and Fisher, 1986).

The anthropological principle that a phenomenon is always embedded within a larger frame, and cannot be understood outside of its context, corresponds to the basic semiological assumption that a sign (let us substitute *variable*) has no inherent significance; its meaning arises from its opposition to other signs, from its position in a sequence of signs, and from its relationship with other signs within the discourse or, in anthropology, the cultural scene. For example, in a study of the father figure in a matrilineal society (Corin, 1971), it became apparent that the significance of the father could not be defined *a priori* and could be understood only in relation to the positions of the maternal uncle and the patrilateral grandfather. The significance of the father was revealed only by an analysis of the positions occupied by these various figures in a variety of rituals concerning basic life transitions: birth, adolescence, marriage, funerals, and the like.

Furthermore, the anthropological assumption that meanings are always culturally constructed parallels the semiological postulate of nonequivalence between signs and reality. Following Pierce (1978), semiologists acknowledge that a sign is never equivalent to reality and never exhausts reality; it always represents reality from a particular angle, determined by the conceptual frame of the interpreter and by the shared knowledge of the community of interpreters. The more distant the interpreters' conceptions and values from the world in which the observed phenomena are embedded, the greater the risk of misinterpreting the phenomena.

Identification and interpretation of signs or variables, therefore, must be contextual in two senses: signs and variables always exist within a frame that influences their significance, and we as interpreters always occupy a specific cultural frame that influences our observations, identifications, and interpretations of phenomena. This will be especially salient when we discuss the sociopolitical ramifications of the construction of meaning. The French philosopher and hermeneutician Paul Ricoeur (1986) has spelled out the methodological implications of this position. He warns against the danger of a "naive" and empathic understanding of phenomena, which tends to reflect the researcher's personal and ideological convictions. Ricoeur proposes pursuing "scientific" understanding by way of hermeneutical interpretation, which seeks to discover the internal structure of phenomena through systematic structural analysis.

Such an interpretive approach to the determinants of health and disease would involve a process of "bracketing" our own personal, professional, and cultural world view in order to grasp the categories significant in the others' world and their specific role in the production of health. This does not mean that cultural categories are only and entirely culturally relative; that would render impossible any kind of cross-cultural dialogue and research. Anthropology has always been interested in universals as well as cultural variations. The real challenge is not to take our definitions of variables as *a priori* universal, but rather to aim at discovering universal principles through dialogue, and through comparisons between our own and others' representations of phenomena. This is illustrated by Kleinman's comparison between the Western notion of depression and what the Chinese call neurasthenia. Both phenomena share some common characteristics revealed by the use of a standard instrument; they are, however, integrated into different meaning frames in the two cultural contexts and are embedded in different bodily experiences.

Meaning and Context: Toward a "Thick" Description of Health Determinants

In order to decipher how a specific cultural feature (such as a cockfight) condenses basic elements of the symbolic frame, the social structure, and the cultural concept of the person, Geertz (1983) advocates a "thick" description of cultural phenomena. Similar perspectives are also emerging from a series of epidemiological studies. Let us look at a few gender studies and cross-cultural comparisons to illustrate the point.

Gender Issues

Gender differences in morbidity and mortality have led to numerous discussions of the respective roles of biological and psychosocial variables as determinants of health. While women's longer life expectancy has often been explained by invoking biological factors, a substantial increase in male-female differences between 1964 and 1975 suggests that there are other influences associated with gender-related behavioral patterns (Mechanic, 1978). In the area of psychiatric disorders, the most impressive gender differentials involve the relative prevalence of various types of disorders (Dohrenwend, 1975). In the early 1980s, the Ecological Catchment Area (ECA) Study (Robins et al., 1991) confirmed that, though the global rate of active disorders is the same for men and women, the mode of presentation varies according to gender: alcohol abuse and antisocial personality are expressed more among males, and somatization disorders, obsessive-compulsive disorders, and major depressive episodes more among women. The authors of the ECA Study do not comment on factors responsible for the observed differences, and one cannot rule out the hypothesis that they express biological differences. Other writers have noted that the relative prominence of specific disorders among men and women mirrors gender-specific role expectations and social rules governing the expression of emotion.

It has also been observed that comparable stressful situations elicit different reactions from men and women. Epidemiological data suggest that widowhood and divorce are more detrimental to men than to women, as manifested by relative mortality rates (Mechanic, 1978; Smith et al., 1988). This finding has been explained by hypothesizing that the benefits derived from marriage vary according to gender; men gain from marriage in the realm of social relationships and wives in the sphere of financial resources. Divorce or widowhood would therefore have a different impact on men than on women due to the loss of different types of resources (Gerstel et al., 1985). This hypothesis is congruent with studies showing that within the conjugal couple, women act as key mediators of social relationships, especially with regard to close links (Corin, 1984). The Alameda County Study has also shown that the types of social relationships beneficial to health differ according to gender: marriage is more advantageous for men than for women, while contacts with friends and relatives and involvement in community groups are more beneficial for women than for men (Berkman and Syme, 1979).

Gender-related health data, therefore, indicate the existence of gender specificities that seem to be related to the roles and values associated with gender in contemporary societies. Traditional gender studies have described differing socialization processes for boys and for girls, in line with the social roles, values, and expectations associated with each gender. Cross-cultural studies indicate that this social elaboration of gender differences is not a purely "natural" process and varies from culture to culture.

In a recent research project involving a dozen countries, Williams and Best (1990) found both similarities and differences in gender-related notions of the perceived self, the ideal self, and sex-role ideologies. Among the cross-cultural similarities is a general tendency for men's ideal and perceived selves to be stronger and more active than those of women. The authors also observed a general tendency for the perceived and ideal self-descriptions of women to include more features culturally associated with men, while the self-descriptions of men less frequently integrate features culturally associated with women; generally speaking, women self-descriptions tend to be more "androgynous" than men's. The most pervasive intercountry differences involve sex-role ideology, defined as "the person's view of the proper role relationships between men and women, scaled along a traditional/male dominant to modern/egalitarian dimension." The authors observe that prevailing sex-role ideology is related to the differences between men and women with regard to what the authors call the "affective meaning" of their self-concepts (both perceived and ideal), or their relative strength, activity, and favorability. In more traditional countries, men's and women's self-concepts and ideal self-concepts tend to be more highly differentiated in terms of affective meaning; the sex-role ideology is also more traditional. They also note, however, that sex-role ideology is not related to the average masculinity or femininity of self-concepts when these notions are defined from within the culture, thus calling into question the cross-cultural validity of the authors' notion of sex-role ideology. The overall pattern of findings suggests that, with increasing modernity, differences decrease between the self-perceptions of men and women, and the discrepancy increases between how individuals view their real selves and their ideal selves or their selves as they would like them to be. The authors characterize these two patterns, both characteristic of Western societies and the Western concept of ideal personhood, as positive.

Their conclusions and their emphasis on certain findings at the expense of others exemplify a tendency prevalent in cross-cultural psychological research, namely, to treat Western representations of reality as the gold standard of judgment, not because of explicit prejudice against other cultures but because of bias embedded in methodological choices and because the authors have not made an effort at "decentration" from their own cultural frame.

Recent research favors a less dichotomous approach to gender relationships, considered as ongoing interactional processes between men and women, and also among women and among men (Gerson and Peiss, 1985). The notion of "separate gender spheres" is replaced by that of boundaries circumscribing complex structures of commonalities and differences in gender-based experience. This approach highlights the dynamic quality of the structure of gender relations and allows for the possibility of permeable boundaries. The notion of negotiation supplements that of domination, and draws attention to the ways women and men bargain for privileges and resources. Gender consciousness is understood as an emerging process that develops dialectically through social relations between the sexes.

How this gender negotiation is constrained by collective influences is not explored in Gerson and Peiss's study (1985). It is better illustrated in a study by Mirowsky (1985) on the association between marital power and depression, which found each spouse to be less depressed if marital power was shared to some extent. Marital power was coded to indicate the wife's dominance, the husband's dominance, or equality in making the major decisions. The study found both spouses to be less depressed if marital power is to some extent shared. Increased marital power only reduces expected depression up to a point; beyond that point, it is counterproductive and actually increases depression. This finding confirms an equity model of the relationship between depression and marital power. The data also indicate that this subtle equilibrium is affected by collective values in that the optimal level of relative marital power—the level associated with the lowest depression rate—is higher for men than for women. The higher the husband's earnings, the higher is the level of husbands' relative marital power associated with both spouses' lowest depression scores; wives' earnings do not have an influence. The more traditional the wives' sex-role beliefs, the higher is the level of husbands' marital power which is associated with the fact that wives have the lowest depression.

Hochschild (1979) offers an interesting approach to the collective processes that frame the interactions and negotiation between genders. She considers ideology as an interpretive framework with two aspects: "framing rules" that ascribe definition or meaning to situations, and "feeling rules" that indicate which feeling is appropriate in a given situation. In a context of rapid social change, the content of rules loses its clarity due to conflicts and contradictions between contending sets of rules: "feelings and frames are deconventionalized, but not yet reconventionalized" (Hochschild, 1979, p. 568).

Gender-related data thus cast a spotlight on the kind of social context men and women live in, on how it evolves in the course of individual lives, on the social and personal values and expectations attached to it, and on the range of constraints that impinge on it. As these few examples illustrate, if we are to interpret studies focused on individuals complementary research is required on the social and cultural context that underlies observed differences. It seems equally important to try to specify the positions that individuals occupy within a changing scene, and to observe how personal and historical circumstances combine to protect groups and individuals, or to render them fragile.

Cross-Cultural Comparisons

Cardiovascular diseases

A classic example of cross-cultural variation in disease prevalence is the study by Marmot et al. (1975) of cardiovascular disease among Japanese men. The authors sought to examine the potential contribution of socioenvironmental factors to differing rates of cardiovascular disease observed in the United States, where the rate is especially high, and in Japan where it is especially low. They therefore examined the association between the relative Americanization of Japanese and rates of cardiovascular disease by comparing Japanese living in three settings—Japan, Hawaii, and California. In order to examine the protective influence of the Japanese culture, they attributed to individuals scores of exposure to Japanese culture on the basis of their exposure to Japanese culture during childhood and of adult social involvement with other Japanese. The results demonstrated both intergroup and intragroup differences associated with Americanization: Japanese people in Japan demonstrated significantly lower levels of cardiovascular disorders than those in Hawaii, and Japanese in Hawaii lower levels than those living in California. The more culturally traditional men had a lower prevalence of coronary heart disease than nontraditional men. These differences persisted after controlling for dietary preference and for other known biological risk factors such as blood pressure and cholesterol levels.

In order to better understand the influence of culture on cardiovascular diseases, the authors then analyzed Japanese culture for well-known risk and protective factors. They described traditional Japanese culture as characterized by a high degree of social support, as being associated with close-knit social groups, and with restraint on individual competitiveness in favor of loyalty to the organization. These interpretations remain hypothetical, and the picture they draw of Japanese society may lack nuance and obscure certain complexities of Japanese society. For example, the alleged lack of competitiveness should be reconciled with the recent complaint by the Japanese National Council on Education Reform in 1986 about excessive competition in entrance examinations (Lock, 1991). In an interesting article on "adolescent dissent" in Japan, Margaret Lock notes that "despite its commitment to equality, the school system is intensely competitive and in recent years appears to have become even more so" (Lock, 1991, p. 513). More generally, she contrasts idealistic depictions of harmonious and nurturant socialization practices, which are in keeping with the established cosmological and political order, with actual socialization practices, by using descriptions of socialization practices offered by many Japanese who emphasize its disruptions and discontinuities. For Lock, both positions offer a partial view and must be situated within a broader historical frame; in this context it becomes clear that the Japanese conception of education and enlightenment has always involved tension between diverging philosophies of what life represents in this society. One could conclude that intercultural differences are difficult to interpret solely on the basis of the variables considered significant in Western epidemiological studies. In this case, it also appears important to take into account basic differences in philosophies of life and of personhood, which could deeply influence people's involvement in, and experience of, daily life. The findings of Marmot et al. (1975) call for additional studies, which could reinforce the strength of their conclusions and explore the social and cultural features of Japanese society more systematically. Potentially relevant cultural variables could be identified by scrutinizing intrasociety variation and by expanding the range of cultures under consideration.

Schizophrenia

Comparative research on schizophrenia over the last two decades has raised challenges to current conceptions about the disease and its evolution. The World Health Organization has sponsored two large studies on prevalence and incidence rates of schizophrenia and on its evolution in a range of developed and developing countries. In the 1970s, the International Pilot Study on Schizophrenia (IPSS) (Sartorius et al., 1978; World Health Organization, 1979) found that a larger proportion of schizophrenic patients in developing countries (India, Nigeria, Columbia) experienced favorable outcomes after 2 years than in developed countries (Denmark, U.S.A., U.K., U.S.S.R., Czechoslovakia). It is interesting that sociodemographic and clinical variables known to predict outcome in the West did not explain intersite differences. The authors concluded that much of the variance in the course and outcome of schizophrenia may be due to factors not yet identified. Cultural and social variables were not systematically studied, and the authors could only conjecture about those responsible for the variation (Cooper and Sartorius, 1977; Sartorius et al., 1978). Recently published results from the 5-year follow-up reinforce the original conclusions regarding the better outcome of schizophrenia in developing countries (Leff et al., 1992).

A second study, The Determinants of Outcome of Severe Mental Disorders research project, which was undertaken to confirm the trends identified by the IPSS (Sartorius et al., 1986), provided a more valid picture of the incidence rate of schizophrenia in each country and tested a number of hypotheses concerning social and cultural factors associated with differential courses in schizophrenia. As in the study of cardiovascular disease among Japanese, the authors restricted their investigation to social and cultural variables known for their predictive potential in Western societies, specifically life events (Day et al., 1987) and expressed emotion (Wig et al., 1987; Leff et al., 1990).

The study of life events aimed at discovering whether the onset of schizophrenia is preceded by an increase in stress-provoking life events during the months immediately preceding the episode. The authors constructed the WHO Life-Event-Schedule (LES) to document changes that could be considered stress-provoking for an average member of the patient's social group of origin. The instrument was developed in close collaboration with investigators native to each country, for purposes of cross-cultural comprehensiveness. Several items were assigned alternative threshold-rating criteria adapted to the differing cultural conditions of different countries. The data reveal that there were striking similarities in rates of stressful life events preceding the onset of schizophrenia in six of the nine sites (Aarhus, Denmark; Cali, Columbia; Honolulu and Rochester, U.S.A.; Nagasaki, Japan, and Prague, Czechoslovakia). The remaining three sites, in developing countries (Agra and Chandigarh, India; and Ibadan, Nigeria), were significantly different. Although the authors controlled for possible methodological biases, complementary analysis revealed difficulties in applying the LES in these two countries, as well as the existence of real differences; the two Indian and the Nigerian sites reported significantly lower event rates before the onset of the disease.

According to the main investigators, in these cultures "the instruments never achieved the same comfortable, common sense quality reported in the developed countries." The Chandigarh investigators remained particularly doubtful about the applicability of certain operational criteria. The investigators comment on the dilemma of balancing culturally specific applicability with the requirements of cross-cultural comparability. It is clear from their discussion, nevertheless, that they favor cross-cultural comparability and consider similarity a criterion of validity.

A study performed in Nigeria with a different instrument (Gureje and Adewunmi, 1988) found results similar to those of WHO. Among Nigerian schizophrenic patients, the onset of illness did not appear to be preceded by an increase in stressful life events. This study included a control group. The only significant observation was that the control subjects had experienced more events in the month preceding the interview; differences were largely accounted for by male control subjects who mentioned family members' household moves. In Nigeria, therefore, the onset of schizophrenia seemed to be preceded by a low frequency of life events. Among the authors' hypotheses is that rapid culture change could precipitate schizophrenia even if it cannot be categorized as a life event. The lack of stressful family-related events could signify a meager social-support network, a situation which could render patients more susceptible to the disturbing influence of social change.

Similarly, the chief collaborating investigator from Agra, India, in the WHO study suggested that in a context of extreme social conditions associated with rapid culture change (such as disruption of extended family, migration of husbands and fathers, collapse of community structures and questioning of the traditional forms of authority and legitimacy) and a "fatalistic" philosophy of life, events could appear very diffused and thus go unacknowledged as events. In Nigeria, WHO investigators also noted the problems associated with the difficulty of pinpointing illness onset and general unfamiliarity with this kind of investigation. One could hypothesize further that perceptions of such notions as time flow and "event" vary culturally, which may severely compromise the validity, in non-Western cultures, of an investigation based on the scoring of life events.

The other factor examined in the Determinants of Outcome project is the cluster of attitudes expressed by family members toward schizophrenic patients, attitudes referred to in the literature as "expressed emotion" (EE) (Wig et al., 1987; Leff et al., 1990). In Western societies, frequent critical comments, general hostility, and overinvolvement have been shown to be associated with relapse among schizophrenics. The WHO study rated expressed emotion in two samples of relatives of first-onset patients in Aarhus, Denmark, and Chandigarh, India; its predictive value was assessed at follow-up 1 and 2 years later.

The study found striking intercultural differences in the global and relative importance of EE components individually and in combination (Wig et al., 1987). For example, Indian relatives expressed much less criticism and emotional overinvolvement than British and Danish relatives, even after adjustment for possible underrating of emotional overinvolvement in India. In India, general hostility associated with the belief that the patient is responsible for his or her disturbed behavior was not invariably associated with high levels of criticism, as it has been shown to be in Western cultures. The authors comment that hostility is probably subject to different social constraints than is criticism in India, which needs to be understood in the context of a general "attributional style." Finally, a surprisingly high number of Chandigarh relatives scored high on both critical comments and warmth, a combination rarely encountered among Anglo-American families. The number of positive remarks was also significantly lower in India. The peculiarities of these data suggest that rules for expressing emotions and the very meanings of the attitudes measured differ with the milieu.

At the 1-year follow-up in India, a dramatic reduction was apparent in each of the components of expressed emotion (negative and positive), and on the global index, especially in the rural sample where no relative scored high on expressed emotion. This pattern of reduction has rarely, if ever, been documented in research among Anglo-American families. Regarding the predictive value of expressed emotion at the 1-year follow-up, statistically significant associations were found only between hostility and relapse and between a generally high expressed-emotion score and relapse. At the 2-year follow-up (Leff et al., 1990), the global expressed-emotion index during the initial interview did not predict relapse in schizophrenics; the only significant association was between initial hostility and subsequent relapses. Generally speaking, relatives showed considerable acceptance of symptoms of schizophrenia; they seemed to have come to terms with the fact that the patient suffered from an illness and had learned not to be provoked by the patient's irritability. Neuroleptic drugs played an insignificant role in the aftercare of these patients and could not be held responsible for the lower rates of relapse in India.

The authors cannot explain why hostility emerged as the key component of expressed emotion in the Indian families, and they invite research on the nature of emotional relationships in Indian culture. They also conclude that the low relapse rate of Chandigarh patients cannot be fully explained by the effects of hostility or of expressed emotion; they acknowledge that they did not identify a single comprehensive explanation, though the tolerant and accepting attitudes of family members seemed to contribute to favorable prognoses.

In light of their own study of Mexican-Americans and a careful review of cross-cultural data, Jenkins and Karno (1992) deplore the kind of naturalization of the EE concept found in the literature. They assert that the nature of EE is culture-specific, and that culture influences the family response to an ill relative. Culture provides a system of interpretation and a vocabulary of expression, assigns meaning to kin relations, and prescribes codes for the identification of rule violation.

As this body of research on culture and schizophrenia reveals, the utilization of standardized and reliable methods of data collection has enhanced the value of comparative studies on schizophrenia and confirmed the existence of cross-cultural variation in its course. These studies also demonstrate the limitations of classical epidemiological designs; findings suggest that the meanings of key variables can vary with the context.

Anthropologists and culturally sensitive psychiatrists (Kleinman, 1988; Fabrega, 1989) have suggested that cultural studies of schizophrenia should look beyond the factors associated with the onset and course of the disorder to examine how the very experience of the illness is intimately shaped by cultural conceptions of self and by subjectivity. Among the symptoms of schizophrenia are an alteration in self-others boundaries, distorted bodily feelings, and difficulty distinguishing between perceptions originating internally and those originating in the external world. These symptoms blur the boundaries between self, others, and the supernatural world; interpersonally, behaviors and symptoms associated with schizophrenia evoke a range of reactions and expectations, and these differ from culture to culture.

A Cultural Approach to Determinants of Health

Consideration of the determinants of health from a cultural perspective requires a "thickening" of one's understanding, which in turn requires exploration of alternative methodological avenues. Let us focus on the stress-research model which describes the risk and protective factors that indicate the impact of stress on individual health; this will reveal the way an interpretive approach can enrich this model with the aim of deepening the application of this paradigm through an interpretive approach.

Stress and Meaning

Human beings do not live in a purely objective world in which objects and events possess an inherent and objective significance. Objects and events are imbued with meanings that vary with individuals, times, and societies. Meaning emerges from a network of associations; objects and events do not merely signify themselves but also evoke associations from the context of personal and collective histories through the system of meanings and symbols of which they are part.

In stress research, the issue of meaning has been addressed most directly in relation to the concept of life events. Two aspects of this discussion possess special interest from a cultural perspective. The first concerns the relative importance of subjective and "objective" meaning: Is an event significant for a given individual because of the affective connotations it possesses, or is its significance related to the degree of objective adaptation it requires? Authors favoring the first option have designed a set of complementary questions aimed at describing various subjective facets of an event: its positive or negative value, its degree of predictability, and the perceived importance of the domain to which it belongs. Those in favor of the second option have aimed instead at attributing an objective and standard weight to each event on a list, based on a judgment of the amount of disruption normally entailed by the event; the positive or negative significance of the event for the individual is considered of little value in predicting its potential health consequences. Both positions recognize that events are not equivalent and have to be described in more specific terms. They differ, however, in their conception of meaning.

The second noteworthy theme concerns the scope of the frame one must consider in order to assess the significance of an event: Is its meaning contained within the event itself and its subjective or objective connotations, or is its meaning only grasped within a larger biographical frame?

The Patterning of Events in a Life-History Context

The well-known scale of life events designed by Holmes and Rahe (1967) is a prototype of the objective and event-bound approach to the significance of life events. The scale provides a score by combining the standard stress scores associated with each event reported. The universal character of the score normatively attributed to each life event, however, has been questioned by several authors (Dohrenwend, 1973).

In Britain, by contrast, Brown and Harris (1978) have designed an approach that combines objectivity and individual specificity in rating the degree of stress associated with a particular life event. Rather than relying on subjective description of the significance of an event, the authors have designed a lengthy qualitative interview aimed at exploring its context. Each event is then rated on 28 dimensions describing various aspects of its objective impact on the life of the person. The best predictors of depression are long-term threats and events that directly involve the person being rated; threat of loss also increases the predictability of depression. Compared to an 11 percent risk of developing depression after any severe event, 32 percent of the women who experienced a severe event involving a loss developed depression by the 1-year follow-up (Brown and Harris, 1989).

Two features of more recent work by Brown and Harris are of special interest. First, the authors have extended the definition of loss to integrate its symbolic dimension. This expanded definition includes, for example, the loss of a beloved idea, which can encompass both the disruption of one's expectations about someone's commitment, faithfulness, and trustworthiness, and an event that leads one to question such qualities in oneself, or that challenges one's identity. In a study the authors undertook in Camberwell England (Brown and Harris, 1989), they noticed that only one third of the reported loss events involved actual loss of a person; 56 percent of these events involved the loss of a cherished idea that could be expected to entail a direct threat to the person's sense of self-worth.

The other noteworthy feature of Brown and Harris' work is their use of operational methods to describe how a particular event is integrated into a chain of related events that modifies its meaning. To this end, they have developed the concept of "matching events," or events that acquire their pathogenic significance from their association with something else in the person's life. Three types of matching events are described. The first category encompasses severe events within a sphere of high commitment for the person (as assessed in a previous interview), such as a husband's infidelity for a woman highly committed to marriage. Women who experience this kind of matching event were three times more likely to develop depression than women who experience a comparable severe event not involving an area of commitment. The second kind of matching involves an event in a sphere where marked difficulties were noticed at the first interview; for example, a husband's leaving home in a context of marital disputes over his heavy drinking and violence. A threefold increase in the risk of developing depression was observed with this kind of matching event. When one considers the proportion of women at risk of being depressed after experiencing a severe event, it was one for 2.7 among women who had experienced one of these two kinds of matching events and only one for 4.5 among women who had experienced any other kind of severe events. The third type of matching involves events associated with a role conflict documented during the first interview; in such cases, the relative risk of depression is 43 percent compared to 18 percent for women experiencing a severe event not associated with role conflict. In Brown and Harris' work, the notion of "matching" thus replaces the "additivity" implied by most life-event scales; it accounts for the fact that a single event of sufficient severity can be critical in the development of psychiatric disorders. It remains to be seen how much of the meaning of individual life events is accounted for by immediate circumstances within the life of the individual, and to what degree meaning is framed by a larger context.

Brown and Harris also considered the influence of the individual's whole life. People with a childhood history of death or separation from parental figures appear to be especially vulnerable to the impact of life events. Extending their analysis of "matching events," the authors speculate that life events tend to be associated with certain key events or nuclear scenes that organize them along certain structures. They also postulate that an early experience of separation generates a general feeling of helplessness, as well as constituting a basic "script" that absorbs later scenes of life, and frames future reactions to stressful events and circumstances. Depression, which is associated with a general feeling of helplessness, would therefore be likely to develop as a reaction to later threatening life events.

One can postulate that life events also derive their meaning from the particular weight and value they possess in a given society. As the Nigerian study (Gureje and Adewunmi, 1988) on the association between the onset of schizophrenia and life events indicates, the notion "event" must be broadened to include more pervasive potentially stressful conditions, as well as their concrete repercussions in a particular society.

Brown and Harris' work evokes the "semantic network" described in medical anthropology by Good (1977) in his attempt to formalize the study of the meanings associated with illness in Iranian society. For the members of a given culture, illness condenses a network of personal and collective symbols, as well as meanings, motives, and feelings anchored both in individuals' lives and in the culture. The last section of this paper will discuss how the notion of collective "organizing experience" (Corin et al., 1990) that was developed in the context of a research project conducted in Québec can be considered a particular history-sensitive version of Good's semantic network.

Epidemiological research provides several examples of studies that demonstrate the social and cultural framing of the significance of an event. We will consider two main lines of research: studies performed in a context of cultural change, due either to acculturation or to migration, and analyses of the influence of macrosocial conditions.

A Cultural Web of Significance

Studies of the consequences of culture change for the health of a population have shown that these consequences vary with different categories of people, and suggest that the significance and stressful potential of the new situation differ accordingly. Interpreting observed differences requires more in-depth information about community life.

A study by Kunitz and Levy (1986) of the prevalence of hypertension among elderly Navajo is illustrative. Among the women, hypertension was consistently associated with acculturation to the dominant American society, as measured by educational level attained, having gone to a boarding school off the reservation, and fluency in the English language. Among women only, hypertension was also significantly associated with isolation. By contrast, among the men, off-reservation residence for at least 1 year was significantly associated with a low prevalence of diagnosed hypertension. This finding runs parallel with the finding by DeStefano et al. (1979) that within traditional Navajo society young adult men have a higher rate of hypertension. This pattern of data suggests that traditional Navajo culture could be a risk factor and source of stress for men, while acting as a protective factor for women.

A review of ethnographic data indicated that young adult men occupy a marginal position within a matrilineal and matrilocal society. In offering them escape, migration would thus be beneficial for men; wage work would be perceived by them as opening up new life opportunities. By contrast, the situation of women appears much more secure in the traditional society. Mother-daughter bonds are particularly significant in this society, where women typically remain in their family of origin after marriage; they also retain decision-making rights regarding their property. For women, therefore, involvement in the modern educational system and wage work may signify the loss of a secure context and render them more vulnerable to hypertension.

In this example, intragroup differences must be understood in the context of gender-related social roles and life characteristics. Ultimately, they can only be understood in relation to kinship rules, lines of authority, and marriage regulation. These cultural features shape the meaning of daily life and, at least in part, determine the stressful potential of culture change.

The same kind of social process is illustrated in the prospective longitudinal research by Salmond et al. (1989) on people migrating from a subsistence economy on an atoll in the Pacific to an urbanized Western lifestyle in New Zealand. His 14-year follow-up data revealed a puzzling specific association: among high-status men, those who subscribed to nontraditional values had significantly higher blood pressure than those who adhered strongly to traditional values. The author hypothesizes that men who experience conflict between their status and their private values have elevated blood pressures. This cultural dissonance within the person would promote vulnerability to elevated blood pressure.

Culture change is not restricted to objective transformations affecting concrete conditions of life; it also involves deep cognitive changes at the level of values and self-perceptions. Research conducted in the context of immigration has similarly led Murphy (1987) to conclude that the degree of match or mismatch between the original cultural background and the resettlement conditions plays a significant role in migrants' adaptation. Each culture develops ways of enabling individuals to be satisfied with their physical and social environments. Changes brought about by migration may be well prepared for by cultural conditioning and may correspond closely with initial expectations and values; alternatively, they may conflict quite markedly with cultural expectations. For example, the material rewards offered by migration may compensate for the hardship of this migration for societies which favor material success and competition, but not for societies which promote strong social bonds and collective embedding within extended family networks. Hence, the impact on health of changes associated with migration may be mediated by the meaning they possess within the cultural frame of the country of origin. This observation does not preclude the necessity of paying attention to conditions in the host country that accentuate the hardships of migration, but it does direct attention to the complex interaction between the objective and subjective worlds, and between reality, expectations, and values.

The Sociocultural Framing of Meaning

The studies we have examined so far try to identify pathways of meaning that define or mitigate the stressful potential of culture change. Other studies have focused on the ways macrosocial forces frame the meaning of the collective world in which individuals live.

Pearlin (1989) has developed an approach to stress that in certain respects parallels that of Brown and Harris, but in which the network of associations among stressors is viewed as framed by powerful macrosocial forces rather than by personal biography. According to Pearlin, primary stressors give rise to secondary stressors; both in turn interact with role strains, and it is largely through these interactions that the social context structures people's activities, relationships, and experience. They also interact with "ambient strains" like poverty, chronic illness, and neighborhoods characterized by crime and violence. Pearlin argues that a sequential approach to life events must be superseded by observation of the ways that events and strains converge in people's lives. Few events occur at random or in a vacuum; most can be traced back to the system of social stratification and to the place occupied by the individual within the system. Social institutions are characterized by arrangements of statuses and roles that persist throughout time; they form structural arrangements in people's lives and are the source of repeated experiences that may result in stress. Pearlin asserts that values mediate the effects of an experience by regulating its meaning and its importance, but does not pursue this idea in depth, being more interested in the system of social stratification as such.

In an epidemiological survey known as the Stirling County Study, Leighton and his collaborators (1959) sought to understand how certain sociostructural features of a remote rural Canadian community are associated with a certain kind of cultural environment, characterized by the degree of consensus achieved around values, meaning, and shared sentiments. The authors were particularly interested in how the social "integration" or "disintegration" of communities is associated with the prevalence of mental-health disorders. Their study's originality lies in their decision to pursue research simultaneously at the levels of the community and the individual. Intensive in-depth studies of the community used a combination of ethnographic observations, interviews with key informants, and analysis of existing statistics; meanwhile, epidemiological data on the prevalence of mental-health problems were collected through a random community survey, interviews with general practitioners, and analysis of hospitalization data. The authors hypothesized that the social and cultural environment influences various aspects of a person's life—ideas, feelings, conscious motives, defenses, and the like—each of which is directly related to mental health. The study demonstrated that social disintegration is directly related to the prevalence of psychiatric disorders. This general finding was later replicated among the Inuit and in Nigeria (Leighton,

1969). The authors hypothesize that social disintegration undermines consensus around social values and symbols, which maintain what they call "common sentiments." People forced to live in a context characterized by disorder and chaos have to strive to maintain their inner equilibrium, and such striving would be associated with a higher prevalence of mental-health disorders.

Dressler's studies of culture change are more directly informed by a sociostructural perspective. Thus he assumes that the transformation of culture has an impact on the social structure of relationships and involves social differentiation; its impact would be manifested by differential access to material goods and to sources and symbols of prestige, which play an important role in the framing of social identity. Dressler (1982, 1985) considers "lifestyle" an important marker of the place an individual occupies within the new system of positions, and defines it as the symbolic aspect of social class and modernity status. "Lifestyle stress" would result from the conjunction between low economic status and a high material lifestyle; it is hypothesized to undermine social identity. According to Dressler, culture change is not pathogenic in itself. Adaptation to modern life is problematic only when individuals lack access to the economic resources necessary to sustain their aspirations to a modern lifestyle. This hypothesis was tested first in St. Lucia in the eastern Caribbean (Dressler, 1982, 1985) and later in other contexts, such as a southern black community (Dressler and Badger, 1985).

Over the last decade, medical anthropologists and cultural psychiatrists committed to an interpretive frame have explored the social origins of disease and the ways that macrosocial forces translate into local structures of power and interact with cultural features and bodily processes in the production, expression, and management of disease (Kleinman, 1981, 1986). In a study of neurasthenia in China, Kleinman found that local systems of explanation and traditional values helped to shape the meaning, experience, and manifestations of the disorder. Specifically, the general disruption brought about by the Cultural Revolution constitutes an overarching frame of meaning, encompassing discrete events in individuals' lives and in part determining both the occurrence and the significance of these events. Relying on a combination of epidemiological data and intensive interviews with patients, their families and health-care providers, Kleinman illustrates how macrosocial forces are reflected in micro-depressogenic systems, and how they can lead to demoralization, distress, and despair. To this general analysis, the author has recently added what he calls "personal webs of significance." He reproaches anthropology for being "experience-distant" and for objectifying the illness experience and delegitimizing the human experience of suffering thus participating in the same process of professional transformation as medicine or psychiatry. He argues that one must focus on local worlds: "the local context that organizes experience through the moral resounding and reinforcing of popular cultural categories about what life means and what is at stake in living" (Kleinman and Kleinman, 1991, p. 293).

The key challenge for this line of research is to identify the links and articulations between the macrosocial context, cultural codes, and the ways that such codes are used by individuals (Bibeau, 1988). For example, Kleinman's (1986) interpretation of the high prevalence of a diagnosis of "neurasthemia" in China mentions the general tendency of Chinese patients, families, and doctors to express and to interpret suffering in physical terms. This would reflect the influence of traditional conceptions of psychological and physical disease, a long-established tradition among Confucian scholar-bureaucrats to claim illness to explain withdrawal from dangerous political situations or individual strategies, to justify repeated failure, or to obtain relief from heavy obligations imposed by the sociopolitical system.

The Cultural Dimension of Support and Coping

The Relativity of Social Support

The quantitative approach to social support does not capture the way social support operates in real life, nor the complexity of the reality it signifies. It is clear that in real life, stressors and social support are closely related phenomena, which interact with each other. Important life events and changes, such as bereavement, loss of job, moving, and debilitating illness, have direct effects on the social life of the person and on the availability of social support. The question is not only to what degree external social support can prevent adverse consequences, but also to what degree life changes affect or undermine key sources of support. The answer varies from context to context.

Bereavement is interesting to consider from this perspective. In African societies, mourning rituals are a unique opportunity for the community to gather and spend time with the bereaved. Collective dances, sharing of beverages, and lengthy palavers serve to strengthen community ties. In India, by contrast, a woman who loses her husband also loses her social identity and is not supposed to survive, or at least to continue to lead a normal life. In the first case, mourning rituals strengthen social support; in the second case, one has to wonder who is culturally entitled to offer support in these circumstances and what such support would consist of.

Quantifications of social support only capture a limited interpretation of a person's social embeddedness and of what he or she perceives as supportive. In a study of the association between social support and mental health, controlling for the level of stress, Biegel and his collaborators (1982) found that the relative importance of various dimensions of social support differs according to the group. Among the lowest socioeconomic group, members of ethnic communities, and the elderly, a feeling of global attachment for one's neighborhood had the greatest effect on mental health, regardless of level of stress. Its effect was greater than direct support from family, friends, or co-workers, or indirect support measured by social interactions with neighbors and participation in organizations. By contrast, in the higher socioeconomic group and among nonethnic and younger populations, the relative importance of the various components of social support varies with the level of stress. "Neighborhood attachment," however, is not often included in social-support scales.

What has value as support can vary according to situations, categories of people, contexts, and cultural values. In a study of the kind of social support associated with good mental health for recently widowed women and women returning to school, Hirsch (1981) demonstrated that adaptation to new circumstances in life requires a specific type of social support characterized by loose connections within a social network, while in other circumstances a densely connected social network appears to be more supportive.

The social and cultural embeddedness of social support is also well illustrated by Dressler's studies. In a southern black community (Dressler, 1985), the support of extended family tended to be associated with a lower rate of mental health symptoms and therefore beneficial for men, both directly and as a mediator in stress situations; this finding corresponds with what we know about the importance of the extended-family structure in this community. Among 17- to 35-year-old women, by contrast, more support from extended kin was associated with more mental-health symptoms. In explanation, the author notes the high psychological cost incurred by young women who receive family support. Young women in this community are closely watched; if they receive kin support, they are expected to follow advice strictly, which can impose heavy obligations.

Generally speaking, social support is inscribed within a larger set of exchanges, which can facilitate the circulation of help but which also entails exacting expectations and duties. This network of communication and exchanges needs further examination. It has been studied largely in connection with the elderly, for whom social support received from children can reinforce a sense of dependence and undermine self-esteem, as well as triggering feelings of helplessness (Lee, 1985; Corin, 1986). Wentowski (1981) describes the complex strategies resorted to by elderly people in order to retain a sense of reciprocity in social exchanges, in spite of their growing need for support. One such strategy the author calls "delayed reciprocity," whereby services provided years ago entitle the elderly to support from those they helped in the past.

In the studies by Brown et al. (Brown and Harris, 1978; Brown and Prudo, 1987), the protectiveness and vulnerability value of traditionality in a rural community in the Outer Hebrides illustrates further the collective dimension and relativity of social support. The authors undertook a comparative study of psychiatric disorders among 18- to 65-year-old women in Camberwell, an inner-city working-class South London borough, and in two Gaelic-speaking rural populations in North Uist and Lewis in the Outer Hebrides. The comparison revealed that the overall rate of psychiatric disorders was higher in Camberwell than in North Uist due to the overall prevalence of depressive cases. However, anxiety disorders were unexpectedly high in the Outer Hebrides. In the latter milieu, the variable associated with high rates of psychiatric disorders was a two-factor index of women's involvement in traditional life (regular churchgoing and crafting). The most traditional women had a lower rate of depression but also, quite unexpectedly, a much higher rate of anxiety and phobic disorders. This finding suggests that a traditional way of life has a simultaneously protective and fragilizing impact on women.

To explain this phenomenon, the authors invoked Durkheim's distinction between two aspects of traditional societies: *réglementation*, or social regulation, and *intégration* or social cohesiveness and supportiveness. They hypothesized that integration protects against depression and that the repressive aspect of regulation is associated with anxiety. In this Outer Hebridean society, they considered involvement in crafting an index of integration, and churchgoing an index combining integration, social support, and regulation. In this Calvinist society, religion is associated with the threat of hell and with strictly regulated day-to-day religious practices. The authors hypothesized that crafting and churchgoing are associated with low rates of depression and that churchgoing is associated with high rates of anxiety.

The results yielded only partial confirmation of this hypothesis. As expected, both crafting and churchgoing were associated with a low rate of depression, but crafting emerged as the main contributor to the high rate of anxiety. Women's discourse revealed that the salient aspect of religious beliefs was not social regulation but ethical guidance for behavior, and support, purpose, and direction in the wake of adversity. It was more difficult to explain why the aspect of integration mediated by crafting had a fragilizing impact with regard to anxiety and phobic disorders. The authors' observation that many cases of chronic anxiety and phobic disorders seemed to have developed right after the death of a close relative, usually a parent, and seemed to be concentrated among women who had lived with the dead relative, invited closer examination of the possible role of women's "attachment style." The authors speculated that the social environment fostered dependency among women in their youth by discouraging them from individuating, separating, or acquiring a sense of self-confidence, and by emphasizing loyalty to the family of origin. This pattern was later reinforced, they hypothesized, by the limited range of social roles for women and by intense commitment to the family of origin. An index of social contacts with kin was in fact associated with crafting and not with churchgoing.

One of the most interesting aspects of Brown's study is its attempt to explore the relationships among cultural values, social roles, behaviors, and subjective experiences. Specific aspects of regulation and integration appear to interact to produce both a certain type of vulnerability, specific to this setting and associated with a feeling of hopelessness, and a sense of protection against the hazards of life.

The Collective Dimension of Coping

Coping strategies can be defined as characteristic ways of contending with one's circumstances. Coping scales aim to characterize coping strategies along a few dimensions, such as activity versus passivity, or in terms of the relative weight given to emotion, cognition, or action. The stability of coping strategy remains controversial; some authors view it as a stable individual trait while others suggest that it can be situation-specific. The possibility that individual approaches in part reflect collective influences needs more in-depth study. Empirical studies suggest three complementary ways to consider this issue.

First, collective norms influence the meaning associated with a given situation, as well as reactions to it, and must be considered an integral part of the situation: "How a problem is defined greatly determines what is done to solve it" (Goodhart and Zautra, 1982, p. 251). This definitional process compares and contrasts the event with normative standards associated with groups or individuals of reference. Events like pregnancy, widowhood, and unemployment function as markers of transitions that may be collectively connoted as positive or negative. For instance, losing one's job has a different meaning at age 30, when it is likely to be an unfortunate incident, and at 55 when it may be interpreted as a sign of aging. Depending on the culture, aging may be regarded as a new stage of life oriented toward interiority and spiritual growth, or toward increased authority within the extended family, or it may be associated with a loss and a decline.

Second, individual coping strategies also vary by culture, as does the protective value of specific coping styles. A study by Murakami (1983) on coping responses associated with stress among Japanese Americans and Caucasian Americans aged 65–75 years old, reviewed by Marsella and Dash-Scheuer (1988), illustrates the cultural grounding of coping strategies. The results indicate that Japanese Americans tend to utilize social support to cope with health problems, and rely more on go-between and avoidance strategies to resolve family problems; Caucasian Americans rely more on personal responsibility for their health and on active personal problem solving in the face of family problems. Increased use of coping mechanisms appears to be associated with high overall life-satisfaction for Caucasians but not for Japanese. According to Murakami, the Japanese style of coping is explained by the value placed on suppression of personal feelings, by general reliance on the family for support, and by the norm of accepting one's circumstances in life.

Third, individual coping strategies must be viewed in the context of the collective coping strategies that are part of the general culture or represent culturally specific ways of confronting difficult situations. The culturalization of childbirth exemplifies collective coping strategies. Thus, many traditional societies recognize a "fourth trimester" of gestation, which ensures that infant and mother remain in close skin-to-skin physical contact; this practice appears to promote infant survival and neurological development (McElroy, 1990).

Various aspects of cultural and community life provide ways to face difficult situations. The transposition to new environments of traditional ways of coping, their potential for adaptation, and their impact on individuals' lives remain poorly understood. One of the rare studies of this topic was conducted on Samoan migrants to northern California (Janes, 1986). According to the author, the collective strategies observed in this new environment can be understood as a direct transposition of old coping strategies, possibly undermined by the transformations of the larger society. In traditional Samoan society, people benefit from three support systems: the localized kin descent group, an important source of support and affiliation in daily life; diffuse kinship networks, which involve an elaborate set of exchanges and obligations; and church congregations, an organizational unit of utmost importance in all areas of life. All three structures have persisted in new settings in California, and play central roles in receiving and helping new migrants. This support system suffers, however, from growing socioeconomic constraints and is challenged by the appeal of Western values. The system is undergoing progressive erosion in the face of the transformation of social life as a kind of commodity, especially the monetarization of Samoan institutions and sources of prestige. Involvement in church and kin affairs now has a paradoxical character: on the one hand, it sustains strong community values and provides avenues for satisfying individual needs; on the other hand, active participation in both institutions is expensive and thus could act as a potential stressor. This hypothesis was partly tested by the construction of an index of "status inconsistency," which revealed that individuals with relatively high status but limited access to the resources necessary to demonstrate one's prestige appear to suffer the most severe stress, as measured by blood-pressure levels.

As for collective coping strategies, a few anthropological studies suggest that cultural rituals and beliefs may play an important role in framing individuals' reactions to adversity. The transformative quality of the complex elaboration of personal grief and guilt through mourning rituals has been described in various cultural contexts (Mahaniah, 1979; Good and Good, 1988). In studies conducted in Sri Lanka, Obeyesekere (1985) hypothesized that painful motives and emotions likely to lead to depression in the West are transformed into publicly accepted sets of meanings and symbols through what he calls "the work of culture." This process is grounded in the congruence between the emotions associated with loss and bereavement and the Buddhist view of the world and of the person in the world. Rituals such as "the meditation of revulsion" provide forms for cognitive channelling and expression of these personal feelings, and help people to view their feelings with enough detachment to transcend them.

Another form of collective coping involves the framing of mental-health symptoms and the experience of illness. Kleinman's study (1986) in China was aimed at understanding why neurasthenia is the most common diagnosis of neurotic patients in China, while in the West it is virtually unheard-of. This diagnosis was very popular in Western countries in the nineteenth century, but has since been replaced by diagnoses of depression, anxiety, hysteria, and stress-related psychophysiological reactions. While affective disorders have a clear psychological/emotional connotation, neurasthenia, defined as a "chronic, functional disease of the nervous system" (Beard (1881), in Kleinman, 1986), has a vague organic connotation. It conveys neither the stigma attached to mental illness nor personal accountability for the associated physical correlates of emotional illness. Kleinman wondered whether the prevalence of neurasthenia in China represented a diagnostic trend, a specific subjective experience, or real variations in the experience of symptoms under the influence of culture.

On the basis of his study, Kleinman attributes patients' emphasis on the somatic aspects of their problems to a combination of factors: cultural norms that sanction somatization but stigmatize psychologization; the "positive uses" and benefits available to a person suffering from a physical disease; and medical practitioners' failure to recognize the psychosocial aspect of illness behavior and their endorsement of their patients' views about acceptable modes of expressing symptoms. Case histories illustrate how access to social support depends partly on a person's ability to adopt the culturally acceptable idiom of distress. Manifestations of distress are part of an ongoing negotiation with one's workplace, family, and other local contexts; otherwise, they can entail rejection and exclusion. Similar processes have been described in Western cultures, associated with social class (Mechanic, 1978), ethnicity (Dohrenwend, 1966; Kleinman, 1988; Kirmayer, 1989), and aging (Corin, 1985).

In conclusion, an interpretive perspective clearly opens new avenues for understanding the collective dimension of the experience of stress. Studies involving culture change and immigration reveal with particular clarity the cultural dimension of adaptation and of reactions to stress. They indicate that adaptation does not develop in a vacuum, and that the connotations, impact, and degree of transformation associated with new situations depend on the cultural framing of roles, values, expectations, and strategies—variables that can themselves evolve within the passage between different societal environments. The individual experience is framed by, and helps to frame, such a changing environment. And the possibilities of adaptation also depend on macrosocial forces that give rise to stressful circumstances and events that constrain or support reorganization.

Meaning and Power: The Macrosocial Construction of Health Determinants

According to Bibeau (1988), two main trends in anthropological research indicate the possible emergence of a new frame of thought: one stresses the importance of context, history, and practices in the interpretation of cultural codes, while the other tries to connect phenomenological and existential perspectives with the study of cultural semiological codes and macroscopic contexts. Few studies inspired by this challenging agenda have yet been published.

The fact that health problems are not distributed at random and tend to be concentrated among specific groups or communities is well recognized in epidemiological research. The factors influencing this differential distribution cannot be fully understood without taking into consideration collective influences and processes such as cultural norms and values, structures of prestige and authority, rapports of domination and exploitation. The preceding section has shown that variables are embedded within cultural frames that give them shape, define their significance, and modulate their influence. It also spelled out the importance of examining how macrosocial forces influence the risk of exposure to stressors and the meanings associated with specific stressors.

We must go further in this direction, and identify more precisely the way macrosocial forces—such as political organization, economic development, or social structure—can undermine the foundations of a society, its culture, and the ability of its members to experience the world positively. When macrosocial forces become a critical determinant of cultural life, the process of defining the significance of a situation can become a medium of confrontation, and its appropriation by the dominant group can reinforce imbalances in the positions of the participants and promote the process of domination. The position adopted by researchers, administrators, and health-service providers can thus assume a crucial importance.

The Situation of Canadian Native Groups

Let us first examine the dramatic example of native groups in Canada. The exceptional accumulation of health hazards and problems among these groups may be considered a sign of a more general deterioration of collective life. Epidemiological data (Manson et al., 1989; Earls et al., 1990) show that they have poorer health status and shorter life expectancy than the general population. Alcohol abuse contributes significantly to 5 of the 10 leading causes of death among most tribes. The average suicide rate among American Indians and Alaskan natives in 1980–1982 was 1.7 times that of the population as a whole. For the age groups 10–14, 15–19, and 20–24, the corresponding figures were 2.8, 2.4, and 2.3. Canadian data for Indians and Inuit are comparable (Grescoe, 1981): the infant-mortality rate is four times the national average, and average age at death is 24 years younger than that of the general population. Between ages 20 and 29, death by violence is almost four times more common than among whites. Problems associated with beer and wine, and with less-publicized gas-sniffing by children, are tremendous.

The general living conditions of this population are likewise worse than for the rest of the population. Average income is considerably lower than the national average ($13,678 versus $19,917), and twice as many Indians/natives (27.5 percent) are below the poverty line. The unemployment rate is twice the national average. This accumulation of risk factors has many negative consequences for health status. The main impact, however, on the health and living conditions of American and Canadian native peoples appears to be a global demoralization. Leighton and his collaborators describe the negative impact of social disintegration on mental health in similar terms. Grescoe, in his paper on Canadian Indians and Inuit, quotes the National Indian Brotherhood's warning: "the worst effects of such an existence under these conditions are apathy, alcohol and drug abuse, and finally, a high rate of suicide" (1981, p. 111).

Certain particulars of these morbidity and mortality data are of special concern, and indicate the depth of the damage to the collective identity. The high rate of suicide among youth, the increasing tendency for youthful suicides to occur in clusters and predominantly among males, the rise of such self-destructive behaviors as gas-sniffing, and the overall prevalence of family and intragroup violence all indicate the collapse of a collective frame of meaning within which people, and especially youth, can find a place and project their existence into the future.

In such a context, it appears crucial to attempt to understand how a set of "structuring conditions" (see page 298) affects the collective experience of what "being an Indian" means rather than to limit investigation to a search for discrete etiological variables. In their review of the literature on youth suicide, Manson and his collaborators (1989) identify a range of individual risk factors and collective influences. Those who take their lives typically belong to tribes with loose social structures that are undergoing rapid socioeconomic change and that emphasize individuality rather than conformity. The authors refer to Hochkirchen and Jilek's hypothesis (1985) that "culture conflict and concomitant problems in identity formation are believed to produce a chronic dysphoria and anomia, which render Indian youth vulnerable to suicidal behavior during periods of acute stress" (Earls et al., 1990, p. 587). In their own longitudinal study of American Indian students, the authors noticed that an important risk factor for suicidal ideas was having relatives or friends who had committed or attempted suicide; quite surprisingly, high peer support was also related to greater risks of suicide. One gets the impression that among youngsters suicide has become a mode of expressing distress, fury, provocation, or protest, and is a metaphor for the ongoing destructive process in the cultural group. At first glance, the association between individualization and risk of suicide seem difficult to explain. One might have expected that individualistic Native cultures would have prepared their members well to confront Western ways of life. It is possible that the traditional parameters of individuality are at odds with those associated with modern life, or that the constraints associated with modern society do not allow Native people to achieve their individual potential.

Dramatic variations from tribe to tribe also invite examination of how relatively uniform conditions associated with whites' conquest of America have given rise to different experiences, which have generated different patterns of reactions. The preexisting cultural matrix and its degree of flexibility may have played an important role in varying adaptation of different tribes to culture change.

A comparable broadening of perspectives must also occur at the level of interventions. One cannot confine oneself to acknowledging deficiencies and to transforming vulnerable populations in "at-risk groups"; to do so would risk accentuating the powerlessness of the target communities and therefore reinforcing the problem rather than alleviating it. What is needed is a thorough understanding of the dynamics of vulnerability and protection in such communities, as well as an attempt to create or reinforce processes of meaning construction that could be appropriated by the people themselves. In discussion of suicide among American Indians and Alaskan natives, numerous preventive interventions targeted at potential suicide victims and suicide risk factors were described (Earls et al., 1990). Nearly three-quarters of the programs reviewed are "promotional in nature, seeking to ensure the continued well-being of Indians/native people by enhancing their psychosocial strengths and coping resources." The authors comment that by and large, Indian/Native communities press for essentially promotional approaches which hold appeal because of their nonstigmatizing aspect and emphasis on the collectivity, but that interventions of this nature require long periods of time before one can expect to observe outcomes.

In this context, it might be valuable to describe the collective strategies elaborated by "successful" tribes, and to sort out what is due to circumstances of contact, what to differential access to resources, and what to inner cultural dynamics.

That a community-centered perspective on intervention requires broadening the definition of goals and strategies of action is well illustrated by Grescoe's quotation from Dr. Charles Simpson of Victoria, former chairman of an Indian health committee for the British Columbia Medical Association: "Health cannot come without self-respect. Self-respect in a group cannot occur without political awareness. The development of political awareness is a turbulent process and has its own priorities—health is not high on that list. Land is. Land claims are top priority in the (Indians') political awareness program" (in Grescoe, 1981, p. 122). Validating native cultural values might also significantly enhance a sense of collective identity and, through it, personal identity. In the context of the most recent (1992) constitutional debates in Canada, the leader of the First Nations Assembly, Ovide Mercredi, claimed the right to ancestral lands not only to reclaim past history but also to provide a possible future for the new generations.

Community Frames: Structuring Conditions and Organizing Experiences

Corin et al. (1990) used ethnographically oriented methods to describe core characteristics of community life, and their association with perceptions, interpretations, and reactions pertaining to mental health, in six communities in a remote area of Quebec. We defined a range of areas to be systematically documented through interviews with key informants, the interviews were to be supplemented by 5–6 months of field observation in each community. The areas documented were intended to qualify the community life in relation to three main axes: integration-disintegration, competence-dependence, and openness-closedness. We chose two communities in each of the locally dominant economic sectors: lumbering, agriculture, and mining.

Analysis of the data reveals that the three axes do not have the same relevance in all communities. Of the three axes, one appeared to be specifically salient in the organization of the collective life of each community; cultural and social life is organized around a few key features that manifest its particular history and a general mode of reacting to historical constraints and challenges. We used the term *structuring condition* to refer to objective external events and realities and their influence on the formation of the socioculture. Each community builds its own individuality around some founding communal experience, or *organizing experience*, which shapes the morphology and architecture of the socioculture. The organizing experience has a mediating function, manifesting the influence of sociohistorical conditions and imposing meaning and value while maintaining the sociocultural individuality of the group.

We elicited and reconstructed case histories of local people identified by key informants as presenting 10 kinds of mental-health problems, described behaviorally and in local terms. The case histories we elicited provided access to prevailing popular systems of signs, meanings, and practices in the area of mental health—that is, how the community perceives, interprets, and reacts to mental-health problems. Analysis revealed that the narratives collected in a given locality were constructed around a limited number of key themes whose configuration of meaning appeared to characterize that locality.

Comparison of the two levels of data indicated similarities, or cross-references, between the core organizing elements of the system of signs, meaning, and actions, and the key features of a community's social and cultural life—or, to put it another way, between the macrosocial context, the cultural frame, and individual experiences. For example, in a farming village characterized by population decline and a very high rate of dependence on welfare benefits, narratives about people with mental-health problems are organized around three themes: (1) precariousness, or susceptibility to seeing one's social and personal life destroyed by a tragic accident with severe mental and physical consequence (echoing the difficulties arising from life conditions and from the norms of exploitation imposed by large companies on workers); (2) the image of their milieu as a "nest," which expresses a key collective strategy by which people construct a mirage of a cohesive and supportive social environment in spite of contradictory evidence, leading to denial of the existence of cases of depression and emphasis on the tragic personal consequences of the very unusual cases of isolation; (3) excess or outburst, which cross-cuts most narratives and echoes companies' excessive demands on workers. Personal excess also seems to be positively valued as the only possible way to remain in touch with the male cultural values of autonomy and strength. The general distrust of professional services and the very low rate of service utilization have to be understood within this context: the community either takes care of the problems or radically excludes people who become "un-seen" in collective discourses and practices. Cultural analysis indicates how these features, which are manifest in the prevailing way of describing, interpreting, and reacting to mental-health problems, are related to the global collective challenges of survival faced by farming communities in the remote region of Abitibi, and how they reflect more specific local circumstances and values. These findings have pragmatic implications for the management of mental-health problems—for instance in choosing which problems to target and finding culturally and socially acceptable strategies of action (Corin et al., 1990).

A parallel analysis of statistics on utilization of mental-health services revealed that underutilization of mental-health services is associated in certain communities and for certain categories of people with the presence of a strong network of social support and, in other cases with isolation or marginality that prevents contact with these services. On the other hand, high utilization of mental-health services appeared in some cases to characterize the best socially supported people. It appeared mandatory that service providers be aware of the varying significance of the utilization or lack of utilization of professional services. If underutilization is associated with a general lack of support, special outreach strategies could be appropriate; if it seems to be explained by the presence of a social-support system, one has to consider how long informal helpers can continue their action or if they need some kind of complementary support; if underutilization seems to correspond to an unexpectedly low rate of problems, it would be interesting to examine which preventive strategies seem to be involved. In a given community, the explanatory factors associated with under- or overutilization can vary for different categories of persons, and the professional strategies of action should vary accordingly.

The dynamics of the use of social support and formal resources also appears to vary with community characteristics. The more fragile the community, for example, the more defensive are its members about professional help and the more reluctant to use it. It became clear that targeting these communities as "at-risk" could reinforce their marginalization and undermine the coping strategies they have established. Though some kind of intervention was clearly needed, it had to be provided in such a way as not to accentuate existing problems.

Conclusion

We have looked at the cultural dimension of the determinants of health from a variety of perspectives, ranging from culturally sensitive epidemiological surveys, to in-depth community studies and reconstruction of illness narratives embedded in complex social and cultural webs. These diverse studies suggest the following thoughts on further research in this area.

First, studies should explore the interaction between collective and individual processes in an attempt to describe how social and cultural frames interact with personal biographies and how they contribute to shaping life experiences. Conversely, what takes place in individual lives and what surfaces in personal and interpersonal systems of meaning also sheds light on collective processes.

Second, we need to develop meaning-centered research methods for dealing with problems of health and with the network of circumstances associated with them. New designs and approaches should honor the qualitative and "thick" nature of meaning while attempting to systematize its study. Research should aim at examining how meaning is grounded in culture, shaped by history, framed by context, and reinterpreted and used by individuals to articulate their own experiences.

Third, the awareness that people in modern societies live in a plurality of worlds should be more fully acknowledged in research designs in the arena of health. Diversity and multiplicity contribute to the construction of philosophical and existential attitudes regarding life, death, and suffering. This pluralism contends with homogenizing forces also associated with modern life. We need to understand better how this dialectic functions in the arena of health and how it impinges on health and disease.

Fourth, the main challenge for future research is to develop linkages between different research paradigms and methods, and between quantitative and qualitative approaches. This may be accomplished by designing double-level strategies, by alternating between them, or by means of a temporary "decentration" from one's usual perspective. Progress in this area could be a matter less of technique than of attitude. One challenge for future research is to design methods and instruments both culturally

relevant and appropriate for comparison. Berry (1969) has proposed starting with potentially universal concepts (such as "support") but defining them provisionally, then
examining their local significance in a particular society, and reexamining the first definition and transforming it according to the local formulation. The examples of collective forms of social support provided above illustrate how the notion of support has to
be broadened beyond what is currently measured in scales of social support. At a
methodological level, this process would involve much more bidirectional collaboration than usual between epidemiologists and anthropologists.

Finally, this chapter has drawn attention to the political challenges associated with
the definition of meaning, and has outlined the radical reorientation of a new action-
geared philosophy called for by a meaning-centered and politically sensitive style of
intervention.

References

Beard, G. M. 1881. *American Nervousness.* New York: G.P. Putnam.

Berkman, L. F., and L. Syme. 1979. Social networks, host resistance and mortality: A nine-year
follow-up study of Alameda County Residents. *Am. J. Epidemiol.* 109:186–204.

Berry, J. W. 1969. On cross-cultural comparability. *Int. J. Psychol.* 4:119–128.

Bibeau, G. 1988. A step toward thick thinking. From webs of significance to connections across
dimensions. *Med. Anthropol. Q.* 2:402–416.

Biegel, D. E., A. J. Naparstek, and M. M. Khan. 1982. Social support and mental health in urban
ethnic neighborhoods. In D. E. Biegel and A. J. Naparstek (eds.), *Community, Social
Support and Mental Health,* pp. 21–36. New York: Springer.

Brown, G. W., and T. O. Harris. 1978. *Social Origins of Depression: A Study of Psychiatric Disorder in Women.* London: Tavistock.

Brown, G. W., and T. O. Harris (eds.). 1989. *Life Events and Illness.* New York: Guilford Press.

Brown, G. W., and R. Prudo. 1987. Psychiatric disorder in a rural and urban population: Life
events, social integration and symptom formation. In E. Corin, S. Lamarre, P. Migneault,
and M. Tousignant (eds.), *Regards anthropologiques en psychiatrie,* pp. 111–149. Montréal: Édition du GIRAME.

Cooper, J., and N. Sartorius. 1977. Cultural and temporal variations in schizophrenia: A speculation on the importance of industrialization. *Br. J. Psychiatry* 130:50–55.

Corin, E. 1971. Le père comme modèle de différenciation dans une société clanique matri-
linéaire (Yansi, Congo-Kinshasa). *Psychopathologie Africaine* 7:185–224.

Corin, E. 1984. Manières de vivre, manières de dire: Réseau social et sociabilité quotidienne des
personnes âgées au Québec. *Question de culture. La culture et l'âge* 6:157–186.

Corin, E. 1985. Définisseurs culturels et repères individuels: Le rapport au corps chez les personnes âgées. *Int. J. Psychol.* (special issue on Symbol and Symptom) 4-5:471–500.

Corin, E. 1986. The relationship between formal and informal social support networks in rural
and urban contexts. In V. W. Marshall (ed.), *Aging in Canada. Social Perspectives,* 2nd
edn., pp. 167–394. Markham, Ont.: Fitzhenry & Whiteside.

Corin, E., G. Bibeau, J.-C. Martin, and R. Laplante. 1990. *Comprendre pour soigner autrement.*
Montreal: Presses de l'Université de Montréal.

Crapanzano, V. 1992. *Hermes' Dilemma and Hamlet's Desire. On the Epistemology of Interpretation.* Cambridge, MA: Harvard University Press.

Day, R., J. A. Nielsen, A. Korten, G. Ernberg, K. C. Dube, J. Gebhart, A. Jablensky, C. Leon, A.
Marsella, M. Olatawira, N. Sartorius, E. Strömgren, R. Takahashi, N. Wig, and L. C.

Wynne. 1987. Stressful life events preceding the acute onset of schizophrenia: A cross-national study from the World Health Organization. *Cult. Med. Psychiatry* 11:123–206.

DeStefano, F., J. L. Coulehan, and M. K. Wiant. 1979. Blood pressure survey on the Navajo Indian Reservation. *Am. J. Epidemiol.* 109:335–345.

Dohrenwend, B. P. 1966. Social status and psychological disorder: An issue of instance and an issue of method. *Am. Soc. Rev.* 31:14–34.

Dohrenwend, B. P. 1973. Life events as stressors: A methodological inquiry. *J. Health Soc. Behav.* 14:167–175.

Dohrenwend, B. P. 1975. Sociocultural and social-psychological factors in the genesis of mental disorders. *J. Health Soc. Behav.* 16:365–392.

Dressler, W. W. 1982. *Hypertension and Culture Change. Acculturation and Disease in the West Indies*. New York: Redgrane.

Dressler, W. W. 1985. Psychosomatic symptoms, stress and modernization: A model. *Cult. Med. Psychiatry* 9:257–286.

Dressler, W. W., and L. W. Badger. 1985. Epidemiology of depressive symptoms in black communities. *J. Nerv. Ment. Dis.* 173:212–220.

Earls, F., J. I. Escobar, and S. M. Manson. 1990. Suicide in minority groups: Epidemiologic and cultural perspectives. In S. J. Blumenthal and D. J. Kupfer (eds.), *Suicide Over the Life Cycle*, pp. 571–598. Washington, DC: American Psychiatric Press.

Fabrega, H. 1989. On the significance of an anthropological approach in schizophrenia. *Psychiatry* 52:45–65.

Geertz, C. 1983. *Social Knowledge*. New York: Basic Books.

Gerson, J., and K. Peiss. 1985. Boundaries, negotiation, consciousness: Reconceptualizing gender relations. *Social Problems* 32:317–331.

Gerstel, N., C. K. Riessman, and S. Rosenfield. 1985. Explaining the symptomatology of separated and divorced women and men: The role of material conditions and social networks. *Social Forces* 64:84–101.

Good, B. J. 1977. The heart of what's the matter. The semantics of illness in Iran. *Cult. Med. Psychiatry* 1:25–58.

Good, B., and M.J.D. Good. 1984. Toward a meaning-centered analysis of popular illness categories: "Fright-illness" and "heart distress" in Iran. In A. J. Marsella and G. M. White (eds.), *Cultural Conceptions of Mental Health and Therapy*, pp. 141–166. Dordrecht, Holland: D. Reider.

Good, M.J.D., and B. J. Good. 1988. Ritual, the state, and the transformation of emotional discourse in Iranian society. *Cult. Med. Psychiatry* 12:43–63.

Goodhart, D. E., and A. Zautra. 1982. Assessing quality of life in the community: An ecological approach. In A. Jeger and R. S. Slotnick (eds.), *Community Mental Health and Behavioral Ecology. A Handbook of Theory, Research and Practice*, pp. 251–290. New York: Plenum.

Grescoe, P. 1981. A nation's disgrace. In J. Coburn, C. D'Arcy, P. K. New, and G. M. Torrance (eds.), *Health and Canadian Family. Sociological Perspectives*, pp. 109–122. Canada: Fitzhenry & Whiteside.

Gureje, O., and A. Adewunmi. 1988. Life events and schizophrenia in Nigerians. A controlled investigation. *Br. J. Psychiatry* 153:367–375.

Hirsh, B. J. 1981. Social networks and the coping process: Creating personal communities. In B. H. Gotlieb (ed.), *Social Networks and Social Support*, pp. 149–170. Beverly Hills, CA: Sage.

Hochkirchen, B., and W. Jilek. 1985. Psychosocial dimensions of suicide and parasuicide in Amerindians of the Pacific Northwest. *J. Operational Psychiatry* 16:24–28.

Hochschild, A. R. 1979. Emotion work, feeling rules and social structure. *Am. J. Soc.* 85:551–575.

Holmes, T. H., and R. H. Rahe. 1967. The social readjustment rating scale. *J. Psychosomatic Res.* 11:213–218.

Janes, C. R. 1986. Migration and hypertension: An ethnography of disease risk in an urban Samoan community. In C. R. Janes, R. Stall, S. M. Gifford (eds.), *Anthropology and Epidemiology*, pp. 175–211. Dordrecht, Holland: D. Reidel.

Jenkins, J. H., and M. Karno. 1992. The meaning of expressed emotion: Theoretical issues raised by cross-cultural research. *Am. J. Psychiatry* 149:9–21.

Kirmayer, L. 1989. Cultural variation in the response to psychiatric disorders and emotional distress. *Soc. Sci. Med.* 29:327–339.

Kleinman, A. 1981. *Patients and Healers in the Context of Culture*. Berkeley, CA: University of California Press.

Kleinman, A. 1986. *Social Origins of Distress and Disease. Depression, Neurasthenia and Pain in Modern China*. New Haven: Yale University Press.

Kleinman, A. 1988. *Rethinking Psychiatry. From Cultural Category to Personal Experience*. New York: Free Press.

Kleinman, A., and J. Kleinman. 1991. Suffering and its professional transformation: Toward an ethnography of interpersonal experience. *Cult. Med. Psychiatry* 15:275–301.

Konner, M. 1991. The promise of medical anthropology: An invited commentary. *Med. Anthropol. Q.* 5:78–82.

Kunitz, S. J., and J. E. Levy. 1986. The prevalence of hypertension among elderly Navajos: A test of the acculturation stress hypothesis. *Cult. Med. Psychiatry* 10:97–121.

Lee, G. R. 1985. Kinship and social support of the elderly: The case of the United States. *Aging and Society* 5:19–38.

Leff, J., N. N. Wig, H. Bedi, D. K. Menon, L. Kuipers, A. Korten, G. Ernberg, R. Day, N. Sartorius, and A. Jablensky. 1990. Relatives' expressed emotion and the course of schizophrenia in Chandigarh. A two-year follow-up of a first contact sample. *Br. J. Psychiatry* 156:351–356.

Leff, J., N. Sartorius, A. Jablensky, A. Korten, and G. Ernberg. 1992. The international pilot study of schizophrenia: Five-year follow-up findings. *Psychol. Med.* 22:131–145.

Leighton, A. H. 1959. *My Name Is Legion: Foundations for a Theory of Man in Relation to Culture. The Stirling County Study of Psychiatric Disorders and Sociocultural Environment*, Vol. 1. New York: Basic Books.

Leighton, A. H. 1969. A comparative study of psychiatric disorder in Nigeria and rural North America. In S. C. Plog and R. B. Edgerton (eds.), *Changing Perspectives in Mental Illness*, pp. 179–199. New York: Holt, Rinehart & Winston.

Littlewood, R. 1992. Humanism and engagement in a metapsychiatry. Review of Arthur Kleinman "Rethinking Psychiatry: From cultural category to personal experience." *Cult. Med. Psychiatry* 16:395–405.

Lock, M. 1991. Flawed jewels and national disorder: Narratives on adolescent dissent in Japan. Festschrift for George DeVos. *J. Psychohistory* 18:507–531.

Mahaniah, K. M. 1979. L'élément social et thérapeutique de rites funéraires chez les Kongo du Zaïre. *Psychopathologie Africaine* 15:51–79.

Manson, S. M., J. Beals, R. Wiegman-Dick, and C. Duclos. 1989. Risk factors for suicide among Indian adolescents at a boarding school. *Public Health Rep.* 104:609–614.

Marcus, G., and M. Fisher. 1986. *Anthropology as Cultural Critique*. Chicago: University of Chicago Press.

Marmot, M. G., S. L. Syme, A. Kagan, H. Kato, J. B. Cohen, and J. Belsky. 1975. Epidemiological studies of coronary heart disease and stroke in Japanese men living in Japan, Hawaii and California. Prevalence of coronary and hypertensive heart disease and associated risk factors. *Am. J. Epidemiol.* 102:514–525.

Marsella, A. J., and A. Dash-Scheuer. 1988. Coping, culture, and healthy human development. A research and conceptual overview. In P. R. Dasen, J. W. Berry, and N. Sartorius (eds.), *Health and Cross-Cultural Psychology. Toward Application.*, pp. 162–178. Beverly Hills, CA: Sage.

McElroy, A. 1990. Biocultural models in studies of human health and adaptation. *Med. Anthropol. Q.* 4:243–265.

Mechanic, D. 1978. *Medical Sociology. A Comprehensive Text*, 2nd edn. New York: Free Press.

Mirowsky, J. 1985. Depression and marital power: An equity model. *Am. J. Soc.* 91:557–592.

Murakami, S. 1983. *Quality of Life Among Senior Citizens from Different Ethnocultural Traditions.* Unpublished doctoral dissertation, University of Hawaii, Honolulu.

Murphy, H.B.M. 1987. Migration, culture and our perception of the stranger. In E. Corin, S. Lamarre, P. Migneault, and M. Tousignant (eds.), *Regards anthropologiques en psychiatrie*, pp. 77–86. Montreal: Édition du GIRAME.

Obeyesekere, G. 1985. Depression, Buddhism and the work of culture in Sri Lanka. In A. Kleinman and B. Good (eds.), *Culture and Depression*, pp. 134–152. Berkeley, CA: University of California Press.

Pearlin, L. I. 1989. The sociological study of stress. *J. Health Soc. Beh.* 30:241–256.

Pierce, C. S. 1978. *Écrits sur le signe.* Paris: Le Seuil.

Ricoeur, P. 1986. *Du texte à l'action. Essais d'herméneutique, II* Paris: Le Seuil, Collection Esprit.

Robins, L. N., B. Z. Locke, and D. A. Regier. 1991. An overview of psychiatric disorders in America. In L. N. Robins and D. A. Regier (eds.), *Psychiatric Disorders in America. The Epidemiologic Catchment Area Study*, pp. 328–366. New York: Free Press.

Salmond, C. E., I. A. Prior, and A. F. Wessen. 1989. Blood pressure patterns and migration: A 14-year cohort study of adult Tokelauans. *Am. J. Epidemiol.* 130:37–52.

Sartorius, N., A. Jablensky, and R. Shapiro. 1978. Cross-cultural differences in the short term prognosis of schizophrenic psychoses. *Schizophr. Bull.* 4:102–113.

Sartorius, N., A. Jablensky, A. Korten, G. Ernberg, M. Anker, J. E. Cooper, and R. Day. 1986. Early manifestations and first contact incidence of schizophrenia in different cultures. *Psychol. Med.* 16:902–928.

Singer, M. 1990. Reinventing medical anthropology: Toward a critical realignment. *Soc. Sci. Med.* 30:179–187.

Smith, J. C., J. A. Mercy, and J. M. Conn. 1988. Marital status and the risk of suicide. *Am. J. Public Health* 78:78–80.

Wentowski, G. J. 1981. Reciprocity and the coping strategies of older people: Cultural dimensions of network building. *Gerontologist* 21:600–609.

Wig, N. N., D. K. Menon, H. Bedi, A. Ghosh, L. Kuipers, J. Leff, A. Korten, R. Day, N. Sartorius, G. Ernberg, and A. Jablensky. 1987. Expressed emotion and schizophrenia in North India. *Br. J. Psychiatry* 151:156–173.

Wiley, A. S. 1992. Adaptation and the biocultural paradigm in medical anthropology: A critical review. *Med. Anthropol. Q.* 6:216–236.

Williams, J. E., and D. L. Best. 1990. *Sex and Psyche. Gender and Self Viewed Cross-Culturally.* Newbury Park, CA: Sage.

World Health Organization. 1979. *Schizophrenia. An International Follow-Up Study.* Chichester: John Wiley.

10

The Role of Medical Care in Determining Health: Creating an Inventory of Benefits

JOHN P. BUNKER, HOWARD S. FRAZIER, and FREDERICK MOSTELLER

Average life expectancy for citizens of industrial countries has increased from approximately 45 to 75 years during this century, a gain assumed by many to be largely the result of advances in medical care. This assumption has been called into question by a number of observers (Carlson, 1975; Illich, 1976; McKinlay and McKinlay, 1977; McKeown, 1979). Others have argued for the good that medicine does (McDermott, 1978; Beeson, 1980; Levine et al., 1983; Anderson and Morrison, 1989); in most instances these views are unsupported by measurements of benefits, although in one study lower regional death rates were found to be associated with higher Medicare expenditures (Hadley, 1982). Today most observers agree that the causes of increased longevity include, in addition to medical care, improvements in nutrition, housing, sanitation, occupational safety, and lifestyle. If we wish to allocate effort and material resources to achieving further increases in life expectancy, we need to distinguish among these determinants and to estimate the magnitude of their separate effects.

The purpose of this chapter is to initiate that process. We will first estimate the contributions of specific medical interventions, preventive and curative, to increasing life expectancy in the United States. We will next consider medical interventions directed at improving the quality of life. An increase in life expectancy is not the only valued outcome of medical care. Indeed, most medical effort is directed at improving the quality of life, and it is for the relief from symptoms that patients most frequently seek medical assistance. Even so, the methodology of assessment is less well developed and the relevant data are less readily available for such interventions than for those aimed at increasing life expectancy.

We have developed an inventory of the medical services currently provided in industrial countries that make the greatest contributions to increased life expectancy and improved quality of life. Our purpose is to inform decision makers of outcomes that have been achieved by medical services. The inventory also identifies unresolved health-related problems that are amenable to resolution on the basis of present knowledge, if resources are allocated to appropriate medical care.

Estimating Gains in Life Expectancy and Improvements in Quality of Life

To estimate gains in life expectancy attributable to a specific disease and attributable to a preventive or curative service, we used several approaches. For certain diseases we could base our estimates on governmental investigations of the anticipated effect of eliminating the disease altogether. This approach takes account of the process of a disease as it attacks a cohort year by year. For several conditions (heart disease, cerebrovascular disease, pneumonia), we extrapolated from National Center for Health Statistics estimates of gains in "expectation of life due to elimination of specified causes of death" (National Center for Health Statistics, 1988). More precise estimates could be made for heart disease and cerebrovascular disease by adjusting the 1988 life table for the age-specific 40-year decline in mortality published in *Health, United States, 1991* (National Center for Health Statistics, 1992).

For many other diseases the 40-year changes in mortality are only reported in a single age-adjusted rate, precluding a full life-table estimate. Approximations could nevertheless be made by assigning a proportion of the overall increase in life expectancy to a reported decrease in the mortality rate for each condition. For example, the age-adjusted death rate for pneumonia and influenza fell from 26.2 per 100,000 in 1950, to 13.7 in 1989, a reduction of 12.5 per 100,000. During the same period the age-adjusted death rate from all causes fell from 840.5 to 523.0 per 100,000, a difference of 317.5, and life expectancy rose by 7.1 years. As a first approximation, the fall in the death rate for pneumonia and influenza can be calculated to have contributed $(12.5/317.5) \times 7.1$, $= 0.28$ years, or about 3 months. Such a "back of the envelope" approximation when applied to age-adjusted death rates for diseases of the heart and for cerebrovascular disease gave answers within 10 or 20 percent of those based on the standard life table, as described in greater detail in the appendix.

For some conditions no such basis was available, and we accepted estimates of improvements in life expectancy from other sources (even though in some the method of calculation was not described). In the text we give, where we can, an idea of the information that helps us make the estimate. The references to our data sources accompany Tables 10–1 to 10–3.

Our estimates of improvements in life expectancy use different baselines for different conditions and treatments; the choice of baseline depends on when an effective treatment became available or, in some instances, when reliable data became available. For instance, the improvement in life expectancy attributable to smallpox vaccination can be traced to the middle of the nineteenth century, appendectomy to the beginning of the present century, treatment of diabetes to the introduction of insulin in 1921, and the sharp decline in maternal mortality to the introduction of antibiotics and wider use of blood transfusions by mid-century. Estimates of increases in life expectancy for patients with heart disease, hypertension, and pneumonia, on the other hand, are based on mortality data available only from 1950 to the present. Thus any earlier gains will have been missed.

Some conditions for which we have estimated increases in life expectancy are interdependent: for instance, treatment of hypertension may be responsible for some of the gain we attribute to the medical treatment of ischemic heart disease and of diabetes. The prophylactic administration of aspirin should account for some of the gain in the treatment of hypertension. Less obviously related interactions may also occur: the patient who is spared death from heart disease may be at increased risk of death from other causes. Such "competing risks" are a persistent problem that a deeper analysis based on better data might try to address.

A number of offsetting risks are incorporated in the life expectancy calculations. They include increases in mortality attributed to respiratory neoplasms and chronic obstructive pulmonary disease from 12.8 and 4.4 per 100,000, respectively, in 1950, to 40.3 and 19.4 in 1989. Human immunodeficiency virus infection, appearing for the first time in 1987 data, was responsible for 8.7 deaths per 100,000 in 1989. The loss of life expectancy attributable to these conditions which we estimate to be slightly more than a year, offset about a fifth of the gains in life expectancy that we list below.

Accuracy of Life-Expectancy and Quality-of-Life Calculations

We provide some discussion about our intent and the accuracy of the data given on extension of life, the number of people involved, and the benefits received by the population. The reader will appreciate that estimating the number of people affected by a disease or symptom is attended by many uncertainties. Diagnoses can be mistaken, and methods of gathering data are often inadequate, despite decades of effort, national and international, to improve them. Similar shortcomings characterize data about relief of symptoms, cure of disease, and cause of death. When we calculate the numbers of people who benefit from particular procedures, we combine these uncertain figures in ways that lend considerable uncertainty to the final numbers. It will help if the reader keeps in mind that we are trying to produce rough estimates of the number of U.S. residents affected favorably by a specific type of medical care. How many people need access to care, and what are the benefits of care? A striking example of the numbers of those who would benefit is that nearly every sighted adult will benefit at some time from the use of corrective lenses. The type of benefit will include visual acuity adequate to drive, to read, to carry on with employment, and to recreate.

We are especially sensitive to the point that at some stage in many assessments we have to estimate—guess—what fraction of an improvement or benefit results from various changes in society and what fraction from medical care. These estimates are best guesses, not conservative or liberal estimates, and other students differently informed might make substantially different estimates. Since a best guess may not be a good guess; readers may want to ask themselves how interpretations would change if our estimates were altered by 10 or 20 percent in either direction. These uncertainties seem to be in the nature of this kind of work.

We have not tried to develop formal methods of assessing uncertainty in our estimates, but we are familiar with unpublished evidence (Alpert and Raiffa, 1969) that people who make these kinds of estimates are usually overconfident about the accuracy of their guesses.

Selection of Data for Analysis

The conditions for analysis were chosen on the following basis. For the life-table analyses we chose conditions that fulfilled the following criteria: death rates for the condition have fallen (National Center for Health Statistics, 1992); relevant treatment has been shown, usually in randomized trials, to be efficacious; and the prevalence of the condition, together with the two previous criteria, creates an impact on life expectancy of at least 1 day when the effect is spread across the U.S. population.

Developing estimates of the effects of medical care on quality of life is more difficult than for life expectancy. For our present purposes, we take quality of life to be roughly the same as the state captured by the terms "health status" and "well-being." The difficulty in measuring the effects of medical care on quality of life persists, despite improvements in definitions and in measuring instruments directed at both generic and condition-specific attributes of quality of life, and an enlarging base of relevant data. We focus attention on quality of life because, increasingly, medical care is sought and delivered in the expectation that it will improve not the length of life but rather the quality of that life. The conditions to be evaluated were chosen primarily from the most recent estimates from the National Health Interview Survey listing of chronic conditions (Adams and Benson, 1991); they were chosen on the basis of incidence and prevalence, and of efficacious treatment, evidence for which was strong but usually not based on randomized trials.

The Role of Medical Care in Extending Life: Clinical Preventive Services

The U.S. Preventive Services Task Force, in its *Guide to Clinical Preventive Services* (1989), reviewed the evidence for the efficacy of screening for 47 medical conditions, counseling to prevent disease and promote health, childhood and adult immunizations; and aspirin, postmenopausal estrogen replacement and postexposure prophylaxis of a group of infectious diseases. Limiting its endorsement to services having clear experimental evidence of efficacy, the Task Force recommended routine screening for only six conditions, childhood immunizations, and counseling to prevent tobacco use.

Screening

Four of the recommended screening procedures are for conditions that affect life expectancy.

1. The Task Force recommends that blood pressure be measured regularly in all persons aged 3 and above. Treatment of moderate and severe hypertension is clearly efficacious; the efficacy of screening will depend on the correct prescription of treatment and on patient compliance. Hypertension may occur in as many as 58 million Americans, of whom an estimated 10 million adults are moderate or severe hypertensives. We estimate that an increase in life expectancy of 5–6 months since 1950 can be attributed to the treatment of hypertension. It is unclear how much of this gain should be credited to population screening, and how much to incidental case-finding during examination and treatment of other medical conditions; we tentatively credit 1.5–2 months to population screening (Table 10–1) and 3.5–4 months to incidental case-finding (Table 10–2).
2. The Task Force recommends that all women over 40 receive an annual clinical breast examination and that mammography be performed every 1–2 years from age 50 to 75. The decrease in mortality from breast cancer for women aged 50 and above who receive annual breast examinations and mammography may be as great as 20 percent. This is roughly equivalent to an increase in life expectancy of 5 years for 50-year-old women otherwise destined to die of breast cancer and of 1.5 months for all women aged 50. These advances are not reflected in increases in national life expectancy, however, for they have been entirely offset by increases in the incidence and national death rate of breast cancer. Even so, screening for breast cancer and appropriate treatment appear to have prevented an even greater rise in the national death rate from breast cancer.
3. The Task Force also recommends Papanicolaou testing for cervical cancer every 1–3 years with the onset of sexual activity. For the estimated 1.4 percent of women destined to develop cancer of the uterine cervix, Papanicolaou testing every 3 years beginning at age 20, with appropriate curative treatment at the time of diagnosis, is estimated to increase their life expectancy by 10–15 years. For all women, screening for cervical cancer every 3 years increases life expectancy by 96 days (Eddy, 1990). Between 60 and 90 percent of women are reported to have been screened within the past 3 years (Muller et al., 1990); we thus

estimate that two thirds of this potential has been achieved, for an increase in women's life expectancy of 2.0 months, which is the equivalent of 1.0 month for the population as a whole.

4. Screening for high blood cholesterol is recommended by the Task Force on the basis of the association between high blood levels and coronary atherosclerosis, and of the ability of cholesterol-lowering drugs to reduce the incidence of coronary artery disease in asymptomatic persons. Taylor and his associates (1987), having modeled the published evidence, estimate a gain in life expectancy from a lifelong program of cholesterol reduction for low-risk persons aged 20 to 60 years of from 3 days to 3 months. For persons at high risk, they estimate a gain of from 18 days to 12 months. Neither the Task Force nor Taylor takes notice of the repeated failures to demonstrate an increase in life expectancy resulting from the reduction in coronary artery disease, a subject of considerable current scientific controversy (Manson et al., 1992; Ravnskov, 1992). Until this controversy is resolved we will not designate screening for cholesterol as a life-extending service.

5. After publication of the *Guide to Clinical Preventive Services* the efficacy of screening for colorectal cancer was reported in a randomized study of fecal occult-blood testing (Mandel et al., 1993). Annual testing of 50 to 80-year-old men and women was found to decrease the 13-year cumulative mortality from colorectal cancer by 33 percent; but there was little if any benefit for individuals screened only every 2 years. Reducing by one third the age-adjusted death rate attributed to colorectal cancer (13.6 per 100,000 in 1989) would amount to an increase in life expectancy of about 1 month. Several other trials are in progress; until their results are available, we will credit annual screening with the potential to increase life expectancy by 2.0 weeks and will assign half of this increase to clinical preventive services and half to clinical curative services.

Counseling

In recommending cessation counseling for all smokers, the Task Force cites a recent meta-analysis of 39 clinical trials that found cessation rates averaging about 8 percent after 6 months and 6 percent after 1 year. The key elements of effective counseling appear to be consistent and repeated advice to stop smoking, a specific "quit date," and a follow-up contact or visit. Taylor and colleagues (1987) estimate additional life expectancy after quitting smoking as 2 years for a 60-year-old woman to 6 years for a 20-year-old man. If one third of the population now smokes, if counseling is followed by a 6 percent drop in the number of smokers, and if an average increase in life expectancy of 4 years (48 months) is assigned to a middle-aged person who stops smoking, cessation counseling could increase the average life expectancy of the population by about 1 month ($1/16 \times 1/3 \times 48$). We assign this gain only to the "potential" column of Table 10–1 because we do not know what proportion of smokers currently receive counseling. This potential may well be an underestimate, since it ignores the possible effects of repeated counseling.

Immunizations

Infectious disease, the most common cause of death in childhood at the beginning of the century, has become rare as a cause of death today. In 1900 the annual death rates for diphtheria, measles, and pertussis were 40, 13, and 12 per 100,000 respectively; by 1960, there were no deaths reported for diphtheria, and only 2 and 1 per 100,000 for measles and pertussis respectively. Most of the drop in death rates from measles and pertussis occurred before the introduction of their respective vaccines or of antibiotics (McKeown, 1979). Thus we can assign credit only to diphtheria antitoxin and immunization for the drop in mortality, equivalent to an increase in life expectancy of approximately 10 months.

Death rates from poliomyelitis and tetanus before the introduction of immunization were lower, varying between 0.4 and 1.8 per 100,000 for poliomyelitis between 1920 and 1950, and for tetanus between 0.7 and 1.7 in the 1920s and 1930s. The virtual elimination of both diseases following implementation of immunization represents an increase in life expectancy of about 3 weeks for both combined. (Prevention of the paralytic complications of poliomyelitis is discussed in a later section.)

Smallpox represents a special case, since immunization has been practiced for 200 years. Nevertheless, deaths continued to be attributed to smallpox until the early 1930s, peaking at 6.5 per 100,000 in 1902, with a smaller peak of 0.9 per 100,000 in 1924. It is estimated that before the introduction of vaccination more than 10 percent of all deaths were caused by smallpox. In eighteenth-century England one-third of all deaths in childhood were attributed to smallpox. Smallpox usually occurred in epidemic form; in 1752, for example, more than 30 percent of the population of Boston became infected, with mortality of more than 30 percent among those infected. The increase in life expectancy for the vaccinated individual otherwise destined to contract smallpox we estimate as approximately one third of his or her remaining life expectancy, perhaps 10 to 20 years. McKeown (1979) credits 1.6 percent of the decline in mortality in Great Britain over the past century to smallpox vaccination, equivalent to a 3- to 6-month increase in life expectancy. We thus credit an increase of 3–6 months in life expectancy to vaccination against smallpox and its worldwide eradication in 1977.

What conclusions can we draw about the contribution of immunization practices to health today? Measles offers a case in point. While death attributed to measles is rare in the United States, the recent marked upsurge in measles in unvaccinated preschool children in the inner city raises the specter of a resurgence of measles-related deafness and mental retardation (Hersh et al., 1992), which we will discuss in a later section. Waning confidence in immunization gives added cause for concern. Koplan and colleagues have explored the potential effect of curtailment of pertussis vaccination

(1979). Using decision analysis, they predicted that there would be a 71-fold increase in cases and an almost 4-fold increase in deaths.

Adult Immunizations

Ten thousand or more excess deaths have been documented in each of 19 influenza epidemics between 1957 and 1986, and more than 40,000 people have died in each of several recent epidemics; pneumococcal disease accounts for about 40,000 deaths each year (Burman et al., 1985; Williams et al., 1988). Pneumonia and influenza together accounted for 76,550 deaths in 1989, and hepatitis-B is estimated to account for 5,000 deaths annually.

The *Guide to Clinical Preventive Services* recommends pneumococcal vaccine at least once and influenza vaccine annually to everyone aged 65 and older and to certain high-risk groups, and hepatitis-B vaccine to high-risk groups. Gardner and Schaffner (1993) estimate that implementation of these recommendations will prevent 9,800 deaths per annum from influenza and 20,640 deaths from pneumococcal infection, equivalent to increases in life expectancy of about 3 and 6 weeks respectively. They also estimate that universal immunization of infants with hepatitis-B vaccine, in addition to the immunization of high-risk groups, could prevent 4,050 deaths annually, equivalent to an increase in life expectancy of 1.5–2 weeks.

Chemoprophylaxis

The *Guide to Clinical Preventive Services* recommends that estrogen therapy be considered for asymptomatic women at increased risk of osteoporosis. Evidence from observational and uncontrolled studies indicates that estrogen replacement is associated with a decreased rate of fractures. Overviews of observational studies also estimate a reduction in coronary artery disease of 44 percent (Manson et al., 1992; Stampfer and Colditz, 1991; Stampfer et al., 1991). These benefits are partly offset by an increased risk of endometrial cancer and possibly of breast cancer. Several careful analyses of the potential risks and benefits of estrogen-replacement therapy have concluded that its life extending benefits outweigh by a large margin the risk of death from cancer of the uterus or breast. Estimates of the net increase in life expectancy of hormone replacement therapy vary from approximately 3 weeks to 6 months, depending on choice of hormones, length of treatment, and whether prior hysterectomy has been performed (Weinstein and Tosteson, 1990; Daly et al., 1992). For postmenopausal women receiving combined estrogen and progestin for 15 years or longer, these authors estimate, life expectancy is extended by 3 months. Approximately half of postmenopausal women in the United States are currently receiving hormone replacement. On the basis of current usage and the assumption that combined estrogen and progestin are taken for at least 15 years, we assign a current increase in life expectancy for all women of 1.5 months and a potential increase of 1.5 months if all postmenopausal women were so treated.

The *Guide* also recommends that low-dose aspirin be considered for men aged 40 and over who are at increased risk for myocardial infarction (MI). The evidence supporting this recommendation comes from a very large, randomized, placebo-controlled, double-blind trial in healthy men that demonstrated a decrease in risk of both fatal and non-fatal MI in those taking aspirin but failed to show a significant decrease in cardiovascular mortality (Steering Committee of the Physicians' Health Study Research Group, 1989). The Antiplatelet Trialists' Collaboration (1994) gives data on the protective effect of aspirin in preventing myocardial infarction, stroke, and death among high risk patients. These data do not translate readily into extensions of life expectancy. However, for high risk patients they show for men and women reductions of about one-third in non-fatal myocardial infarction, about one-third in non-fatal stroke, and about one-sixth in vascular death. Overall mortality was significantly reduced. The most common regimen used was medium dose aspirin (75–325 mg/day). Because we are concerned here with effects on life expectancy, we do not include low-dose aspirin prophylaxis in our list of cardiovascular interventions. Because of the size of the favorable effect of aspirin on the risk of MI in the first study, however, and the lack of comparable information about its effects in women, we emphasize the importance of further study of the value of aspirin prophylaxis before it is widely applied to the population of either gender.

Summary of Contributions to Life Expectancy from Clinical Preventive Services

Table 10–1 summarizes the contribution of the clinical preventive services to life expectancy. The next-to-last column suggests that the gain is about 18 months when averaged over the whole population. This gain is small compared to the number of years gained by the afflicted who are saved (shown in column 4). For each treatment the population gain tends to make the contribution look small and thus we may undervalue successful treatment or prevention of rarer diseases.

The column on the far right suggests that more nearly universal treatment with these services might add another 7 to 8 months to the life expectancy of the entire population.

The Role of Medical Care in Extending Life: Clinical Curative Services

Cancer is a major cause of death in the United States. While there have been dramatic improvements in the mortality statistics for a few malignant neoplasms, there is no evidence that medical care has reduced mortality when all cancers are added together. Indeed, the age-adjusted death rates for all malignant neoplasms has risen from 125.3 per 100,000 in 1950 to 133.0 in 1989. This increase is entirely accounted for by the increase in smoking-induced malignancies, primarily lung cancer, for which treatment is particularly unsuccessful. If one excludes lung cancer, as Doll (1992) and Peto et al. (1992) propose, there remains a modest overall improvement for which surgery and medicine might reasonably take credit. After eliminating smoking-associated cancers

Table 10-1 Clinical Preventive Services. Estimated Numbers at Risk and Gains in Life Expectancy for Those Receiving Selected Successful Services, with Gain in Life Expectancy for the U.S. Population and Potential Gain Not yet Achieved.

Clinical Preventive Service	Relevant Population	Individuals Affected by Condition in the Absence of Preventive Service	Gain per Individual Receiving Preventive Service	Proportion of Those at Risk Receiving Preventive Service	Gain in Life Expectancy Distributed Across U.S. Population	
					Current	Potential
Screening for hypertension	All over 3 years	58 million[a] (10 million moderate or severe)	3 months	50%	1.5–2 months	1.5–2 months
Screening for cancer of cervix	Adult women	13,000[b]	96 days	60–90%	2 weeks[c]	1 week[c]
Screening for colorectal cancer	All 50–80	155,000[b]	2 weeks	Unknown	Unknown	1 week
Counseling to stop smoking	Smokers	Smokers (approximately 1/3 of population)[a]	3 months	Unknown	Unknown	1 month
Immunization for diphtheria	All children	40 deaths per 100,000[c]	10 months	73–85% preschool; 97–98% entering school	10 months	0
Immunization for poliomyelitis	All	2500 deaths[b]	3 weeks	73–85% preschool; 97–98% entering school	3 weeks	0
Immunization for tetanus	All	2500 deaths[b]				
Immunization for smallpox	All	NA[d]	3–6 months[e]	Almost all before eradication; almost nobody today	3–6 months	0
Immunization for influenza	All over 65	10,000–40,000 deaths[b]	3 weeks	30%	1 week	3 weeks
Pneumococcal immunization	All over 65	400,000 cases[b]	6 weeks	14%	1 week	6 weeks

Hepatitis-B immunization	All	21,000 cases[b]	1.5–2 weeks	10%	1–2 days	1.5–2 weeks
Hormone replacement	Post menopausal women	8,000 deaths[b]	3 months	50%	3 weeks[c]	3 weeks[c]
Aspirin prophylaxis for heart attack	Men over 40	Appoximately 30% of men	Unknown	Unknown	Unknown	Unknown

a. Prevalence (all cases).

b. Incidence (new cases per annum).

c. Double for single sex.

d. Not applicable following worldwide eradication.

e. Limited to this century only.

Sources:

Hypertension: MacMahon et al., 1990; Collins et al., 1990; Subcommittee on Definition and Prevalence of the Joint National Committee on Detection, Evaluation and Treatment of High Blood Pressure, 1985.

Cancer of cervix: Eddy, 1990.

Colorectal cancer: Mandel et al., 1993.

Counseling to stop smoking: Taylor et al., 1987.

Immunization: Amler and Dull, 1987; *Morbidity and Mortality Weekly Report*, 1986; Gardner and Schaffner, 1993.

Hormone replacement: Daly et al., 1992; Weinstein and Tosteson, 1990.

Aspirin prophylaxis: Hennekens et al., 1988; Steering Committee of the Physicians' Health Study Research Group, 1989.

of the respiratory system, the age-adjusted annual death rate for malignant neoplasms would be 112.5 per 100,000 in 1950 and 92.7 per 100,000 in 1989, an improvement representing 80,000 fewer deaths per year and equivalent to a gain in life expectancy for the entire population of 4 or 5 months. Exclusion of all smoking related cancers would provide a more conservative estimate of net impact of medical care in cancer deaths (Peto et al., 1992).

Dramatic advances have been made in the prevention or delay of death caused by some malignancies, most notably childhood leukemia, the malignant lymphomas, and testicular cancer. There have also been modest decreases in case-fatality rates for cancers of the breast; colon and rectum; and cervix and uterine fundus.

Acute lymphocytic leukemia is the most common cause of cancer death in children. Annual mortality between 1950 and 1954 was 5.3 per 100,000 children ages 0–4, 3.4 for ages 5–9, and 2.3 for ages 10–19; death rates have since fallen progressively, and in the 5-year period 1985–1989 the rates for the same age groups ranged from 1.2 to 1.4. Assuming that the life expectancy of survivors is somewhat lower than for the population as a whole, we assigned a gain in life expectancy of 50 years to surviving children. Because of the low incidence of this disease this amounts to no more than 1 or 2 days increase in life expectancy for the population as a whole. For the same reason, dramatic increases in survival of patients suffering from the malignant lymphomas and testicular cancer fail to translate into substantial increases in life expectancy for the population as a whole.

Case-fatality rates of breast cancer have fallen 25–30 percent in premenopausal women and 20–25 percent in postmenopausal women (Early Breast Cancer Trialists' Collaborative Group, 1992). This improvement is attributed to earlier detection of the tumor, as documented by much smaller size on removal, and to more effective adjuvant hormonal therapy and chemotherapy, as documented by randomized clinical trials. These advances have been offset by a very large increase in the number of diagnosed cases, with the result that there has been no decrease in overall mortality from breast cancer. Indeed, age-adjusted mortality from breast cancer has increased slightly, from 22.2 per 100,000 in 1950 to 23.0 per 100,000 in 1989.

Age-adjusted death rates attributed to colorectal cancer have fallen from 19.0 per 100,000 in 1950 to 13.6 in 1989. This decrease roughly coincides with the level of improvement reported in randomized trials of radiotherapy and adjuvant chemotherapy, but there is considerable uncertainty about interpretation of the trials (Sleven and Gray, 1991; Taylor and Northover, 1990), and much of the improvement is thought to be due to changes in diet. We credit medical care with half of the improved survival, amounting to 2 weeks of increased life expectancy for the population as a whole, and the potential for an additional 2 weeks, one of which was assigned to screening (p. 314) and Table 10–1.

Cancer of the cervix is virtually 100 percent curable if detected early by screening. The annual age-adjusted death rate has fallen from 10.2 per 100,000 American women in 1955–1957 to 3.1 in 1985–1987 (American Cancer Society, 1991), a gain in life expectancy of about 2 months for women only, or 1 month for the population as a whole. The remaining mortality reflects the fact that one third of American women are currently not screened for cancer of the cervix and is roughly equivalent to a loss in life expectancy of approximately 1 month. We credit screening followed by surgery with a gain in life expectancy of 2 months, with the potential for a gain of 1 additional month. We assign half of these gains to treatment and half to screening.

In contrast to cancer, survival of patients suffering from heart disease has improved dramatically. Goldman and Cook (1984), reviewing evidence of the efficacy of medical interventions, estimate that 40 percent of the decline in cardiac deaths between 1968 and 1976 could be attributed to medical care, chiefly coronary-care units, treatment of hypertension, and medical treatment of ischemic heart disease.

Goldman and Cook's analysis was limited to an 8-year period; cardiac mortality had already fallen and has continued to fall. The National Center for Health Statistics reports a fall in annual age-adjusted death rates for diseases of the heart from 307.2 per 100,000 in 1950 to 155.9 in 1989. If 40 percent of this fall were the result of medical intervention, this would represent an increase in population life expectancy of nearly 18 months (see the Appendix for details of calculation of life expectancy in heart disease).

The age-adjusted death rate for cerebrovascular disease fell from 88.6 per 100,000 in 1950 to 28.0 in 1989, representing approximately 130,000 fewer such deaths annually and an increase in life expectancy for the whole population of a little more than 1 year. Marked increase in medical control of hypertension during this period, from less than 10 percent of individuals with moderate or severe elevations of blood pressure to approximately 50 percent (Drizd et al., 1986), and a 42 percent reduction in stroke observed in randomized trials of antihypertensive drugs (MacMahon et al., 1990; Collins et al., 1990). This could explain as much as 15–20 percent of the reduction in stroke mortality, with an increase in life expectancy of 2.5–3 months, about a half of the net effect assigned to screening in Table 10–1 and half to treatment in Table 10–2.

Among the most spectacular recent advances in medicine is the treatment of chronic kidney failure or end-stage renal disease by hemodialysis or kidney transplant. In the past, chronic kidney failure was uniformly fatal. Today the life expectancy of a 40-year-old suffering end-stage renal disease is 8.8 years, that of a 59-year-old 4.2 years (U.S. Renal Data System, 1991). These advances have added an estimated 2–3 months to the life expectancy of the population, about 2 weeks of which can be credited to transplantation.

The introduction of insulin in 1921 brought about an abrupt decrease in the death rate for diabetes. Prior to the introduction of insulin the life expectancy of a patient with newly-diagnosed diabetes mellitus was less than 2 years, with all but 5 percent dead by the end of 10 years (Krolewski et al., 1985). Today diabetes is estimated to shorten life by approximately 12 years (National Center for Health Statistics, 1988); the juvenile diabetic survives on average to 50–55 years, the adult-onset diabetic to 60–70 years. The gain of over 50 years in life expectancy at birth for the juvenile diabetic is primarily due to insulin, but the introduction of antibiotics, management of hypertension, and other improvements in management of the complications of diabetes have also contributed. Of the approximately 5.5 million diabetics in the United States, half a million to a million are insulin-dependent; we estimate that almost all are alive today because of advances in medical care. It is considerably more difficult to estimate the gain in life expectancy of the larger numbers of non-insulin-dependent diabetics, since there are no reliable baseline data on their prognosis prior to the introduction of therapy. Our best estimate, given this caveat, is that diabetics gain an average of 25 years of additional life, and that the population as a whole gains 6 months in life expectancy by virtue of medical care of diabetes.

Age-adjusted deaths from pneumonia and influenza have fallen from 26.2 per 100,000 in 1950, to 13.7 in 1989, representing approximately 30,000 fewer deaths per year, and 1 million fewer deaths since 1950, an increase in life expectancy of approximately 3 months for the U.S. population. We credit medical care with all of the increase in life expectancy.

The importance of the introduction of streptomycin in 1948 to treat pulmonary tuberculosis, followed by other effective antitubercular drugs, has been minimized by McKeown and others who point out that the mortality rate from tuberculosis had already fallen by 90 percent (McKeown, 1979). But pulmonary tuberculosis still killed an estimated 40,000 people each year in the United States. Effective treatment further accelerated the decline in mortality to the point that tuberculosis had, until recently, nearly disappeared as a cause of death. Assuming that mortality attributed to tuberculosis would have continued to fall without treatment, McKeown credited 51 percent of the additional improvement to treatment. We accept his estimate and assign an increase in life expectancy of 3 months to medical care.

Deaths from peptic ulcer disease fell from approximately 10,500 per annum in 1965 to 5,500 in 1980 (Fineberg and Pearlman, 1981), equivalent to about 1 month in increased life expectancy. This period witnessed a gradual decline in the incidence and prevalence of peptic ulcer disease, attributable in part to a continuing decrease in the number of male smokers, and in part to the introduction of cimetidine and other histamine blocking drugs. We credit medical care with half of this improvement, or a 2-week increase in life expectancy for the entire population.

How much of the improvement in survival of patients suffering from life-threatening cardiac and pulmonary disease can be attributed to the technologies of the modern intensive-care unit is difficult to determine. Goldman and Cook (1984) estimate that coronary care units may be responsible for saving 10,000 lives per annum, or about one third of the decrease in cardiac deaths that they attribute to medical care. Because their estimate is based primarily on observational data, we accept it with caution, tentatively assigning an increase in life expectancy of 4–6 months. Here, as elsewhere, the reader is reminded to see the Appendix for estimates of the total effects of the multiple treatments for heart disease.

By far the best evidence of the effectiveness of intensive care pertains to newborn infants. Between 150,000 and 200,000 infants (4–6 percent of all newborns) are treated annually in neonatal intensive care units, at least one half of them low-birth-weight infants (Office of Technology Assessment, 1987). The Office of Technology Assessment reports that mortality for infants with birth weights of 1,000 to 1,500 grams fell from 50 to 10 percent over the previous 25 years, and from 90 percent to about 50 percent for infants weighing less than 1,000 grams. Many of these infants fail to survive their first year (about one fifth and two thirds of the respective birth-weight groups) (Buehler et al., 1987), and it is assumed that the surviving infants have a higher incidence of other life-shortening conditions and a greater-than-average death rate in subsequent years. In the absence of more precise survival data, we estimate an increase in their life expectancy of 20–30 years. Given that 1.24 percent of all newborns weighed less than 1,500 grams in 1987 and 1988, the most recent years for which data have been published, their increased life expectancy is roughly equivalent to an increase in life expectancy for the population as a whole of about 3 or 4 months.

Maternal deaths during this century have fallen from 27 per 100,000 women in 1900 to 5.4 per 100,000 in 1940 and to 2 per million in 1987. This represents an increase in life expectancy for women of about 6 months since 1900 and 5–6 weeks since 1940. Improved social conditions may have been responsible for much of the decline in maternal mortality early in the century. The introduction and availability of antibiotics, ready availability of blood transfusions, and an overall improvement in obstetrical and anesthetic care must be credited with the subsequent decline in mortality. We assign women a 1-month gain in life expectancy since 1940 to improved medical care.

Surgery may be undertaken under life-threatening circumstances in which the only goal is to prevent or postpone death. It may also be undertaken in an effort to improve quality of life. All surgery entails a risk to life that must be balanced against life-extending benefits if we are to estimate its net impact on life-expectancy.

Rates of death during and following surgery are reasonably well established, but the number of lives saved is often difficult to determine. Data on improvement in quality of life following specific operations are only beginning to become available; we will examine them in a later section. What is known about the effect of surgery on mortality rates? There is no evidence that geographic areas that perform more surgery have lower death rates (Bunker and Wennberg, 1973; Wennberg and Gittlesohn, 1982). Thus, it is necessary to examine the net effects of individual types of operations or groups of operations.

The greatest surgical potential to save life appears to be in the care of injury. An estimated 90,000 Americans die annually from accidental injury, equivalent to a loss in life expectancy of about 9–10 months. Considerable improvement has already been achieved. The death rate from "accidents and adverse effects" fell from 57.5 per 100,000 in 1950 to 33.8 in 1989, equivalent to an increase in life expectancy of 6–7 months. Much of this improvement is attributable to prevention: improved road safety, a decrease in occupational hazards, improved home safety, and the like. Federally mandated trauma centers have made a contribution, but the centers are poorly funded and it has been estimated that no more than 25 percent of the population is served by such centers (Trunkey, 1990). We estimate that medical care has contributed 1.5–2 months toward the improvement to date, with the potential of a further increase of 3–4 months in life expectancy.

Only a small fraction of all surgery is performed under life-threatening conditions. With the exception of trauma surgery, appendectomy is the only common emergency operation performed for the sole purpose of saving lives; McKeown singled it out as the only medical or surgical intervention that had made a recognizable contribution to the large increase in life expectancy between the mid-nineteenth century and 1971 (McKeown, 1979). As a first approximation, we might accept the mortality rate attributed to appendicitis when it was first recognized as a pathological entity in 1886, prior to the introduction of appendectomy, and from this subtract the average mortality associated with the operation today. McKeown estimated that annual mortality from appendicitis and peritonitis in England and Wales in 1848–1854 was 75 per million, a rate that would amount to approximately 20,000 deaths for a population of 260 million. The mortality rate for appendectomy in the National Halothane Study (Bunker et al., 1969) was 0.54 percent; applied to the nearly 300,000 appendectomies performed each year in the United States, this rate would represent 1,500 deaths, for a net gain in lives saved of about 18,500 per year. If we assume an average age at appendectomy of 20, that the gain in life expectancy is about 60 years, and that the lifetime probability of dying from appendicitis would have been 1 in 200 [18,500 $\times$ 75 $\div$ 260 million], the resulting increase in life expectancy is about 4 months.

The coronary artery bypass graft operation was introduced in 1969, primarily to prevent death in patients suffering from coronary arteriosclerosis. The operation has been widely evaluated in randomized clinical trials, which have shown that only under very limited circumstances does the operation prolong life. Goldman and Cook (1984) estimated that 3.5 percent of the decline in ischemic heart disease mortality rates could be attributed to the bypass operation, amounting to about 3,000 lives saved each year or about 1 month in added life expectancy. (The main benefit of this operation, it is now generally acknowledged, is relief of the pain of angina pectoris and improvement in quality of life.) The Appendix identifies the aggregate effects of cardiac treatments.

Three other widely performed operations—hysterectomy, prostatectomy, and cholecystectomy—have been subjected to intensive observational studies and cost-effectiveness analysis. These analyses indicate that elective hysterectomy may increase women's life expectancy by as much as 2 months or as little as 3 weeks by eliminating the risk of cancer of the cervix and uterine fundus (Korenbrot et al., 1981; Sandberg et al., 1985), that cholecystectomy for asymptomatic gall stones may increase life expectancy by 1–2 weeks (Fitzpatrick et al., 1977), or shorten it by as much as 2.5 weeks (Ransohoff et al., 1983), and that prostatectomy shortens life expectancy by about 1 month (Barry et al., 1988). The net impact of these three elective operations, among the most frequently performed, is less than a week of added life expectancy for the population as a whole.

Hysterectomy for hemorrhage, cholecystectomy for acute cholecystitis, and prosta-tectomy for acute urinary retention are life-saving operations in many or most cases, but they represent a very small proportion of operations and there are no data on their frequency or outcomes. Indeed, there are no reliable data documenting the frequency of emergency surgery in general. While this represents a serious obstacle to assessing the overall life-saving effect of surgery, the contribution of emergency surgery would appear to be relatively small. Only 7 percent of the 856,000 operations for which data were collected in the National Halothane Study were listed as emergencies; many of these were for non-life-threatening conditions, and some—perhaps many—did not succeed in saving life.

We conclude that only a small number of operations make substantial contributions to national life expectancy. We have identified five: appendectomy, hysterectomy, colectomy, coronary artery bypass graft, and kidney transplant. An important point that should be kept in mind is that mortality alone is an insufficient index of surgery's con-tribution to the public's health; quality of life is a more appropriate index with which to judge much of surgery.

Summary of Estimated Increase in Life Expectancy for the Population from Clinical Preventive and Curative Services

Table 10–2 presents the estimated gains from selected curative services. Together they add approximately 3.5–4 years to life expectancy. The 18-month gain for heart disease derives from a collection of technologies rather than a single treatment. Within the framework of medicine as currently practiced, we estimate that an additional year to 18 months might be gained by extending current clinical curative services to more people. Trauma care appears to be a particularly promising component of this extension for further investigation.

All told, Tables 10–1 and 10–2 estimate a gain in life expectancy of about 5 years by the last decade of the century and a potential for adding 2 or 2.5 more years by extend-ing access to therapies already known to be efficacious.

The curative services seem to be making a larger contribution to length of life than do preventive services. In looking for possible errors, one might ask whether we have undervalued gains from immunization and other clinical preventive services or over-valued curative services. We do not consider costs in this paper, but it would be in-structive to compare the cost-effectiveness of preventive and curative services.

The Role of Medical Care in Improving Quality of Life

The quality of life is determined by social, environmental, economic, and occupational factors as well as by health status. Health status is in turn influenced by medical care. Among the components of quality of life, morbidity and disability provide a measur-able connection between medical care and quality of life.

Table 10-2 Clinical Curative Services. For Selected Diagnoses, Estimated Numbers at Risk and Gains in Life Expectancy for Those Receiving Successful Treatment, with Gain in Life Expectancy for the U.S. Population and Potential Gain not yet Achieved.

Condition Treated	Relevant Population	Number at Risk	Gain per Individual Receiving Successful Treatment (years)	Gain in Life Expectancy Distributed Across U.S. Population	
				Current	Potential
Cancer of cervix	Adult women	13,000[b]	21[c]	2 weeks[d]	1 week[d]
Colorectal cancer	All	155,000[b]	12[c]	2 weeks	1 week
Peptic ulcer	All	250,000[b]	10[e]	2 weeks	Unknown
Ischemic heart disease[f]	All	6 million[a]	14[e]	1.2 years	6–8 months
Hypertension	All	58 million[a]	10[e]	3.5–4 months[g]	3.5–4 months[g]
Kidney failure	All	41,000[b]	11[e]	2–3 months	Unknown
Infant respiratory failure	Premature infants	75,000–100,000[b]	20–30[c]	3–4 months	Unknown
Appendicitis	All	273,000[b]	50[c]	4 months	0
Diabetes	All	6 million[a]	25	6 months	Unknown
Pregnancy, puerperal sepsis and/or hemorrhage	Women 15–44	4 million[b]	45	2 weeks[d]	0
Pneumonia & influenza	All	400,000–1,000,000[b]	9[c]	3 months	0
Tuberculosis	All	27,000[b]	15[c]	3 months[h]	Uncertain[h]
Trauma, life-threatening	All	50–65 million[b]	24–38	1.5–2 months	3–4 months

a. Prevalence (all cases).

b. Incidence (new cases per annum).

c. For cancer of the cervix, colon cancer, infant respiratory distress syndrome, and appendicitis, we have made rough approximations based on mean age at death and life expectancy at that age.

d. Double for women.

e. From Table E, "Gain in expectation of life at birth due to eliminating specified cause of death by race and sex, for those who would have died; United States, 1979–81" (National Center for Health Statistics, 1988).

f. Includes coronary-artery surgery, coronary care units, and medical management of heart disease.

g. Impact of treatment of hypertension on stroke and heart mortality contributing about one-half to each.

h. Increased likelihood of poor compliance with treatment regimens and increased frequency of infection with drug-resistant strains of tuberculosis make these estimates speculative and subject to change.

Sources:

Cancer of the cervix and colon: Gloeckler Ries et al., 1990; American Cancer Society, 1991.

Colorectal cancer: Gloeckler Ries et al., 1990

Peptic ulcer: Adams and Benson, 1991; Fineberg and Pearlman, 1981.

Ischemic Heart Disease: National Heart, Lung, and Blood Institute, 1985.

Hypertension: Subcommittee on Definition and Prevalence of the Joint National Committee on Detection, Evaluation and Treatment of High Blood Pressure, 1985; Collins et al., 1990; MacMahon et al., 1990.

Kidney failure: U.S. Renal Data System, 1991.

Infant respiratory distress syndrome: Office of Technology Assessment, 1987; Buehler et al., 1987.

Appendicitis: Graves, 1990.

Diabetes: Adams and Benson, 1991.

Pregnancy: National Center for Health Statistics, 1991.

Pneumonia and influenza, Burman et al., 1985; Williams et al., 1988; National Center for Health Statistics, 1992.

Tuberculosis: Amler and Dull, 1987.

Trauma: Collins, 1990; National Center for Health Statistics, 1992; Trunkey, 1990.

Data collected by the National Health Interview Survey, combined with the size of the nursing-home population, indicate that 35 million people in the United States live with disabling conditions (Adams and Benson, 1991). Data from the Survey of Income and Program Participation, which includes information on functional limitations, work limitations, and receipt of disability benefits from Social Security or the Veterans Administration, indicate that about 46 million people have some type of work or functional limitation (Pope and Tarlov, 1991). Only limited data are available on the magnitude of specific causes of disability, and we have few quantitative data on the potential role of medical care in ameliorating the national burden of disability. Indeed, most data suggest that the numbers of disabled persons are increasing, and it is only in 1993 that evidence has been presented that the prevalence and incidence of chronic disability have begun to decline (Manton et al., 1993).

Medical care improves the quality of life primarily in alleviating pain and suffering, and in ameliorating physical, social, and mental dysfunction. Pain and dysfunction are usually specific, or even unique, to a particular medical condition. To estimate the contribution of medical care, therefore, it is necessary to consider the effects of specific treatments for specific illnesses or conditions (the same approach used to estimate contributions to life expectancy).

Formal, quantitative, condition-specific quality-of-life measurement methods are in an early stage of development, but there is abundant qualitative evidence of the role of medical care in improving function and in relieving suffering. Formal studies have addressed the poor quality of life experienced in chronic illness (e.g., depression, AIDs, arthritis), the positive impact of therapy (e.g., relief of angina pectoris by coronary bypass surgery, improvement of function and relief of pain by hip replacement, relief of depression by mood-elevating drugs), and the trade-off between poorer quality of life and the effort to increase life expectancy.

Impaired functional status, poor mental health, and perceived pain associated with nine common medical conditions were documented in the Medical Outcomes Study. Each condition reflected a unique profile among the several indices of quality of life (Stewart et al., 1989; Tarlov et al., 1989). Hypertension had the least overall impact; congestive heart failure, myocardial infarct, and gastrointestinal disorders the greatest. Depression was found to impair function as much as or more than the other eight conditions (Wells et al., 1989).

Impaired functional status, poor mental health, and pain are the major complaints for which individuals seek relief from medical care. Severe pain caused by acute illnesses such as appendicitis, myocardial infarct, and renal colic, and by serious injury, is relieved by successful treatment. Increasingly, the pain and suffering associated with chronic illness preoccupies the medical professions, and documentation of successful intervention is beginning to be compiled. Table 10–3 lists a selection of conditions for which medical care has profoundly improved the quality of life; a more complete list awaits more formal documentation and analysis.

Unipolar depression (as distinguished from bipolar or so-called manic depression) is a condition characterized by high prevalence, high morbidity, and high aggregate cost. It affects an estimated 10.5 million adults at any one time, and 8–12 percent of males and 20–26 percent of females at some point in their lives. Half of those who recover from an episode of major depressive disorder will have at least one recurrence. An episode of major depression typically lasts 6 months or more in the absence of therapy. Effective treatment with antidepressive drugs, psychotherapy, or electroconvulsive therapy is, in principle, readily available and is effective in 70–80 percent of patients, but more than half of all persons with major depressive disorder receive no treatment, and half of those who are treated receive treatment in ineffective amounts (Boyd and Weissman, 1981; H.S. Frazier, unpublished manuscript).

Arteriosclerotic heart disease, a serious threat to life, is also associated with profound disturbances in quality of life. Coronary artery revascularization, introduced primarily in an effort to reduce the risk of death, has been valuable primarily in relief of the severe pain of angina pectoris and in improving physical function. Eighty percent of patients undergoing coronary artery bypass surgery were afflicted with angina preoperatively. Of these, one half to two thirds are relieved during the 5 years following operation, and one third to one half experience improved physical function (CASS Principal Investigators and Their Associates, 1983). The quality-of-life advantages of surgical over medical care may fade after 5 years, as graft closure accelerates. Of the more than 2 million living men and women who have undergone coronary bypass graft surgery, as few as 12 percent after 5 years, and 5 percent after 10 years are functionally improved and free of pain (Veterans Administration Coronary Artery Bypass Surgery Cooperative Study Group, 1992).

Osteoarthritis, a chronic illness of growing prevalence in the elderly, occurs in an estimated 6 percent of the population as detected by radiological examination, and in 0.5 percent as manifested in pain and physical dysfunction (Lawrence et al., 1989). Total joint replacement to relieve pain and restore function has been one of the great success stories of medical care today. In 1989, 86,000 total or partial hip replacements and 41,000 knee replacements were performed on American men and women 65 and over, at rates of 2.8 and 1.3 per thousand respectively in that age group. Given life expectancy of 17 years at age 65, 3–4 percent of individuals over 65 will undergo replacement of one or both hips, and 1.5–2 percent will undergo replacement of one or both knees. Of the more than 1 million men and women who have undergone total hip or knee replacement, 85–90 report relief of pain and 70–80 percent report functional improvement (Liang et al., 1982).

Other medical conditions for which pain relief is a dominant consideration are terminal cancer, peptic-ulcer disease, gall-bladder disease, migraine, and the operative experience. Over 500,000 American deaths are attributed to cancer each year. Many of these patients are in severe and constant pain (Bonica, 1986; Jacox et al., 1994). It is increasingly agreed that such pain is not necessary, and that analgesics sufficient to control it should be made available.

A 1981 report estimated that about 250,000 Americans develop new peptic ulcers each year (Fineberg and Pearlman, 1981). Peptic ulcers are characterized by pain that is typically epigastric and often severe. They are treated by reducing acid secretion, neutralizing acid with antacids, and most recently by prescribing cimetidine or the more potent drugs ranitidine and famotidine, which block H2-receptors. How much of the recent decline in incidence in peptic-ulcer disease is due to treatment and how much to prevention (e.g., by stopping smoking) is not clear.

Before the age of 65 an estimated 20 percent of the population will suffer one or more acute attacks of cholecystitis of sufficient severity to justify removal of the gall bladder. While cholecystectomy in patients harboring asymptomatic gallstones is now generally considered unjustified, it can profoundly improve the quality of life of patients who suffer repeated attacks of debilitating biliary colic (Bates, 1991; Thistle et al., 1984).

Migraine, a disorder with many manifestations in addition to headache, can be profoundly disabling. Though poorly understood, it can often yield to medical care. Oliver Sacks, in *Migraine: Understanding a Common Disorder* (1985), asserts that "headache is the commonest complaint that patients bring to physicians, and migraine is the commonest functional disorder by which patients are afflicted." Sacks estimates that "common migraine" headache occurs in 5–20 percent of the population and that 1–2 percent suffer the more debilitating classical migraine. According to a mail survey (Stewart et al., 1992) 18 million females and 5.6 million males currently suffer from severe migraine headaches, and 8.7 million females and 2.6 million males from moderate to severe disabling headache. A wide spectrum of medications, tailored to individual patients, in combination with a variety of supportive therapies, keeps the majority largely free of pain.

Approximately 22 million operations are performed in the United States annually, nearly one for every ten individuals. Freedom from pain during the operation itself has been routinely available for nearly 150 years, thanks to modern anesthesia, but suffering after surgery has varied from mild to unbearable. Only recently have techniques for relieving perioperative pain, such as self-medication and continuous epidural anesthesia, become available. We estimate that these forms of pain relief are still provided to no more than 25 percent of patients undergoing abdominal or thoracic surgery. They should be made more widely available.

Benign prostatic hypertrophy afflicts almost all men, in varying degrees, with age. The prostate surrounds the urethra, and as it enlarges can obstruct the flow of urine. In as many as 5 percent of men 70 years of age and older it enlarges to the point that urination is completely obstructed, requiring urgent medical and surgical care, usually including surgical removal of all or part of the prostate. The majority of men, however, experience only partial obstruction, and the medical issue is whether to proceed with prostatectomy for symptomatic relief—that is, to improve the quality of life. Fowler and colleagues (1988) reported that 93 percent of severely and 79 percent of moderately symptomatic patients experienced subjective improvement in the quality of life after surgery, but for men with lesser symptoms the quality of life was well served by "watchful waiting."

A 1981 report to the Congress on handicapped people (Office of Technology Assessment, 1981) reported that there are "11,415,000 blind and (at least moderately) visually impaired people; 16,219,000 deaf and hearing impaired people; 1,995,000 speech-impaired people; 1,532,000 people affected by paralysis; 2,500,000 people with upper extremity impairments (not including paralysis); and 358,000 people with the absence of major extremities . . . Overall, 67 percent of the impairments are found in the categories of blind and visually impaired and deaf and hearing impaired."

Few medical innovations have such a substantial and broad contribution as eyeglasses and contact lenses. The major refractive errors are easily diagnosed and relatively inexpensively ameliorated. Though eyeglasses and contact lenses are largely taken for granted by those who use them—a group that encompasses almost all of the population at one time or another during their lives—without them millions would not be able to read, drive a car, or pursue their occupations and recreations.

In 1980 over 18 million elderly persons suffered from some form of hearing loss, and this number will approximate 25 million in the 1990s (Mulrow et al., 1990). The hearing loss that accompanies the normal aging process can be ameliorated, however, with the standard hearing aid. In a randomized study of elderly veterans with impaired hearing, 82 percent of whom reported adverse effects on the quality of life and 24 percent of whom were depressed, those who received a hearing aid experienced highly significant improvements in social and emotional function, communication skills, cognitive function, and relief from depression (Mulrow et al., 1990).

Finally, though we have not included the benefits of diagnosis in our table, it is worth noting that accurate diagnosis alone can enhance quality of life. Patients often experience anxiety if their symptoms suggest a life-threatening disease. When the physician can assure the patient that the problem is minor or temporary, anxiety is relieved. Some evidence suggests that, even when the news is bad, patients become less anxious and set about making the best of it.

Summary of Contributions of Medical Care to Quality of Life

Table 10–3 gives some notion of the numbers of people in the United States who have benefited from various medical interventions intended to improve their quality of life. As the table documents, millions of people have gained relief from pain and improvement of function from therapeutic drugs, surgery, medical management, and medical devices. These cures and ameliorations represent much of what we buy with our medical budget. Those who have not experienced a handicap or limitation of activity tend to underestimate its effect on the person afflicted. But the miseries of depression, shortness of breath, angina, creaky and painful joints, severe pain, disabling headaches, major indigestion, urinary difficulties, toothache and sore gums, fuzzy vision, faulty

Table 10-3 Quality-of-Life Benefits. Effects of Treatments for Selected Conditions, Estimated Numbers at Risk and Gains in Quality of Life for Those Receiving Treatment.

Condition/Symptoms	Number at Risk	Lifetime Risk	Treatment	Magnitude of Relief in Treated Patients	Proportion Treated
Unipolar depression	10.5 million[a]	8–12% men, 20–26% women	Drugs, ECT, psychotherapy	70–80%	<50%
Ischemic heart disease and angina	6 million[a] 150,000–200,000[b]	10–15% men, 3–5% women	Coronary artery revascularization; drugs	50–66% for 5 years	Unknown
Osteoarthritis pain, joint dysfunction	joint replacements 86,000 hip[b], 41,000 knee[b]	3–4% hip, 1.5–2% knee	Joint replacement	85–90% pain relief; 70–80% functional improvement	Unknown
Terminal cancer (severe pain)	450,000–475,000[a]	30%	Analgesic drugs	Nearly complete relief	40–50%
Peptic ulcer (severe pain)	250,000[b]	10–15% men, 4–15% women	H2-receptor-blocking drugs	80–90% healed in 4–8 weeks	Unknown
Gallstones with biliary colic	0.5–1 million[b]	9% men, 27% women	Cholecystectomy	67% pain relief at 2 years	Unknown
Migraine (severe)	18 million women, 5.6 million men[a]	10–15%	Medication	50–75% relief	Unknown
Post-operative pain	22 million operations[b]	90%	Epidural anesthesia; self-medication	Nearly complete relief	<25%
Benign prostatic hypertrophy	125,000[b]	20–45%	Prostatic resection, drugs, etc.	79–93% relief of symptoms	Unknown
Osteoporosis and fracture	1 million[b] (women)	10–12% by age 65, over 20% at 80	Hormone replacement therapy; calcium	20% reduction in fractures in 1st 2 years, then 60% reduction	50%
Poliomyelitis with paralysis	All	0.5–1% prior to 1950	Vaccine	Nearly complete protection	74% pre-school, 98% entering school
Nonfatal stroke	1.9 million	5% by age 70	Treatment of hypertension	50% reduction in incidence	50%
Asthma	10 million[a]	5–10%	Medication	Relief of dyspnea, cough and wheezing	50%
Myopia and presbyopia	All but the blind	Nearly 100%	Lenses	Visual acuity adequate for most activities	Nearly all at some time
Cataract	6 million[a]	5–10%	Lens removal; intraocular implant	75–95% improvement in visual acuity	Unknown

Health Condition	Prevalence / Incidence	Lifetime Risk	Treatment	Relief of Symptoms	Proportion Treated
Impaired hearing	18 million elderly[a]	35–50%	Hearing aid	Improved social function and communication	Unknown
Trauma	50–65 million[b]	Nearly all	Surgical correction, rehabilitation	Restoration of function, pain relief, improved appearance	Unknown

Dental Health Condition	Lifetime Risk	Treatment	Relief of Symptoms	Proportion Treated
Cavities	80%	Fillings	Pain relief, restoration of function	70%
Periodontal disease	20%	Surgery and/or antibiotics	Pain relief, retention of teeth	50%
Edentulism	8% (75% 65 and over)	Dentures and/or implants	Restoration of appearance, speech, ability to eat	Unknown
Malocclusion	54%	Orthodontics	Restoration of appearance, speech, ability to eat	20% if uninsured, 70% if insured

a. Prevalence (all cases).

b. Incidence (new cases per annum).

Sources:

Depression: Boyd and Weissman, 1981; H.S. Frazier, The treatment of unipolar depression, 1993, unpublished manuscript.

Ischemic heart disease and angina: We are not aware of data on the nationwide incidence or prevalence of angina. As an approximation, we assume an incidence of between one half and three-quarters the number of coronary bypass operations, for which angina is a major indication. Over 200,000 bypass operations are performed annually (Feinleib et al., 1989; see also Califf et al., 1989; Winslow et al., 1988; and Alderman et al., 1982).

Osteoarthritis: Lawrence et al., 1989.

Cancer, terminally ill: Bonica, 1986.

Peptic Ulcer: Adams and Benson, 1991; Fineberg and Pearlman, 1981.

Gallstones with biliary colic: Incidence estimated indirectly from prevalence of gallstones and variations in incidence of biliary-tract-related pain reported in patients with previously demonstrated gallstones (Thistle et al., 1984; Ransohoff et al., 1983; Bates et al., 1991).

Migraine: Stewart et al., 1992; Adams and Benson, 1991.

Postoperative pain: Acute Pain Management Guideline Panel, 1992.

Benign prostatic hypertrophy: Over 350,000 prostatectomies are performed annually in the United States. In a nonrandomized group of 318 patients scheduled for prostatic resection, 38% were classified as severely symptomatic (Fowler et al., 1988). We estimate that approximately 125,000 prostatectomies are performed for severe symptoms. The risk of undergoing prostatectomy by age 80 has been reported to vary between 20 and 45% (Wennberg and Gittelsohn, 1982).

Osteoporosis and fracture: Weinstein and Tosteson, 1990; Daly et al., 1992.

Poliomyelitis: Morbidity and Mortality Weekly Report, 1986.

Nonfatal stroke: There are an estimated 1.9 million stroke patients in the United States, with a probability of suffering a stroke by age 70 of 5% (Kannel et al., 1986). About two thirds are nonfatal (Collins et al., 1990).

Asthma: Amler and Dull, 1987; see also Anderson et al., 1981, 1983.

Myopia and presbyopia: Curtin, 1970.

Cataract: Adams and Benson, 1991; Office of Technology Assessment, 1988; Brenner et al., 1993.

Hearing: Mulrow et al., 1990.

Trauma: Collins, 1990; Trunkey, 1990; National Center for Health Statistics, 1992.

Dental Health: Burt and Eklund, 1992.

hearing, paralysis, and broken bones would add up to a national disaster without the relief we are able to document.

As the column on the far right in Table 10–3 indicates, we are very uncertain about
the numbers of recipients of these various interventions. Nevertheless, it is clear that
much effective care is being given. How much more relief is possible, and at what additional cost, must be left for future inquiry.

We look forward to future summaries that are more complete than Table 10–3, and
to the development of better methods for grading improvements. Current research on
the definition and measurement of quality of life may soon lead to an improved inventory. Verbrugge's research on chronic conditions has already been informative (Verbrugge, 1989). When such inventories are accompanied by better data on the extent of
relief and its costs, a more complete assessment of efforts to improve the quality of life
will be possible.

Tradeoffs Between Quality and Length of Life

Much surgery is intended primarily or in part to improve the quality of life: notable examples include orthopedic joint replacement to relieve pain and improve function, in-
traocular lens implantation to improve vision, hysterectomy to relieve severe dysmen-
orrhea, and cochlear implants to improve hearing. All surgery, together with the
necessary anesthesia, entails some risk of death or complication. In some cases the
risks are large, and the potential benefits may or may not be large enough to justify
the risks. In many, perhaps most, cases, however, the risk is small, the anticipated benefit relatively large, and the trade-off therefore favorable—a potentially large improvement in the quality of life in exchange for a small loss in life expectancy.

Other medical interventions may entail a trade-off in the opposite direction: a risk of
a poorer quality of life in exchange for increased life expectancy. Immunization, for
example, may entail slight risks of serious side effects but protect against infectious
disease that could lead to death. Measles vaccination is accompanied by encephalitis
(inflammation of the brain) at a rate estimated at between 1 in 87,000 and less than 1 in
a million; this rate is less than one thousandth of that which occurs in measles itself
(Bloch et al., 1985). Following the introduction of measles vaccine in 1963, the nearly
500,000 cases of measles that had occurred annually fell to a low of 1,497 in 1983,
preventing an estimated 17,400 cases of mental retardation over a 20-year period.
However, there has since been a gradual and accelerating increase in measles incidence; 18,193 cases were reported in 1989, predominantly among unvaccinated
preschool children in inner cities (Hersh et al., 1992).

The risk of paralysis following the administration of live oral poliovirus vaccine is
estimated to be approximately 1 in 3 million. (Inactivated poliovirus vaccine appears
to be free of this risk but may provide less immunity.) Before the introduction of polio
vaccine, there were more than 20,000 cases of paralytic poliomyelitis annually in the

United States. In the past decade there have been fewer than 25 cases a year (Morbidity and Mortality Weekly Report, 1986).

The risks of rubella vaccine appear to be even smaller than those of other vaccines, while the quality-of-life benefits are equally large. Rubella in the past has occurred in epidemics; the one in 1964 resulted in 20,000 cases of congenital rubella syndrome (deafness, blindness, and mental retardation) in the newborn infants of infected mothers. Rubella vaccine was licensed in 1969. Only 221 cases of rubella were reported in 1988, and only 6 cases of congenital rubella syndrome were reported in 1987 (Morbidity and Mortality Weekly Review, 1989). As with measles, however, relaxation in compliance with vaccination has been followed by a resurgence of congenital rubella syndrome in the 1990s (Lee et al., 1992).

Trade-offs of poorer quality of life for increased life expectancy characterize several spheres of patient care, notably chronic renal failure treated by hemodialysis; breast cancer, colon cancer, and other malignancies treated with adjuvant chemotherapy; and hypertension treated by drugs with unpleasant side effects (Croog and Levine, 1989).

Adjuvant chemotherapy in the treatment of breast cancer has typically been accompanied by fatigue, hair loss, nausea, job loss, marital stress and failure, and other profoundly unpleasant side effects, with modest gains in the probability of survival (Meyerowitz et al., 1979; Mosteller and Falotico-Taylor, 1989; Fallowfield, 1990). Yet the majority of women treated "claimed they would recommend participation in a similar program to a friend" (Meyerowitz et al., 1979). Recent advances in the treatment of breast cancer have reduced the negative quality-of-life burden, but there remains considerable disagreement among physicians about the justification for chemotherapy in treatment of breast cancer and other cancers for which the gains in survival may be small or undocumented.

The side effects of antihypertensive drugs (unsteadiness, weakness, impotence, and difficulty with sleep) have been a significant obstacle to the control of blood pressure in hypertensive patients (Croog et al., 1986). Told that they have a "disease" but experiencing no symptoms, many patients are averse to taking medication that causes unpleasant symptoms. The introduction of new and equally effective drugs, relatively free of side effects and tailored to individual responses, has recently improved patient compliance and control of blood pressure (Wassertheil-Smoller et al., 1991).

Discussion and Conclusions

We have several objectives in describing this study. First we want to illustrate a method for quantifying the improvement in life expectancy resulting from the application of one or a package of interventions to a particular condition. The method is dependent upon the prior collection of accurate information on the efficacy of the interventions, a requirement that cannot yet be met in the case of some important conditions and treatments. We call attention here to several circumstances that affect the validity and precision of our estimates. For example, the prolongation of life due to the treatment of hypertension can be initiated by active screening programs to discover hypertensives, on the one hand, or by incidental discovery of hypertension in the course of managing unrelated complaints, on the other. The assignment of medical benefit to either method of case finding is somewhat arbitrary, although the overall incidence of hypertension, however discovered, has a more secure empirical basis.

Another source of approximation in the assignment of benefits stems from the interactions among different conditions and treatments. For example, the discovery and treatment of hypertension is reflected in a decline in cerebrovascular and kidney diseases. More frequent discovery and management of hypertension also reduces the burden of heart disease, but estimates of the extent of the reduction are confounded by concurrent improvements due to better diet and more exercise.

We also note that we have not included in our estimates of the benefits of preventive services those due to lifestyle changes that depend on individual initiative rather than interventions by credentialed care-givers. We omit these important lifestyle changes in order to avoid giving medical care credit for improvements that can be availed of outside the system for professional medical care. We have chosen to restrict our application to conditions of high prevalence, a risk of fatal outcome, and treatment of proven efficacy for a component of the population of the United States of America.

Our second objective is to discover what the results of the method can tell us about the problems in, or opportunities for, the deployment of resources to improve health. What do the results tell us about successful programs, unmet needs, and unrealized potential? Several points deserve emphasis.

We stress once again the critical importance of the results of systematic, ongoing assessment of medical technology, where technology is used in the broadest sense. Knowledge of efficacy, effectiveness, cost, and impact are not the sole determinants of policy decisions, but they powerfully inform our choices.

Our results in Tables 10–1 and 10–2 show some unanticipated effects. The effects of preventive measures on life expectancy achieved as of 1990 (roughly 18–19 months) are less than half as great as the prolongation of life from curative measures (roughly 44–45 months). We do not argue for deemphasis of preventive interventions simply because their impact is less; rather, we urge that curative interventions not be ignored in competition with prevention for available resources. Studies of the cost-effectiveness of a portfolio of preventive compared to curative services would be especially useful here.

We note also the unrealized potential for preventive services in the cases of hypertension (estimated at 1.5–2 months from programmatic screening), counseling regarding smoking cessation (1 month, but possibly much more), and immunization against pneumococcal pneumonia (1.5 months).

The unrealized potential of curative interventions includes packages of services for heart disease as noted above (6–8 months), treatment of hypertension in reducing stroke (1–1.5 months), and the size of the estimate of unrealized potential for treatment of trauma (3–4 months).

Our third objective is to support the growing recognition that health status and well-being, or quality of life, are coming to have at least equal importance with life expectancy in the evaluation of health care by its recipients. Our analysis both of life expectancy and of quality of life is anchored in an approach through individual conditions, the effects of which are then aggregated. In the case of life expectancy, the aggregation may confront problems of data quality, but because the aggregation occurs on a single outcome variable, many problems are simplified.

Assessing quality of life is substantially more complicated. Two decades of work by others have done much to define and organize a set of basic components of global quality of life in the realm of social functioning, physical mobility, capacity for self-care, mental health, and pain. These generic measures permit some comparisons of quality of life across condition-intervention pairs, or the gain in generic measures with time after intervention. Where more specificity is required, condition-specific measures may be added in what amounts to a trade-off between aggregation and generality on the one hand, and sensitivity and relevance on the other. Our belief is that recourse to either generic or condition-specific measures should be determined by the purpose of the description, and that both types of measures have an important place.

In Table 10–3, for example, comparisons across conditions require a method for weighting the impact on quality of life of repeated, short episodes of disability as in asthma, or with chronic, unremitting pain as in metastatic cancer. That decided, the investigator may design a data acquisition system to capture the time/intensity measure and the qualitative generic measure. In the case of chronic conditions, the choice of a generic measure would be influenced by the condition-intervention pair under study and the purpose of the study. For example, the generic measure of performance in social role could be used across the conditions of unipolar depression and terminal cancer in studying treatment with mood-elevation drugs. Table 10–3 shows that large groups in need of treatment are receiving it, but also that many are not.

Our fourth objective is to point out that the need for information on the outcome variables of efficacy and effectiveness, and measures of altered quality of life, can only increase as resources become more constrained, technology proliferates, and health care emphasizes functional status and well-being over simple survival. Organizing the relevant information for the use of physicians and their patients could be achieved by developing and routinely updating an inventory of condition-intervention pairs such as we have illustrated here. Such data might most appropriately be incorporated into the routinely published reports of the Public Health Service. An inventory of this type is urgently needed to assist social institutions (such as the Oregon Medicaid project) in making the value judgements involved in setting priorities and allocating resources.

Appendix: Estimation of the Contribution of the Fall in Death Rate from Heart Disease to Increased Life Expectancy 1950–1989

1. Estimation from Abridged U.S. Life Tables

For selected conditions *Health, United States, 1991* (National Center for Health Statistics, 1992) provides death rates per 100,000 resident population by 10-year age intervals for selected years beginning in 1950. Table 33 provides these for heart disease. The abridged life table for 1988 (U.S. Department of Health and Human Services, 1991) gives the number of deaths from all causes of a cohort of 100,000 born alive by 5-year intervals, and the number remaining alive at the beginning of each age interval. By combining each pair of 5-year intervals we matched the 10-year intervals of Table 33; we then adjusted the age-specific 40-year declines in deaths for diseases of the heart per 100,000, for the number remaining alive in the 1988 life table at each 10-year age interval. These adjusted deaths were then fitted to the size at each age interval of the "stationary population" on which the calculation of life expectancy is based. Using this procedure we calculated that the decrease in death rate for diseases of the heart between 1950 and 1989 was responsible for an increase in life expectancy of 3.49 years, of which 40 percent was divided equally between treatment of ischemic heart disease and screening and treatment of hypertension in Tables 10–2 and 10–1, respectively.

2. Estimation from Age-Adjusted Death Rates

For most diagnoses, death rates from 1950 to 1989 are given as a single age-adjusted number. To test the reliability of limiting the basis on which to estimate changes in life expectancy to age-specific death rates, we compared this approach to the results of the calculation based on life-tables. The age-adjusted death rate for all causes fell from 840.5 in 1950 to 523.0 in 1989, a decrease of 317.5; for diseases of the heart it fell from 307.2 to 155.9, a decrease of 151.3. Life expectancy during the same period rose 7.1 years. The drop in age-adjusted death rate for diseases of the heart contributed just under half of the fall in the death rate for all causes ($151.3/317.5 = 0.48$), which, multiplied by 7.1, yields 3.41 years as a first approximation of the increase in life expectancy attributable to diseases of the heart.

3. Estimation for U.S. Life Tables Eliminating Certain Causes of Death

A second approximation of gain in life expectancy from the fall in death rate attributable to heart disease was made by extrapolating the National Center for Health Statistics life tables of the gain in life expectancy that would occur by "eliminating specified causes of death" (National Center for Health Statistics, 1988). Elimination of all "diseases of heart" from the 1979–1981 life table was estimated to increase life expectancy by 5.79 years. The age-adjusted mortality from diseases of the heart was 202.0 per

100,000 at that time and fell to 155.9 in 1989, a fall of just under 25 percent. If eliminating all deaths from heart disease at a time when the death rate was 202.0 would increase life expectancy by 5.79 years, then a fall of 151.3 (307.2 in 1950 to 155.9 in 1989) should increase life expectancy by $\frac{3}{4} \times 5.79$ years $= 4.34$ years [or, more precisely, $155.9/202.0 \times 5.79 = 4.47$].

Estimations of the increase in life expectancy resulting from the fall in the death rate from cerebrovascular diseases 1950–1989, approximated as above, were: 1.44, 1.34, and 1.35 years.

Acknowledgments

This study was supported in part by a grant from the New England Medical Center, Inc., through the auspices of the Henry J. Kaiser Family Foundation. It was first presented at a conference supported by the New England Medical Center, Inc., through the auspices of the Henry J. Kaiser Family Foundation and held at the Harvard School of Public Health on October 14, 1992, and appeared in an abbreviated version in Bunker, Frazier, and Mosteller, 1994.

The plan for this study was conceived at the Henry J. Kaiser Family Foundation in Menlo Park, California in November, 1988, at a small conference attended by Paul Beeson, John Bunker, Alain Enthoven, Jacob Feldman, Sol Levine, Frederick Mosteller, Ralph Schaffarzick, Peter Schlenzka, Adam Seiver, and Alvin Tarlov; many of their suggestions, as well as their published work, contributed to our investigations. We are indebted to them and to many others from whom we sought advice. An early planning grant was supported by the Commonwealth Fund.

Lester R. Curtin, Chief of the Statistical Methods Section, National Center for Health Statistics, provided valuable guidance in the preparation of estimates of life expectancy. Marie McPherson and Elisabeth Burdick provided day-to-day assistance in the preparation of the manuscript and tables. Alexia Antczak-Bouckoms prepared the data on dental health for Table 10–3. Jennifer Falotico-Taylor made valuable contributions to an earlier draft. Alvin Tarlov and Sol Levine have provided continuous encouragement.

References

Acute Pain Management Guideline Panel. 1992. *Acute Pain Management: Operative or Medical Procedures and Trauma. Clinical Practice Guideline.* AHCPR Pub. No. 92-0032. Rockville, MD: Agency for Health Care Policy and Research, Public Health Service, U.S. Department of Health and Human Services.

Adams, P. F., and V. Benson. 1991. Current estimates from the National Health Interview Survey. National Center for Health Statistics. *Vital Health Stat.* 10(181).

Alderman, E. L., L. Fisher, C. Maynard, M. B. Mock, I. Ringqvist, M. G. Bourassa, G. C. Kaiser, and M. J. Gillespie. 1982. Determinants of coronary surgery in a consecutive patient series from geographically dispersed medical centers: The Coronary Artery Surgery Study. *Circulation* 66(suppl. 1) I6–I15.

Alpert, M., and H. Raiffa. 1969. *A Progress Report on the Training of Probability Assessors.* Cambridge, MA: Harvard School of Business Administration.

American Cancer Society. 1991. *Cancer Facts and Figures—1991.* Atlanta, GA: American Cancer Society.

Amler, R. W., and H. B. Dull. eds. 1987. *Closing the Gap: The Burden of Unnecessary Illness.* New York: Oxford University Press.

Anderson, H. R., P. A. Bailey, J. S. Cooper, and J. C. Palmer. 1981. Influence of morbidity, illness label, and social, family and health service factors on drug treatment of childhood asthma. *Lancet* 2:1030–1032.

Anderson, H. R., P. A. Bailey, J. S. Cooper, J. C. Palmer, and S. West. 1983. Morbidity and school absence caused by asthma and wheezy illness. *Arch. Dis. Child.* 58:777–784.

Anderson, O. W., and E. M. Morrison. 1989. The worth of medical care: A critical review. *Med. Care Rev.* 46:121–155.

Antiplatelet Trialists' Collaboration. 1994. Collaborative overview of randomised trials of antiplatelet therapy. I. Prevention of death, myocardial infarction, and stroke by prolonged antiplatelet therapy in various categories of patients. *Brit. Med. J.* 308:81–106.

Barry, M J., A. G. Mulley, F. J. Fowler, and J. E. Wennberg. 1988. Watchful waiting vs immediate transurethral resection for symptomatic prostatism: The importance of patients' preferences. *J.A.M.A.* 259:3010–3017.

Bates, T., S. R. Ebbs, M. Harrison, and R. P. A'Hern. 1991. Influence of cholecystectomy on symptoms. *Br. J. Surg.* 78:964–967.

Beeson, P. B. 1980. Changes in medical therapy during the past half century. *Medicine* 59:79–99.

Bloch, A. B., W. A. Orenstein, H. C. Stetler, S. G. Wassilak, R. W. Amler, K. J. Bart, C. D. Kirby, and A. R. Hinman. 1985. Health impact of measles vaccination in the United States. *Pediatrics* 76:524–532.

Bonica, J. J. 1986. Past and current status of pain research and therapy. *Semin. Anesth.* 5:82–99.

Boyd, J. H., and M. M. Weissman. 1981. Epidemiology of affective disorders. *Arch. Gen. Psychiatry* 38:1039–1046.

Brenner, M. H., B. Curbow, G.A.Q. Chase, J. C. Javitt, M. W. Legro, and A. Sommer. 1993. Vision change and quality of life in the elderly: Response to cataract surgery and treatment of other chronic ocular conditions. *Arch. Ophthalmol.* 111:680–685.

Buehler, J. W., J. C. Kleinman, C. J. Hogue, L. T. Strauss, and J. C. Smith. 1987. Birth weight-specific infant mortality, United States, 1960 and 1980. *Public Health Rep.* 102:151–161.

Bunker, J. P., W. H. Forrest Jr., F. Mosteller, and L. D. Vandam (eds.). 1969. The National Halothane Study: A study of the possible association between halothane anesthesia and postoperative hepatic necrosis. Washington, DC: Government Printing Office.

Bunker, J. P., and J. E. Wennberg. 1973. Operation rates, mortality statistics, and the quality of life. *N. Engl. J. Med.* 289:1249–1251.

Bunker, J. P., H. S. Frazier, and F. Mosteller. 1994. Improving health: Measuring effects of medical care. *Milbank Q.* 72:225–258.

Burman, L. A., R. Norrby, and B. Trollfors. 1985. Invasive pneumococcal infections: Incidence, predisposing factors, and prognosis. *Rev. Infect. Dis.* 7:133–142.

Burt, B. A., and S. A. Eklund. 1992. *Dentistry, Dental Practice, and the Community*, 4th edn. Philadelphia: W.B. Saunders.

Califf, R. M., F. E. Harrell, K. L. Lee, J. S. Rankin, M. A. Hlatky, D. B. Mark, R. H. Jones, L. H. Muhlbaier, H. N. Oldham Jr., and D. B. Pryor. 1989. The evolution of medical and surgical therapy for coronary artery disease. *JAMA* 261:2077–2086.

Carlson, R. J. 1975. *The End of Medicine*. New York: Wiley.

CASS Principal Investigators and Their Associates. 1983. Coronary Artery Surgery Study (CASS): A randomized trial of coronary artery surgery; survival data. *Circulation* 68:939–950.

Collins, J. G. 1990. Types of injuries by selected characteristics: United States, 1985-87. National Center for Health Statistics. *Vital Health Stat.* 10(175).

Collins, R., R. Peto, S. MacMahon, P. Hebert, N. H. Fiebach, K. A. Eberlein, J. Godnin, N. Qizilbash, J. O. Taylor, and C. H. Hennekens. 1990. Blood pressure, stroke, and coronary heart disease, 2. Short term reductions in blood pressure: Overview of randomized drug trials in their epidemiological context. *Lancet* 335:827–838.

Croog, S. H., S. Levine, M. A. Testa, B. Brown, C. J. Bulpitt, C. D. Jenkins, G. L. Klerman, and G. H. Williams. 1986. The effects of antihypertensive therapy on the quality of life. *N. Engl. J. Med.* 314:1657–1664.

Croog, S. H., and S. Levine. 1989. Quality of life and health care interventions. In H. E. Freeman and S. Levine (eds.). *Handbook of Medical Sociology*, pp. 508–528. Englewood Cliffs, NJ: Prentice-Hall.

Curtin, B. J. 1970. Myopia: A review of its etiology, pathology, genesis, and treatment. *Surv. Ophthalmol.* 15:1–17.

Daly, E., M. Roche, D. Barlow, A. Gray, K. McPherson, and M. Vessey. 1992. HRT: An analysis of benefits, risks and costs. *Br. Med. Bull.* 48:368–400.

Doll, R. 1992. Are we winning the war against cancer? A review in memory of Keith Durant. *Clin. Oncol. (R. Coll. Radiol.)* 4:257–266.

Drizd, T., A. L. Dannenberg, and A. Engle. 1986. *Blood Pressure Levels in Persons 18–74 Years of Age in 1976–1980, and Trends in Blood Pressure from 1960–1980 in the United States.* Vital and Health Statistics, Series 11, No. 234. DHHS Pub. No. (PHS) 86-1684. Washington, DC: U.S. Government Printing Office.

Early Breast Cancer Trialists' Collaborative Group. 1992. Systemic treatment of early breast cancer by hormonal, cytotoxic, or immune therapy: 133 randomized trials involving 31,000 recurrences and 24,000 deaths among 75,000 women. *Lancet* 339:1–15, 71–85.

Eddy, D. M. 1990. Screening for cervical cancer. *Ann. Intern. Med.* 113:214–226.

Fallowfield, L. 1990. *The Quality of Life: The Missing Measurement in Health Care.* London: Souvenire Press.

Feinleib, M., R. J. Havlik, R. F. Gillum, R. Pokras, E. McCarthy, and M. Moien. 1989. Coronary heart disease and related procedures: National Hospital Discharge Survey Data. *Circulation* 79(suppl. 1): I13–I18.

Fineberg, H. V., and L. A. Pearlman. 1981. *Benefit-and-Cost Analysis of Medical Interventions: The Case of Cimetidine and Peptic Ulcer Disease.* Case Study No. 11. Congress of the United States, Office of Technology Assessment. Washington, DC: Goverment Printing Office.

Fitzpatrick, G., R. Neutra, and J. P. Gilbert. 1977. Cost-effectiveness of cholecystectomy for silent gallstones. In J. P. Bunker, B. A. Barnes, F. Mosteller, (eds.), *Cost, Risks, and Benefits of Surgery*, pp. 246–263. New York: Oxford University Press.

Fowler, F. J., J. E. Wennberg, R. P. Timothy, M. J. Barry, A. G. Mulley, Jr., and D. Hanley. 1988. Symptom status and quality of life following prostatectomy. *JAMA* 259:3018–3022.

Gardner, P. and W. Schaffner. 1993. Immunization of adults. *N. Engl. J. Med.* 328:1252–1258.

Gloeckler Ries, L. A., B. F. Hankey, B. K. Edwards. 1990. *Cancer Statistics Review 1973–1987.* Division of Cancer Prevention and Control, National Cancer Institute, NIH Publication No. 90-2789. Bethesda, MD: National Institutes of Health.

Goldman, L., and E. F. Cook. 1984. The decline in ischemic heart disease mortality rates: An analysis of the comparative effects of medical interventions and changes in lifestyle. *Ann. Intern. Med.* 101:825–836.

Graves, E. J. 1990. *1988 Summary: National Hospital Discharge Survey.* Advance Data from Vital and Health Statistics, No. 185. Hyattsville, MD: National Center for Health Statistics.

Hadley, J. 1982. *More Medical Care, Better Health?* Washington, DC: Urban Institute Press.

Hennekens, C. H., R. Peto, G. B. Hutchison, and R. Doll. 1988. An overview of the British and American aspirin studies. *N. Engl. J. Med.* 318:923–924.

Hersh, B. S., L. E. Markowitz, E. F. Maes, A. W. Funkhouser, A. L. Baughman, B. I. Sirotkin, and S. C. Hadler. 1992. The geographic distribution of measles in the United States, 1980 through 1989. *JAMA* 267:1936–1941.

Illich, I. 1976. *Medical Nemesis: The Expropriation of Health*. New York: Random House.

Jacox, A., for the Management of Cancer Pain Guideline Panel. 1994. Management of Cancer Pain. Clinical Practice guideline No. 9. AHCPR Publication No. 94-0592. Rockville, MD: Agency for Health Care Policy and Research, Public Health Service.

Kannel, W. B., and T. J. Thom. 1986. Incidence, prevalence, and mortality of cardiovascular diseases. In J. W. Hurst (ed.), *The Heart: Arteries and Veins*, 6th edn., pp. 557–565. New York: McGraw-Hill.

Kannel, W. B., T. J. Thom, and J. W. Hurst. 1986. Incidence, prevalence, and mortality of cardiovascular diseases. *The Heart*, 6th edn. New York: McGraw-Hill.

Koplan, J. P., S. C. Schoenbaum, M. C. Weinstein, and D. W. Fraser. 1979. Pertussis vaccine: An analysis of benefits, risks and costs. *N. Engl. J. Med.* 301:906–911.

Korenbrot, C., A. B. Flood, M. Higgins, N. Roos, and J. P. Bunker. 1981. *Elective Hysterectomy: Costs, Risks, and Benefits*. Case Study No. 15, Congress of the United States, Office of Technology Assessment. Washington, DC: Government Printing Office.

Krolewski, A. S., J. H. Warram, and A. R. Christlieb. 1985. Onset, course, complications, and prognosis of diabetes mellitus. In A. Marble, L. Krall, R. F. Bradley, A. R. Christlieb, and J. S. Soeldner, (eds.). *Joslin's Diabetus Mellitus*, 12th edn, pp. 251–277. Philadelphia: Lea & Febiger.

Lawrence, R. C., M. C. Hochberg, J. L. Kelsey, F. C. McDuffie, T. A. Medsqer, Jr., W. R. Felts, and L. E. Shulman. 1989. Estimates of the prevalence of selected arthritic and musculoskeletal diseases in the United States. *J. Rheumatol.* 16:427–441.

Lee, S. H., D. P. Ewart, P. D. Frederick, and L. Mascola. 1992. Resurgence of congenital rubella syndrome in the 1990s: Report on missed opportunities and failed prevention policies among women of childbearing age. *JAMA* 267:2616–2620.

Levine, S., J. J. Feldman, and J. Elinson. 1983. Does medicine do any good? In D. Mechanic (ed.). *Handbook of Health, Health Care, and the Health Professions*, pp. 394–404. New York: Free Press.

Liang, M. H., K. E. Cullen, and R. Poss. 1982. Primary total hip or knee replacement: Evaluation of patients. *Ann. Intern. Med.* 97:735–739.

MacMahon, S., R. Peto, J. Cutler, R. Collins, P. Sorlie, J. Neaton, R. Abbott, J. Godwin, A. Dye, and J. Stamler. 1990. Blood pressure, stroke, and coronary heart disease, 1. Prolonged differences in blood pressure: Prospective observational studies corrected for the regression dilution bias. *Lancet* 335:765–774.

Mandel, J. S., J. H. Bond, T. R. Church, D. C. Snover, G. M. Bradley, L. M. Schuman, and F. Ederer for the Minnesota Colon Cancer Control Study. 1993. Reducing mortality from colorectal cancer by screening for fecal occult blood. *N. Engl. J. Med.* 328:1365–1371.

Manson, J. E., H. Tosteson, P. M. Ridker, S. Satterfield, P. Hebert, G. T. O'Connor, J. E. Buring, and C. H. Hennekens. 1992. The primary prevention of myocardial infarction. *N. Engl. J. Med.* 326:1406–1416.

Manton, K. G., L. S. Corder, and E. Stallard. 1993. Estimates of change in chronic disability and institutional incidence and prevalence rates in the U.S. elderly population from the 1982, 1984, and 1989 National Long Term Care Survey. *J. Gerontol*: Soc. Sci. 48:S153–S166.

McDermott, W. 1978. Medicine: The public good and one's own. *Perspect. Biol. Med.* 21:167–187.

McKeown, T. 1979. *The Role of Medicine: Dream, Mirage, or Nemesis?* Princeton, NJ: Princeton University Press.

McKinlay, J. B., and S. M. McKinlay. 1977. The questionable effect of medical measures on the decline of mortality in the United States in the twentieth century. *Milbank Q.* 55:405–428.

Meyerowitz, B. E., F. C. Sparks, and I. K. Spears. 1979. Adjuvant chemotherapy for breast carcinoma. *Cancer* 43:1613–1618.

Morbidity and Mortality Weekly Report. 1986. Poliomyelitis—United States, 1975–1984. 35:180–182.

Morbidity and Mortality Weekly Report. 1989. Rubella and Congenital Rubella Syndrome—United States, 1985–1988. 38:173–177.

Mosteller, F., and J. Falotico-Taylor (eds.). 1989. *Quality of Life and Technology Assessment.* Washington, DC: Institute of Medicine, National Academy Press.

Muller, C., J. Mandelblatt, C. B. Schechter, E. J. Power, B. M. Duffy, and J. L. Wagner. 1990. Costs and effectiveness of cervical cancer screening in elderly women. Congress of the United States, Office of Technology Assessment. Washington, DC: Government Printing Office.

Mulrow, C. D., C. Aguilar, J. E. Endicott, M. R. Tuley, R. Velez, W. S. Charlip, M. C. Rhodes, J. A. Hill, and L. A. DeNino. 1990. Quality-of-life changes and hearing impairment: A randomized trial. *Ann. Intern. Med.* 113:188–194.

National Center for Health Statistics. 1988. L. R. Curtin and R. J. Armstrong (eds.). *United States Life Tables Eliminating Certain Causes of Death. U.S. Decennial Life Tables for 1979–1981, Vol. 1, No. 2.* DHHS Publication No. (PHS) 88-1150-2. Public Health Service. Washington, DC: Government Printing Office.

National Center for Health Statistics. 1991. *Vital Statistics of the United States, 1989, Vol. 1, Natality.* Public Health Service. Washington, DC: Government Printing Office.

National Center for Health Statistics. 1992. *Health United States, 1991.* Hyattsville, MD: Public Health Service.

National Heart, Lung, and Blood Institute. 1985. *Ischemic Heart Disease. Fact Book, Fiscal Year 1985.* Bethesda, MD: National Institutes of Health.

Office of Technology Assessment, Congress of the United States. 1981. *Technology and Handicapped People.*

Office of Technology Assessment, Congress of the United States. 1987. *Neonatal Intensive Care for Low Birthweight Infants: Costs and Effectiveness.* Health Technology Case Study No. 38.

Office of Technology Assessment, Congress of the United States. 1988. *Appropriate Care for Cataract Surgery Patients Before and After Surgery: Issues of Medical Safety and Appropriateness.*

Peto, R., A. D. Lopez, J. Boreham, M. Thun, and C. Heath, Jr. 1992. Mortality from tobacco in developed countries: Indirect estimation from national vital statistics. *Lancet* 339:1268–1278.

Pope, A. M., A. R. Tarlov (eds.). 1991. *Disability in America: Toward a National Agenda for Prevention.* Washington, DC: Institute of Medicine, National Academy Press.

Ransohoff, D. F., W. A. Gracie, L. B. Wolfenson, and D. Neuhauser. 1983. Prophylactic cholecystectomy or expectant management for silent gallstones: A decision analysis to assess survival. *Ann. Intern. Med.* 99:199–204.

Ravnskov, U. 1992. Cholesterol lowering trials in coronary heart disease: Frequency of citation and outcome. *Br. Med. J.* 305:15–19.

Sacks, O. 1985. *Migraine: Understanding a Common Disorder.* Berkeley, CA: University of California Press.

Sandberg, S. I., B. A. Barnes, M. C. Weinstein, and P. Braun. 1985. Elective hysterectomy: Benefits, risks, and costs. *Med. Care* 23:1067–1085.

Sleven, M. L., and R. Gray. 1991. Adjuvant therapy for cancer of the colon: An important step forward. *Br. Med. J.* 302:1100–1101.

Stampfer, M. J., and G. A. Coldtiz. 1991. Estrogen replacement therapy and coronary heart disease: A quantitative assessment of the epidemiological evidence. *Prev. Med.* 20:47–63.

Stampfer, M. J., G. A. Colditz, W. C. Willett, J. E. Manson, B. Rosner, F. E. Speizer, and C. H. Hennekens. 1991. Postmenopausal estrogen therapy and cardiovascular disease: Ten-year follow-up from the Nurses' Health Study. *N. Engl. J. Med.* 325:756–762.

Steering Committee of the Physicians' Health Study Research Group. 1989. Final report on the aspirin component of the ongoing Physicians' Health Study. *N. Engl. J. Med.* 321:129–135.

Stewart, A. L., S. Greenfield, R. D. Hays, K. Wells, W. H. Rogers, S. D. Berry, E. A. McGlynn, and J. E. Ware, Jr. 1989. Functional status and well-being of patients with chronic conditions: Results from the Medical Outcomes Study. *JAMA* 262:907–913.

Stewart, W. F., R. B. Lipton, D. D. Celentano, and M. L. Reed. 1992. Prevalence of migraine headache in the United States: Relation to age, income, race, and other sociodemographic factors. *JAMA* 267:64–69.

Subcommittee on Definition and Prevalence of the Joint National Committee on Detection, Evaluation and Treatment of High Blood Pressure, 1984. 1985. Hypertension prevalence and the status of awareness, treatment, and control in the United States. *Hypertension* 7:457–468.

Tarlov, A. R., J. E. Ware, S. Greenfield, E. C. Nelson, E. Perrin, and M. Zubkoff. 1989. The Medical Outcome Study: An application of methods for monitoring the results of medical care. *JAMA* 262:925–930.

Taylor, I., and J.M.A. Northover. 1990. Adjuvant therapy in colorectal cancer: The need for a mega-trial. *Br. J. Surg.* 77:841–842.

Taylor, W. C., T. M. Pass, D. S. Shepard, and A. L. Komaroff. 1987. Cholesterol reduction and life expectancy. A model incorporating multiple risk factors. *Ann. Intern. Med.* 106:605–614.

Thistle, J. L., P. A. Cleary, J. M. Lachin, M. P. Tyor, T. Hersh. The Steering Committee, and The National Cooperative Gallstone Study Group. 1984. The natural history of cholelithiasis. The national cooperative gallstone study. *Ann. Intern. Med.* 101:171–175.

Trunkey, D. D. 1990. What's wrong with trauma care? *Bulletin of the American College of Surgeons* 75:10–15.

U.S. Department of Health and Human Services. 1991. *Vital Statistics of the United States, 1988: Life Tables*, Vol. 2, Section 6. DHHS Publication No. (PHS) 91-1104. Hyattsville, MD.

U.S. Preventive Services Task Force. 1989. *Guide to Clinical Preventive Services: An Assessment of the Effectiveness of 169 Interventions*. Baltimore: Williams & Wilkins.

U.S. Renal Data System. 1991. 1991 Annual Data Report: Excerpts. Survival probabilities and causes of death. *Am. J. Kidney Dis.* 18:49–60.

Verbrugge, L. M. 1989. Recent, present, and future health of American adults. *Annu. Rev. Public Health* 10:333–361.

Veterans Administration Coronary Artery Bypass Surgery Cooperative Study Group. 1992. Eighteen-year follow-up in the Veterans Affairs Cooperative Study of Coronary Artery Bypass Surgery for Stable Angina. *Circulation* 86:121–130.

Wassertheil-Smoller, S., M. Blaufox, A. Oberman, B. R. Davis, C. Swencionis, M. O. Knerr, C. M. Hawkins, and H. G. Langford for the TAIM Research Group. 1991. Effect of antihypertensives on sexual function and quality of life: The TAIM Study. *Ann. Intern. Med.* 114:613–620.

Weinstein, M. C., and A.N.A. Tosteson. 1990. Cost-effectiveness of hormone replacement. *Ann. N. Y. Acad. Sci.* 592:162–72.

Wells, K. B., A. Stewart, R. D. Hays, M. A. Burnam, W. Rogers, M. Daniels, S. Berry, S. Greenfield, and J. Ware. 1989. The functioning and well-being of depressed patients: Results from the Medical Outcomes Study. *JAMA* 262:914–919.

Wennberg, J. and A. Gittelsohn. 1982. Variations in medical care among small areas. *Sci. Am.* 246:120–134.

Williams, W. W., M. A. Hickson, M. A. Kane, A. P. Kendal, J. S. Spika, and A. R. Hinman. 1988. Immunization policies and vaccine coverage among adults: The risk for missed opportunities. *Ann. Intern. Med.* 108:616–625.

Winslow, C. M., J. B. Kosecoff, M. Chassin, D. E. Kanouse, and R. H. Brook. 1988. The appropriateness of performing coronary artery bypass surgery. *JAMA* 260:505–509.

11

Thinking Strategically About Society and Health

S. M. MILLER

This book has identified a number of social factors that influence health—factors such as race, gender, work, family community, culture, and the national economy. The authors trace the ways in which these factors affect health outcomes directly, indirectly, and in myriad combinations, and identify many facets of health that are shaped by social forces. They also point out important gaps in knowledge and observe that we are far from ready to fashion action plans with any certainty that they will be effective, not to mention politically and economically defensible.

This chapter focuses on such action plans—that is, on shaping the political economy of society and health. In some ways, building a compelling knowledge base is an easier task. Everyone recognizes, to some extent, that health is affected by social conditions—our financial and material resources, how we work and play, the time we have or lack to enjoy and support our families, whether our physical surroundings are reasonably pleasant and hazard-free. We know intuitively as well as intellectually that these aspects of life affect our own and everyone's health, but addressing them seriously seems a hopelessly expensive and long-term proposition.

The hypothesis that economic inequality may be bad for health emerges from virtually every chapter in this book. Although the evidence is still somewhat sketchy (Dutton and Levine, 1989), we will assume here that the proposition is true—that a society that can bring about greater economic parity will be a healthier one. From that premise, we will grapple with the fundamental challenge to a society-and-health perspective: Can the diagnosis that social arrangements may make people sick produce a treatment plan we can trust?

The 3 Rs of the Social Sciences

Since the society-and-health perspective is profoundly critical of the narrow disease paradigm that dominates the health fields, it is obligated to offer an alternative analysis, incorporating but not bounded by the displaced approach. As we have learned from Thomas Kuhn (1962), even clearly inadequate paradigms linger until a more compelling analysis can supplant it. If we are to avoid producing a formless hodgepodge of segmented policies propelled by narrow interests, we need to be guided by an overall vision of what should be done to improve health outcomes.

This will be very difficult to accomplish. We need, first of all, explanations that trace the impact of societal-level influences on the processes that affect functioning. In the case of accidents and injuries, for example, an investigator would have to demonstrate that societally conditioned factors affect their incidence in particular groups. The theme that is proposed here is that inequalities constitute the central though certainly not the sole set of "societally-conditioned factors." Rather than reviewing the enormous number of studies which show that health outcomes are linked to socioeconomic position (many of which are cited earlier in this book), this chapter will offer ways of differentiating between types or sources of inequality that can be useful in thinking about influences on health outcomes. Three broad processes or dynamics, which we can call the social sciences' 3Rs, are involved: resource position, relational position, and relative position.

Resource position points to people's material means. Inadequate resources affect people's well-being. Specifically, poverty is associated with poor health outcomes, including high infant-mortality rates. In Chapter 7, Harvey Brenner links poor health outcomes to unemployment rates; the relationship is due in part to resulting declines in income. Loss of income or chronic low income causes material deprivation; material deprivation affects healthy functioning.

Resources, however, encompass more than wage and salary income. Wealth and pensions contribute to a household's economic position. So do the public and private services (including medical services) available to its members. Formal schooling also significantly affects not only access to jobs but also an increasingly important resource, the ability to navigate a highly complicated and bureaucratized society. Having the financial assets and educational background to invest in and promote the social mobility of one's children is a substantial intergenerational resource transaction.

Such material resources have social-psychological effects on health and on everyday life. The link between deprivation and functioning can be fairly direct, as in the case of household injuries such as fires due to housing inadequacies. Low resources can also have an indirect effect, convincing people that they cannot improve their health by modifying their situation. Deprivation, frustration, low confidence, and fatalism feed on each other. They are not individual defects of character; they are predictable responses to the socially structured experiences of heavy stress and repeated defeats.

Relational position, derived and extended from the pioneering work of Jean Baker

Miller and her colleagues of the Stone Center Theory Group (Judith Jordan, Irene Stiver, and Janet Surrey), involves social roles and connection, the relations among individuals and groups (Miller and Roby, 1970; Miller, 1986; Jordan et al., 1991). The impact of unemployment, for instance, may result as much from the loss of an important social role as from income decline. Transitions, which are frequent occurrences for today's families, may undermine healthy functioning by loosening old connections while new ones are still fragile and strained. As Donald Patrick and Thomas Wickizer discuss in Chapter 3, the lack of effective community bonds means that individuals are not connected in positive ways. Chapter 8 by Jeffrey Johnson and Ellen Hall argues that the strains of working arise not only from specific tasks but also from work settings in which employees are treated as acted-upon objects rather than subjects who are connected in shaping their activities. If resources are households' economic means, relationships can be regarded as their social means.

Respect, or its absence, is a particularly important component of connection (Miller, 1993). Respect yields psychic and material resources; disrespect exacts penalties in both realms. Respected people feel, and are, supported by others, and are thus enhanced in their confidence, effectiveness, and self-respect. Those with whom they interact, whether bureaucrats, police, employers or landlords, are more likely to treat them decently. Respect has many and diverse payoffs. Respected people have access to associations and networks that can help them realize their economic or political objectives. To be disrespected, then, is no mere matter of a social-science status score on a reputational survey; disrespect reverberates through one's public and private life, limiting one's choices and connections. Discrimination on the basis of race—a powerful form of disrespect—still functions as a barrier in American society, as Gary King and David Williams demonstrate in Chapter 4. Disrespect is a burden many experience despite, rather than because of, their personal qualities.

According to the European Community's articulation of its social program, disrespect leads to the exclusion, marginalization, and isolation of particular groups: "The concept of social exclusion is dynamic . . . More clearly than the concept of poverty, understood far too often as referring exclusively to income, the concept of social exclusion highlights the multidimensional nature of the processes whereby individuals and groups are excluded from the social exchanges, practices and rights which are the basis of social integration and identity" (European Community, 1993, p. 3). De Foucauld puts it more succinctly: "Exclusion means the severing of social relationships" (de Foucauld, 1993, p.8).

People like to think that respect is bestowed on the basis of thoughtful assessment of an individual's behavior. In practice, however, we judge and are judged mainly on the basis of economic position and/or identity group (e.g., male or female, Irish, WASP, African-American, Latino, age group, man or woman). Near-constant, automatic disrespect is far different from the occasional affronts we are all likely to experience. Martin Luther King, Jr., asserted that we should be judged not on the basis of our skin color but on the content of our character. That is by no means the standard, however, for most evaluations of "the others." Who we are economically and ethnically has a profound effect on the respect, and thus the self-respect, that we live with and through. And as Diana Walsh, Glorian Sorensen and Lori Leonard show (Chapter 5), gender cannot be ignored in understanding social and economic position.

Both respect and self-respect are thus socially constructed, and both affect fuctioning and well-being. They also influence political outcomes, for mutual respect is a basic ingredient of the social solidarity that is necessary for effective political action to improve the quality of the economy.

Relative position refers to inequalities, that is, differences in power, respect, and material resources among different segments of the population. Poverty is not measured by absolute level of deprivation but by people's comparative position (Miller and Roby, 1970). While it is crucial to recognize and alleviate the acute deprivations inflicted by poverty, inequalities have a deep impact on well-being. Michael Marmot's highly-regarded Whitehall studies of white-collar and managerial employees, for example, strongly suggest that hierarchy at work, which signifies both relative power and respect, influences healthy functioning.

While relative position pertains to both resources and relations, it differs from resource position and relational position in that it stresses comparative standing rather than the sheer quantity of resources or quality of relationships. One can infer from Chapter 6 that it is the disparities that count: whether others have more or less than I have.

Groups that are marginalized, stigmatized, or oppressed recognize their situation by noting what dominant groups have in economic resources, power, or respect that they do not. And in turn some privileged people gain an enhanced sense of well-being from the disadvantages of others.

Meanings and Their Effects

Chapter 9 by Ellen Corin emphasizes the meanings that adhere to behavior and norms. These meanings are important for each of the 3Rs but especially so for relative position. All inequalities are not equally pernicious: the social meanings of an inequality contribute to its effects. It is not just the condition of a group or person that matters: the ways they (and others) interpret their conditions, and live their lives as a consequence of these interpretations, are also fateful for healthy functioning. Such meanings shape the pathways from societal influences to healthy functioning that Sol Levine (S. Levine and D. Dutton, unpublished) stresses.

According to Brenner's analysis of unemployment (Chapter 7), for example, both the material deprivation resulting from loss of income and the related meanings (loss of a key social role) and feelings (awareness of a decline in one's relative standing in the community) are pivotal to declines in healthy functioning. Interpretations of experience are shaped by cultural outlooks, previous experiences, and structural positions. By way of illustration, women, African-Americans, Latinos, and lower- and working-class persons, all of whom are frequent objects of disrespect, are far more likely to be aware of it than are those who dispense it.

Completely wiping out inequalities may not be necessary. (Some may not be pernicious.) Decreasing the net benefit of an inequity, either by decreasing privileged groups' gross gains or by raising the returns to those at the other end, can mitigate the impact of many, if not most, inequalities. This is especially likely to be true if the meanings attached to an inequality subsequently change. The most difficult task may be to recognize the broader societal forces that structure inequalities without neglecting the frames of meaning that mediate reactions to them.

Policy

The pathway to healthy functioning is not exclusively or even mainly through the laboratory, but more and more through society and the economy. Improvements in living standards (such as better nutrition and water systems) have enhanced health worldwide more than have laboratory discoveries. Thus, extending health care may be less important than advancing living standards.

In the 1940s Lawrence K. Frank, a leading proponent of the psychocultural approach to human development that was intellectually popular at the time, gave one of his books the arresting title *Society as the Patient* (Frank, 1948). Today, the society-and-health approach is amassing evidence that society is the illness. Societal pressures and distortions are interfering with healthy functioning. Sen's enlightening and disturbing work on famines underlines the central importance of how a society functions (Sen, 1981). Famines typically result not from bad harvests and resulting dire shortages of food but from economic and political forces that hinder the cultivation, harvesting, and marketing of a supply of food that would be adequate for all. Somalia, where food shipments are blocked and/or pirated by warring factions, is a sad contemporary illustration of Sen's thesis. Ireland in 1846 is another: food was exported to Britain while many Irish starved or migrated (Woodham-Smith, 1962).

Chief among societal pressures and distortions are poverty and inequalities. How do we go about redistributing resources to lessen them? Action plans must focus upstream on economic, industrial, and social policies. The following section stresses policies designed to reduce inequalities and, given the evidence presented in earlier chapters, to improve health. We will look first at policies to reduce resource inequalities and then at policies to minimize relational inequalities.

Reducing Resource Inequalities

A society committed to the reduction of inequalities would seek their prevention rather than their rectification post facto. The aim of policy informed by a society-and-health approach, then, should be to change the original distribution of income and wealth[1] so as to reduce the production of poverty and inequalities, rather than relying exclusively on after-the-fact redistributions. The prevention approach intervenes at an earlier point and lessens, though it does not completely eliminate, reliance on taxation and transfers. An emphasis on prevention is particularly compatible with the society-and-health paradigm, for it can address issues of environmental effects as well as distributive consequences.

Expanding economic resources and distributing them more evenly requires increasing employment, promoting better-paying jobs, reducing the pay and benefits differentials among jobs, and building the assets and return on assets of those doing absolutely and relatively poorly on the wealth dimensions of economic well-being. These goals are typically associated with economic growth and productivity. But general or untargeted growth, calculated as a rise in gross domestic product (GDP), will not necessarily meet the objectives of the society-and-health paradigm. Across-the-board growth may not result in more jobs, or particularly in more jobs open to people with low skills, living in depressed areas, or suffering from racial or gender discrimination.

Growth in the GDP, the number on which most economists and commentators fixate, does not fully determine employment levels and the kinds and qualities of jobs that emerge. The so-called "affluent society" of the 1950s generated considerable poverty and inequality, as did the post-1983 Reagan-era speculative boom. The expansion in the 1980s of the so-called FIRE (finance, insurance, and real-estate) industries generated fewer jobs and more inequalities in wages and wealth than would have resulted from a similar rate of growth in the manufacturing industries. It matters in which industries and regions, and through what means, growth takes place; the same is true of productivity.

In other words, the content or composition of GDP is decisive here: differently arrived at rates of growth could produce varied numbers and types of jobs and affect income and wealth differentially. Growth effects depend on what is produced and how. These patterns also affect the quality of the environment. High rates of economic growth can occur through the rapid exhaustion of natural resources that may damage the environment, auguring poorly for future growth.

The politically acceptable practice in most economic-policy discussions is to overlook the point that there is not just one type of economic growth. Reliance on a single rate of growth averaging the "horses and apples" that make up the gross domestic product obscures the real nature of the economy: different mixes of types of labor, materials, and technology can result in the same rate of economic growth but have differ-

---

1. *Original* refers to pre-tax, pre-transfer distribution. Such distribution, however, is shaped by a variety of governmental policies, including the tax structure, and by responses to them. A distribution is said to be original, then, not because it precedes governmental action but because it is not directly redistributed by governmental programs of taxes and transfers.

ent consequences for economic equality. Even a no-growth society is dynamic, with different mixes resulting in different outputs without any overall increase.

The fundamental questions are: Which parts of the economy do we seek to enlarge, stabilize, or abandon, and how should these goals be pursued? The outcomes of these choices affect people's conditions—and health. Thus a society-and-health perspective suggests that a strong industrial policy is beneficial to health.

The Prose of Industrial Policy

General growth and growth targeted on lessening inequalities need not be incompatible. An economic growth concerned about expanding employment and reducing inequalities requires appropriate economic and regional policies to influence which sectors develop and in what direction. Specifically, do better-paying jobs and new opportunities emerge for those lagging behind? These concerns are anathema to market-indoctrinated economists and to business leaders whose firms would not benefit, but any choice of a growth approach and governmental spending pattern has different consequences for various sectors of the economy. In short, targeted economic growth or industrial policy is constantly practiced. The issues are whether it is pursued openly or covertly and who benefits. What a society-and-health approach calls for is not fortuitous by-products of economic policies, but policies likely to have equality-enhancing outcomes.

A first step is a political-educational effort to raise public awareness that the U.S. government, like other governments, currently has an industrial policy and inevitably shapes the content of GDP. Since the depression of the 1930s, the United States has pursued a clear-cut, though unavowed, industrial policy of promoting military industries, supported in recent decades by government spending that also expanded the construction and health-care industries. A variety of measures (tax deductions for mortgage interest and highway construction) led to the explosion of suburbs. Tax deductions for capital-goods investments have spurred spending in the durable-goods industries. These measures, then, have significantly shaped the employment and growth patterns of the last decades. Like Tartuffe, Moliere's physician who was astonished to discover that he had been speaking prose, we have been experiencing the consequences of industrial policy without recognizing it.

A second step is to promote awareness that the mix of activities that make up the gross domestic product has consequences for employment, income distribution, and productivity. As Bluestone and Harrison (1982) and Harrison and Bluestone (1988) have stressed elsewhere, the character of economic development since the late 1970s has resulted in the emergence of more low-wage jobs. This pattern has caused both poverty and inequalities in household incomes to grow. The resulting "hollowing out of the middle" and the relatively slow growth of well-paying, blue-collar and white-collar jobs, especially for those without a college diploma, contributed to the lopsided income distribution at the end of the 1980s. Widespread awareness of these patterns could provoke public insistence on policies to improve the level and quality of employment and to distribute income and wealth more evenly.

Supplementary Inequality-Reducing Policies

Efforts to influence long-term economic policy should be accompanied by more immediate programs to decrease differentials in pay and benefits and to increase the assets of
those who lack wealth. We will examine three such policies here: (1) a basic package
of benefits attached to all employment, (2) supplementation of low wages, and (3) promotion of worker ownership. Other inequality-reducing policies that do not involve direct governmental money transfers (such as raising the minimum wage) offer some political feasibility. Some, like affirmative action, are more controversial. In addition to
the complexities of fashioning a sensible and comprehensive tax policy, taxation is not
a particularly effective economic or political way to reduce inequalities. Other measures are likely to have a more sustained impact. This view is not an argument against
increasing taxation on those who enjoyed the largesse of the speculative Reagan-Bush
boom years and decreasing taxes on those with low incomes. It is an expression of
skepticism about the political capacity of taxation to achieve and maintain a substantial
reduction of inequalities.

Jobs differ not only in the income and security they offer but also in the so-called
fringe benefits that accompany them. Both public and private (employer-based) benefit
systems affect well-being (Crystal and Shea, 1990). The growth of private benefit systems has increased the urgency of governmental action to reduce inequalities. One way
of reducing differences among jobs is to guarantee that basic benefits, pensions, and
medical care are attached to all jobs. This important step could take the form of governmental programs (such as universal medical benefits) or governmental requirements
that employers provide basic benefits to employees. (Though employer-provided benefits are not currently required, governmental regulations affect how they operate. For
example, federal law protects the portability of pensions when employees leave their
employers.) Whatever health program Congress enacts in the 1990s will probably
serve to reduce this particular inequality among jobs.

In seeking to reduce inequalities, it is important to improve the incomes not only of
the officially-designated poor but also of "the working poor" and those above the
poverty line who nevertheless suffer from low income.[2] One method is the Earned Income Tax Credit (EITC).

The EITC is a form of negative income tax, a device that won the approval of many

---

2. Census Bureau reports acknowledge the limitations of the official poverty line by designat-
ing as "near-poor" those whose incomes exceed the poverty line by only 25 percent. The European Community calculates each country's poverty line as half of its median family income, adjusted for household size. Households with incomes between the official U.S. poverty line and
half of the U.S. median income, adjusted for household size, should at least be regarded as "low-
income," if not as "poor." Some argue that the upper limit of low income should be 80 percent of
median income, adjusted for household size. Indeed, many means-tested programs recognize the
inadequacy of official poverty measures and provide benefits to households with incomes well
above the official poverty line. In sum, the official poverty line does not adequately measure the
numbers who suffer from severe income deficits.

economists but few politicians during the 1960s. In its current form, it is a federal program to increase the number of jobs that provide an income above the poverty level by providing a cash subsidy to low-wage workers with children. Initially, the EITC in effect returned the Social Security taxes paid by low-wage workers. This amount has gradually been increased, and the Clinton administration succeeded in raising the dollar contribution to low-wage workers with children. One current proposal is to peg the payments to the number of children in the household and to rises in inflation (Center on Budget and Policy Priorities, 1993). Constantly increasing the level of the payment would shrink the number of working poor and decrease inequalities.

Even if multiple measures were pursued to equalize the original distribution of income, targeted cash programs would still be needed to aid those with low and poverty-level incomes. Two such targeted programs are children's allowances and public assistance.

Children's allowances, cash payments to families with children, have typically been universal programs in most high-income societies; that is, all families regardless of income have received the allowance. (Some European nations, e.g., Britain, have recently curtailed the universality of the allowance.) The United States has resisted the very idea of children's allowances, but it appears likely to be adopted in the limited and punitive guise of getting at "deadbeat dads." In an experimental program in Wisconsin, the absent parent in one-parent families is expected to contribute a percentage of his (or her) income to the family. The government would strongly pressure the absent parent to pay, to the point of garnishing wages. If the absent parent did not contribute at all or only partially, the government would pay the solo-parent family most of what it should have received from the absent parent. In effect, then, the government would be guaranteeing a minimum income to solo-parent families, a back-door approach to a children's allowance.

Neither absent-parent nor EITC-like programs, however, are likely to lift all families out of poverty or to reduce inequalities. Neither program would help households without children. Nor does EITC, as presently constructed, benefit households in which no one is employed, thus excluding the long-term unemployed and those unable to work because of household responsibilities or disabilities.

Whether or not it is called aid to families with dependent children (AFDC), some form of public assistance is unavoidable despite political rhetoric denouncing its existence. Our goals should be to reduce the need for income-tested assistance by means of economic-policy initiatives, particularly industrial policy, and to help those who need AFDC to move into regular (not necessarily full-time) employment. In an economy with persistent high unemployment and increasing levels of irregular, contingent employment, finding permanent jobs for those with limited skills is exceedingly difficult. Public programs to provide jobs would be very expensive and not well received (at least by those who resist taxation). There is no easy, cheap alternative to public assistance. "Reforming welfare, " as the Clinton administration learned to its chagrin, is costly.

On the other hand, perpetuating the current version of AFDC will fuel anger and disillusionment on the part of taxpayers. Widespread anger at the public-welfare system, even if largely unwarranted, militates against adequate benefits and promotes administrative meanness and inflexibility; recipients routinely experience disrespect and bureaucratic entanglements. Inadequate benefits in turn promote widespread deception: recipients work but do not report their income (Jencks, 1992). A realistic view, then, calls for reducing reliance on public assistance while simultaneously changing it and acknowledging that some use of it is necessary.

Minimizing the need for public assistance requires a realistic set of pro-employment policies and new public spending. Reality, unlike political rhetoric, is expensive. Extensive training to enlarge individuals' job opportunities is costly with an uncertain payoff. It does not assure the availability of jobs for large numbers of public-assistance recipients. To do this, governments will have to offer either public jobs or subsidies to employers to create incentives to hire those deemed less attractive as employees. One alternative is to readopt an "overlap" policy of allowing people to work and receive welfare, an approach discontinued by the Reagan-Bush administrations mainly for ideological reasons. Higher minimum wages would also increase the desirability of working, but might result in the loss of some low-wage jobs.

Economist David Ellwood (Ellwood, 1988) and sociolgist Christopher Jencks (Jencks, 1992), both knowledgeable analysts of the public-welfare system, contend that the general point is that working should offer a decent level of living. Expanding EITC to cover those without children even if they are not in dire poverty would be a valuable first step. Since welfare provides access to Medicaid and relatively few employers who hire low-wage or part-time workers offer health insurance and other benefits, it is crucial that health benefits be provided to all through mandated and at least partially subsidized programs. To make it possible and worthwhile to work, child-care subsidies, transportation arrangements, and other backup supports are also necessary.

Such pro-employment measures, designed to reduce direct public-assistance outlays, are not inexpensive. Reducing the welfare rolls means creating new roles. That cannot be done on the cheap. The likelihood exists that a pro-employment approach to public assistance can win support even if it requires additional spending.

A pro-employment approach should not be pursued in a harsh, inflexible way leading to evasion and stress. Public-assistance recipients who cannot work on a regular basis should not be penalized if they have valid reasons for sustained absence from the labor force. If a large proportion of public-assistance recipients were enabled to give up their heavy reliance on direct public transfers, attitudes toward those unable to enter the labor force in a continuing way would likely soften.

An Educational Solution?

Welfare policy deals with only some of those living in officially designated poverty, and not at all with those above the official poverty line. Even the best possible public-assistance program would reduce income inequalities very little. To do so more effectively calls for improving productivity and expanding the number of good jobs. The widely accepted mantra that more schooling will of itself increase productivity and thus enhance international competitiveness and the number of good jobs is highly questionable. Nevertheless, belief in education-as-productivity, politically popular as it is (since it leaves current economic arrangements untouched), could contribute to lessening inequalities.

Given the concern that a growing proportion of the future labor force will be primarily minority and immigrant groups, generally unprepared for the presumably high-skill requirements of the twenty-first century, investment in the schooling and training of the educationally disadvantaged is likely to increase. Assuming that those at the bottom of the educational ladder advance relative to those above them, some inequalities in both education and income could be narrowed. (The momentum is in the opposite direction: the income gap between high- and low-education jobs has again widened.)

Increased public spending on education does not guarantee a decrease in educational and economic differences. What education-as-productivity may provide is a politically acceptable way of arguing for improving the situation of those who lag behind. Unfortunately, the argument is increasingly voiced in narrow terms, vocational skills and not in terms of a civic outlook based on solidarity and mutual respect.

Assets

Another approach is employee and worker ownership, a realm in which the United States has lagged. Let us look first at the asset dimension of ownership, then at control and participatory dimensions.

Over 7 million workers, according to some recent estimates, participate in Employee Stock Ownership Plans (ESOPs), which provide federal tax subsidies for firms whose employees are offered privileged access to stock ownership. Employee ownership means that employees own stock in the company along with other investors. Such plans have spread mightily because of the federal tax benefits to companies that issue ESOP shares.

Worker ownership, by contrast, means that a cooperative composed of a firm's workers jointly owns the firm. A small but not negligible number of American companies are owned and managed by various kinds of cooperatives.

Both ESOP and worker-owned companies contribute to narrowing the great gap in the distribution of wealth. (Those doing relatively poorly in the distribution of income fare even worse in the distribution of wealth.) By offering a stake in a firm, they provide participants an income-producing asset. (Most households' main asset is their home, which does not usually provide income until it is sold. Even then the proceeds may have to be used to pay for a new home.) Such methods of increasing the assets of wage and salaried workers help narrow enormous wealth inequalities.

Relational Dimensions

The society-and-health approach is not limited to quantitative and qualitative economic improvements. It calls for changes in the social fabric, in people's daily experiences, and in their relationships. If powerlessness, disconnection, disrespect, and hier- archy at home, at work, and in the community are obstacles to healthy functioning, then genuine participation and the promotion of respect and self-respect would con- tribute to healthy functioning.

Social relations are the basic ingredient in community and social support, which many society-and-health analyses consider fundamental explanatory variables (see the chapter by Donald Patrick and Thomas Wickizer.) The policy perspective is to seek positive social relations. Thoughtful assessments of such efforts can also reshape our understanding of causative processes.

Solidarity, a much more widely used word in Europe than here, is a broader term than *community*, which is usually reserved for people who are geographic neighbors and/or socially similar. Solidarity implies mutual concern and responsibility on the part of people who may be socially or geographically distant. More specifically, solidarity (at least in European discourse) signifies concern among those who are doing well for those who are faring poorly. For example, the Swedish solidarity wage policy followed by unions with membership and governmental support improved the wages of low- level workers more than those of higher-paid employees, thus reducing the income gap. The animating spirit was that of "one nation." Somewhat similarly, Britain's anti- inflation policy in the late 1960s was based on the government's increasing transfer benefits to the elderly in return for unions' acceptance of moderate wage gains.

Solidarity is pertinent not only to class but in particular to gender and race relations as they affect healthy functioning. Women, African-Americans, and other so-called minorities have raised disquieting questions about the state of social relations in the United States, including mistreatment of blacks by the police and harassment of women in public and in the workplace. Gender and race have become more significant in discourse and politics. To a large extent, this is due to the current obscuring of class which puts almost all Americans in an omnibus category of "middle class" so that pau- pers and princes are accorded this status.

The keys to building a sense of solidarity are the narrowing of economic distance and the involvement of people in common pursuits. Having already discussed measures to reduce economic differences, we consider the promotion of social interactions. First, widening the scope of local decision-making is likely to encourage more people to par- ticipate in community affairs. Federal- and state-funded programs could require broader-based local participation and self-determination. Community-service programs, with or without governmental support, to which individuals could voluntarily contribute for the good of the locality or the nation could make a difference. President Clinton's beginning of a national service corps for young people is such an endeavor. Edgar Cahn's invention of "service credits" is another way of connecting people (Cahn, 1985). In his Florida experiment, participants' hours of personal or community service (aiding elderly people, providing child care, helping in the public library) are credited to a ser- vice bank, making them eligible for an equal number of hours of service when needed. Such inducements to community solidarity can call forth latent desires for mutual aid.

Social relations have become increasingly politicized as issues of respect: ending discrimination is central, but how women and minorities are treated and talked about are also matters for public concern and action (Miller, 1993). Disrespect on the part of dominant groups creates barriers to the conditions of groups that are negatively viewed. Disrespect leads to exclusion, a prime target of the European Community's social and poverty programs. But the most serious harm it causes may be to the self-respect, self-esteem, and sense of self-efficacy of members of disdained groups.

Others' respect for one's identity group deeply influences group self-respect. The world's evaluation of one's identity group, even if highly distorted, is difficult to escape.

Respect for oneself is not just an interior process of self-will. Low self-respect is, at least in part, imposed. It can also be fateful, weakening the capacity to confront barriers imposed by others' disrespect. Impaired confidence in one's ability to affect one's destiny reduces the effectiveness of members of disdained identity groups. Bravado is not an adequate substitute.

How can public policy bolster group respect and self-respect? There is a need for programs that go beyond promoting individual self-esteem to influencing how social identity groups are viewed and treated. One route is through the schools. For many, schools act as labeling factories that stamp them "rejected," rather than places where they develop their capacities. Such children emerge from school feeling inadequate or "dumb," and find themselves treated as incompetent and barred from good jobs because of their educational deficiencies, lack of school credentials, and/or beliefs about their nontrainability. Spending more money on schools may not be enough in itself, but more funding in conjunction with such effective measures as school-based management, more active parental involvement, peer mentoring, and positive cultural involvements would enable schools to do far more to develop capacities and self-respect.

Multiculturalism, in and out of schools—informed awareness of and contacts with "the others"—on a wide scale is another route to increasing different groups' respect for one another and strengthening the self-respect of historically demeaned groups. Stereotypes flourish on all sides when social distance is great, although those acted upon usually have a more accurate view of those in dominant positions than vice versa (Miller, 1986). Reducing social distance and ignorance are important steps toward group respect and group self-respect.

Respect/disrespect and self-respect are not "natural" phenomena. They are influenced by deliberate and quasi-intentional efforts to inculcate negative attitudes and beliefs. From the point of view of healthy functioning, there is a public interest in doing something about such attitudes.

Improving the income, employment, security, and opportunities of identity groups that have fared badly, thus reducing the inequalities that separate them from more mainstream groups, would enhance the respect accorded them, and their collective self-respect. Our earlier discussion of employee and worker ownership focused only on their resource-enhancing aspects, but there is also some potential for relational enhancement. At present, most ESOPs provide little direct employee influence over company decision making. This situation contrasts with the codetermination requirements in Germany that worker representatives be included in one of the two top governing boards of firms. Broadening mandatory federal requirements to give employee shares more direct influence over decision making would increase the relative power of employees and probably lead to salutary changes in company operations.

Worker cooperatives usually adopt the Rochdale model of one-person one-vote. Facilitating more worker cooperatives would give workers greater control over their destinies. Unfortunately, there is a paucity of research on the broad effects, such as on healthy functioning and participation in other activities, of membership in a workers' cooperative. What complicates such research is that cooperatives are typically established to rescue deeply troubled companies and fear of failure may undermine the benefits of ownership and participation.

With or without ownership rights, greater employee participation in decision making, especially on the part of those in lower-level jobs, would reduce differences in power and influence among jobs and thus reduce stress. Employee involvement plans in large companies range from those that manipulate employees into believing that their wishes and suggestions are influential to that of the General Motors Saturn plant in Tennessee, which is run in close cooperation with local members of the United Automobile Workers Union. Saturn offers a wide scope for employees' participation in executive-office decisions as well as in shop-floor decisions. Public policy could play a role in promoting, financing, and strengthening various modes of worker involvement.

The greatest dangers in non-income approaches to inequality reduction are that they may be used both as substitutes for narrowing economic inequalities (Kaus, 1992) and as sociotherapy, manipulating people to feel better and thus reducing their political will without improving their conditions. In a therapeutic culture with a tax-aversive sensibility, these are real threats. Vigilance is necessary if struggles for respect and self-respect are not to be displaced by "feel-good," "just-say-no" campaigns.

Politics as Policy

In designing policy initiatives that address society-and-health concerns, we have to consider political effectiveness as well as health effectiveness. Unfortunately, the two considerations are likely to pull in opposite directions. Health effectiveness calls for an emphasis on reducing poverties and inequalities, which seem to be prime contributors to unsatisfactory health outcomes. But the deficit-focused political scene is unlikely to embrace greatly increased direct spending on the poor and on efforts to decrease inequalities.

The most promising way to gain support for reducing economic inequalities is to tie such efforts to economic growth and productivity, the two great consensual economic objectives. Reducing poverty and inequalities would improve economic functioning by enhancing the performance of the labor force. Other positive, non health consequences might be reduced crime rates and enhanced community functioning.

An explicit concern with inequalities calls attention to who benefits from economic growth, a question that has considerable divisive potential. The reassuring metaphor that a rising tide raises all ships is tossed overboard. Telling questions are upfront: are inequalities of class, race, and gender widened or narrowed by a particular type of economic growth and change? This outlook may clash with approaches that emphasize rates of economic growth and/or rely on redistributive taxation and transfers to remedy the more glaring poverties and inequalities that lopsided growth may produce.

The underlying theme of policy oriented toward reducing inequalities is a new, expanded understanding of citizenship. It is animated by the hope that deepening and extending the concept of citizenship will improve health outcomes. What does it mean today to be a member of American society? Citizenship is more than the right to vote, equal treatment under the law and access to social programs like health care, income floors, and public pensions. These are the rights of citizenship that British sociologist T. H. Marshall enshrined shortly after World War II (Marshall, 1963). Increasingly, citizenship is recognized as involving the right to opportunity, participation, respect, and social inclusion, including positive interactions.

These are rights that contribute to healthy functioning and a healthy society, and inequalities in exercising these rights should be narrowing. Advocates of the society-and-health approach would not stand alone in advocating the new citizenship. Just as it seeks to expand our understanding of influences on health, a society-and-health approach needs to expand the range of its discourse beyond researchers to include policy makers and activists who are similarly concerned with the current health of American society.

Health Care "Reform"

What are the implications, then, for the discussion of health care reform that President Clinton initiated shortly after assuming office? The most disturbing conclusion is that current proposals are about financing, not about health care. While some argue that universal coverage, if it were enacted, would improve access to medical treatment for those who now lack adequate insurance and would possibly reduce the length of illnesses through earlier medical attention, the general discourse about health at this time is largely about reducing or at least capping the growth of extraordinarily high health expenditures. Consequently, health "reform" is mainly about money and somewhat less about the organization of health services, and is not about broad, preventive measures that would reduce illness and injury and improve healthy functioning.

An indication of the narrow view of health change embodied in on-going discussions is that public health activities and spending are ignored. A reason for that may be that public health expenditures are largely defined as what public health agencies do.

To a considerable extent that now is to provide health care to the medically under-served, the medically indigent. A large part of the health care received by the medically indigent is provided by local public health agencies, particularly preventive services for pregnant women and children. Public health has lost its historically important agenda of promoting community health and is now mainly regarded as providing health care for the poor.

Reshaping health care without rethinking public health is a mistake. The definition of public health should not be restricted to what public health agencies currently do or even to what the classic public health agencies sought to undertake, important as those interventions are. The new public health should be comprehensive in concept and practice. Certainly many organizations—companies and nonprofit agencies as well as governmental bureaus—are involved in promoting public health, and many nonmedical activities contribute to healthy functioning. From the viewpoint of comprehensive public health, the separation between governmental and nongovernmental activities and spending is arbitrary. Similarly, the division in government accounting between what is and what is not a public health measure can be misleading.

Certainly anti-smoking efforts, whether banning smoking in public and in the workplace or requiring cigarette package labels that warn of the ill effects of smoking, are important preventive efforts. Government and business spending to improve air and water contributes to health as do better sewage systems. Business outlays on occupational safety and health under the pressure of legislation and regulation are significant public health measures even though no government money is directly involved. Removing asbestos from school buildings is a public health action even if the local school board pays the bills. Nonprofit watchdog organizations concerned with the quality of food, drugs, or the environment are important public health agencies today.

These and many other public and nongovernmental activities are broad, preventive efforts but are not accorded attention in current thinking about health reform. The general rule should be that actions that have similar effects should be grouped together regardless of their intention or auspices.

Following this rule, the society-and-health approach calls for an even broader understanding of what contributes to the promotion of the public's health. In this perspective, a variety of governmental programs should be regarded, at least in part, as public health actions. For example, the means-tested food stamp program, initiated after the discovery of considerable hunger in the United States, serves to improve nutrition and, subsequently, health. Housing subsidies enhance the living conditions of many, which is an aid to healthy functioning. Brenner's analysis in Chapter 7 would view efforts to decrease unemployment as having, in part, a positive public health effect.

The general point is that indirect or nonmedical measures can enhance health. A good example of the efficacy of indirect measures is what developing nations are discovering—that spreading education and improving the situation of women may do more to lower the birth rate (and improve healthy functioning) than more direct family planning strategems.

The society-and-health approach may run the danger of including and promising too much. Current proposals, as exemplified by those for health finance changes, definitely include and offer too little. The great advantage of the society-and-health perspective is that it is based on a broad, comprehensive view of what contributes to healthy functioning. It is a paradigm breaker, perhaps a paradigm bender or even maker, at a time when an overly introverted view of health prevails. Hell may live in the details, but heaven is in the broad skies.

References

Bluestone, B., and B. Harrison. 1982. *The Deindustrialization of America*. New York: Basic Books.

Cahn, E. 1985. Service credits: The new currency. *Social Policy* 15:56–57.

Center on Budget and Policy Priorities, 1993. *The Clinton EITC Proposal: How It Would Work and Why It is Needed.* Washington, DC: Center on Budget Priorities.

Crystal, S., and D. Shea. 1990. Cumulative advantage, cumulative disadvantage, and inequality among elderly people. *Gerontologist* 30:4.

de Foucauld, J. B. 1993. The need to generate a new public-spiritness. *Poverty 3 Magazine of the European Community* 8:3.

Dutton, D., and S. Levine. 1989. Overview, methodological critique, and reformulation. In J. P. Bunker, D. S. Gomby, and B. H. Kehrer (eds.), *Pathways to Health–The Role of Social Factors,* pp. 29–69. Menlo Park, CA: Henry J. Kaiser Family Foundation.

Ellwood, D. 1988. *Poor Support: Poverty in the American Family*. New York: Basic Books.

European Community. 1993. Toward a Europe of solidarity. *Poverty 3 Magazine of the European Community* 8:1.

Frank, L. K. 1948. *Society as the Patient*. New Brunswick: Rutgers University Press.

Harrison, B. and B. Bluestone. 1988. *The Great U-Turn: Corporate Restructuring and the Polarization of America*. New York: Basic Books.

Jencks, Christoper, 1992. *Rethinking Social Policy: Race, Poverty and the Underclass.* Cambridge: Harvard University Press.

Jordan, J., A. Kaplan, J. B. Miller, I. Stiver, and J. Surrey. 1991. *Women's Growth in Connection: Writings from the Stone Center*. New York: Guildford Press.

Kaus, M. 1992. *The End of Equality*. New York: Basic Books.

Kuhn, T. 1962. *The Structure of Scientific Revolutions*. Chicago: University of Chicago Press.

Marshall, T. H. 1963. *Class, Citizenship, and Social Development: Essays.* Garden City, NY: Doubleday.

Miller, J. B. 1986. *Towards a New Psychology of Women*, 2nd edn. Boston: Beacon Press.

Miller, S. M. 1993. The politics of respect. *Social Policy* 23:44–51.

Miller, S. M., and P. A. Roby. 1970. *The Future of Inequality*. New York: Basic Books.

Sen, A. 1981. *Poverty and Famines: An Essay on Entitlement and Deprivation*. Oxford: Clarendon Press.

Woodham-Smith, C.B.F. 1962. *The Great Hunger: Ireland 1845–1949*. New York: Harper & Row.

INDEX